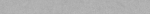

RENAL DISEASE IN THE AGED

RENAL DISEASE IN THE AGED

Jerome G. Porush, M.D.
Professor of Medicine, State University of New York
Health Science Center at Brooklyn; Chief, Division of
Nephrology and Hypertension, Brookdale Hospital Medical
Center, Brooklyn, New York

Pierre F. Faubert, M.D.
Assistant Professor of Medicine, State University of New
York Health Science Center at Brooklyn; Attending
Physician, Division of Nephrology and Hypertension,
Brookdale Hospital Medical Center, Brooklyn, New York

Little, Brown and Company
Boston/Toronto/London

To our wives, Ruth and Jessy

CONTENTS

PREFACE

We decided to write this book because we perceived a need for a comprehensive review of renal disease in the elderly. We understood from the beginning that there might not be, in all instances, sufficient data to suggest that the elderly are different from other adults; it was clear to us, however, that significant literature exists on the elderly, and that it would be possible to extract information about subjects over 60 years of age from the general adult literature. Furthermore, we felt that we had sufficient documented personal experience to add to the existing literature and that by writing this book, we could help fill some gaps in the medical community's knowledge of this important clinical area.

Renal Disease in the Aged represents a synthesis of the literature and our experience. We have included most of the subject matter covered in a standard nephrology text; due to a lack of both specific literature and documented personal experience, some topics receive little attention because we felt that there was little to add. For most subject areas, we summarize the existing information on adults in general and then provide information that is specific to the elderly. In all instances we have been careful to distinguish what we have derived from the literature from what we have learned from our own experience, leaving the reader the option to draw his or her own conclusions when there is a discrepancy. For the most part, we believe we have achieved our goal of producing a comprehensive review of kidney disease, including hypertension, in the elderly.

We want to take this opportunity to thank our close colleagues for supporting us in this endeavor. We also would like to acknowledge gratefully the invaluable assistance of Ruth Porush and Pauline Kleiman, without whom we could not have produced this book. Finally, we would like to acknowledge the encouragement we received throughout from Jane Licht, Executive Editor of Medical Books at Little, Brown and Company.

Pierre F. Faubert
Jerome G. Porush

RENAL DISEASE IN THE AGED

1 ANATOMY AND PHYSIOLOGY

EFFECT OF AGE ON THE ANATOMY OF THE KIDNEY

Like other organs in the body such as the spleen, liver, and brain, the kidneys undergo involutional changes with age [1, 2] (Fig. 1-1 and Table 1-1). The mean total renal area has been estimated to be approximately 55.2 cm^2 with a mean cortical area of 12.7 cm^2 in adult subjects up to the age of 65 years. Both of these parameters decrease significantly in subjects after the age of 65 years [3]. From birth to age 40 the normal human kidney has an estimated 600,000 to 1,200,000 glomeruli [4]. Thereafter, there is a progressive decrease of 30 to 50 percent in the number of glomeruli. Ninety-five percent of the normal population under the age of 50 have less than 10 percent sclerotic glomeruli (range 0 to 7.2 percent). In subjects older than 50 years, the percentage of sclerotic glomeruli increases, with a range of 0.5 to 36 percent, making the distinction between involutional and disease-related sclerosis unclear [5, 6].

In addition to glomerular sclerosis, there is a gradual increase in interstitial fibrosis. The proximal tubular volume of individual nephrons tends to decrease from a mean of 0.076 mm^3 (range 0.030–0.178 mm^3) at 20 to 39 years to a mean of 0.050 mm^3 (0.020–0.120 mm^3) at 80 to 101 years [7]. Since the loss of glomerular mass is proportional to the loss of tubular mass, glomerulotubular balance is, in general, well preserved [8]. On electron microscopic analysis, there is an increase in reduplication and an increase in focal thickening of both glomerular and tubular basement membranes, probably due to the accumulation of type IV collagen [9].

The increase in the percentage of sclerotic glomeruli has been attributed to the protein-rich diet characteristic of modern Western society [10]. This diet, as shown in experiments with rats, induces a state of chronic renal hyperfiltration and hyperperfusion, contributing to progressive glomerulosclerosis and an age-related decrease in glomerular filtration rate. An increase in the function of residual intact nephrons would be expected to lead to an increase in nephron size; however, no significant correlation is found between glomerular area and glomerulosclerosis [11]. Another possible explanation for the progressive increase in sclerotic glomeruli with age is glomerular ischemia secondary to the changes in renal blood flow that occur with age. It has been recently demonstrated that both age and vascular disease correlate independently with the percentage of hyalinized glomeruli in the aged [8]. Indeed, in studies carried out by Hollenberg and associates [12], renal

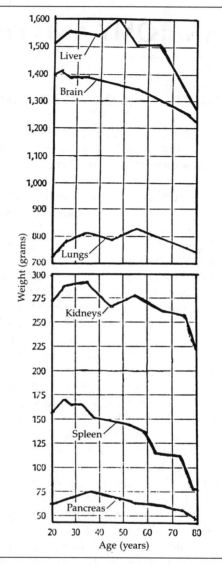

FIGURE 1-1. Organ weight as a function of age. (From Westking D, et al: Morbidity and mortality in the aged. *Hosp Prac* 17:97–99, 1982.)

blood flow declined progressively at a rate of approximately 10 percent per decade, starting after the fourth decade. The mechanism for the decrease in renal blood flow does not appear to be related to a decrease in cardiac output occurring with age but rather is anatomic. Several authors

TABLE 1-1. Mean values of kidney weights and some micromeasuring data in the kidney of whites in various age groups

Age (yr)	Weight of kidneys (g) (144)	Size of glomeruli* (μm) (182)	Cell no. of glomerular tufts (181)	No. of epithelial cells of con- voluted tubules in a given area (125,600 μm²) (100)	Size of epithelial cell nuclei* (μm) (100)
under 39	432.1 ± 36.39 (12)	189.5 ± 1.07 (12)	156.3 ± 4.26 (12)	178.1 ± 6.18 (6)	7.08 ± 0.046 (7)
40–49	388.5 ± 24.49 (23)	186.4 ± 0.86 (25)	133.3 ± 2.66 (25)	159.3 ± 3.71 (15)	6.85 ± 0.028 (14)
50–59	365.8 ± 20.24 (20)	191.9 ± 1.38 (35)	142.3 ± 2.38 (36)	152.4 ± 3.91 (17)	7.07 ± 0.023 (17)
60–69	355.0 ± 13.67 (35)	191.2 ± 0.66 (43)	124.6 ± 1.73 (42)	127.2 ± 2.52 (23)	7.02 ± 0.023 (24)
70–79	327.0 ± 10.89 (32)	189.2 ± 0.65 (42)	121.4 ± 1.89 (41)	120.5 ± 2.77 (23)	7.18 ± 0.023 (22)
above 80	294.9 ± 18.38 (22)	185.1 ± 0.98 (25)	106.4 ± 2.10 (25)	117.9 ± 3.36 (16)	7.27 ± 0.026 (16)

*Square root of value area.
Number of cases examined is indicated in parentheses.
SOURCE: Adapted from Tauchi H, et al: Age changes in the human kidney of the different races. *Gerontologia* 17:87–97, 1971.

have reported fibroelastic hyperplasia of arterioles and of small arteries occurring progressively with age [13, 14]. The changes are more pronounced in the cortical vessels, and, as a consequence, the perfusion pressure is relatively well maintained in the juxtamedullary nephrons.

EFFECT OF AGE ON GLOMERULAR FILTRATION RATE

Since total glomerular filtration rate (GFR) is a function of the number of functioning glomeruli, one might expect it to be decreased in the elderly. In cross-sectional and longitudinal studies reported by Davies and Shock [15], a gradual decrease in GFR was noted with age (Table 1-2). These changes have been confirmed by the longitudinal analysis of Rowe et al [16] (Table 1-3) and Lindeman et al [17].

Based on these data, it has been estimated that after the age of 30 there is a 7.5 to 8 ml/min decline in the GFR per decade. A nomogram has been constructed by Rowe et al [18] to determine the age-adjusted standard creatinine clearance and can be computed for males as follows:

TABLE 1-2. Mean change in GFR and RPF with age

Age (yr)	Inulin clearance (ml/min/ 1.73 m²)	Effective renal blood flow (ml/min/ 1.73 m²)	Filtration fraction (%)
50–59	99.3 ± 15	849 ± 123	21 ± 3
60–69	96.0 ± 26	775 ± 139	22 ± 3
70–79	89.0 ± 20	589 ± 133	26 ± 8
80–89	65.3 ± 20	475 ± 141	23 ± 4

SOURCE: Davies DF and Shock NW: Age changes in glomerular filtration rate: Effective renal plasma flow and tubular excretory capacity in adult males. *J Clin Invest* 29:496–507, 1950. By permission of the American Society of Clinical Investigation.

TABLE 1-3. Age and creatinine clearance

Age (yr)	Creatinine clearance (ml/min/1.73 m²)
45–54	128 ± 2
55–64	122 ± 2
65–74	110 ± 3
75–84	97 ± 3

SOURCE: Rowe JW, et al: The effect of age in creatinine clearance in man: A cross-sectional and longitudinal study. *J Gerontol* 31:155–163, 1976.

creatinine clearance (ml/min /1.73 m²) = 133 − (0.64 × age). For females, multiply the result by 0.93. For instance, a 60-kg male aged 90 years would be expected to have a creatinine clearance of 133 − (0.64 × 90) = 75.4 ml/min/1.73 m². It should be noted that this formula represents only an estimate, and the error inherent can be substantial, since some subjects maintain stable renal function while aging (approximately one-third), and a small number even show an increase [17].

Serum creatinine is the most commonly used marker of kidney function (GFR) in clinical medicine. Kampman et al [19] have demonstrated that the decrease in creatinine clearance that occurs with age is attended by a parallel reduction in daily creatinine excretion, so that there is no change in the serum creatinine level (Table 1-4). As shown by Forbes et al [20], because adult lean body mass declines by 12 kg in males and by 5 kg in females by age 65 to 70, the decrease in creatinine excretion probably reflects a decrease in muscle mass and creatinine production. Thus, the serum creatinine level may be deceiving in the elderly, and for a more meaningful evaluation of kidney function a creatinine clearance or some other measurement of GFR is essential.

Since measurement of creatinine clearance requires a timed urine collection (which is notoriously inaccurate without a bladder catheter), a formula has been developed by Cockcroft and Gault that allows one to calculate the creatinine clearance based on the patient's age, weight, and serum creatinine [21]: Creatinine clearance (ml/min) = (140 − age) × weight (kg)/72 × serum creatinine (mg/dl). For females multiply the result by 0.8. This formula is applicable so long as the patient has stable kidney function and is without severe underlying disease [22]. Using this formula, a good correlation has been found between measured and

TABLE 1-4. Relationship between serum and urine creatinine and creatinine clearance

Age (yr)	Serum creatinine (mg/dl)		Urine creatinine (mg/kg/24 hr)		Creatinine clearance (ml/min/1.73 m²)	
	Male	*Female*	*Male*	*Female*	*Male*	*Female*
40–49	1.10	1.00	19.7	17.6	88	81
50–59	1.16	0.99	19.3	14.9	81	74
60–69	1.15	0.97	16.9	12.9	72	63
70–79	1.03	1.02	14.2	11.8	64	54
80–89	1.06	1.05	11.7	10.7	47	46
90–99	1.20	0.91	9.4	8.4	34	39

SOURCE: Kampman M, et al: Rapid evolution of creatinine clearance. *Acta Med Scand* 196:517–520, 1974.

calculated creatinine clearance in the elderly by Gral and Young [23], Durakovic [24], and Friedman et al [25].

As noted earlier, advancing age is associated with fibroelastic hyperplasia and also with hyalinization of arterioles and small arteries. It has also been found that blood pressure increases with age. The obvious question is whether the decline in renal function with age is mainly a reflection of the increasing blood pressure. Lindeman et al [26] found that at a mean arterial pressure (MAP) of less than 107 mm Hg, no correlation could be found between creatinine clearance and blood pressure. For pressures above that level, however, there appeared to be a negative correlation between creatinine clearance and MAP. Thus the progressive decline in GFR with associated anatomic changes are a function of age per se, but increases in blood pressure might accelerate the decline.

The effects of protein load or intravenous dopamine infusion on functional reserve [27, 28] have not been studied systematically in the elderly; however, it has been noted that after unilateral nephrectomy, patients over 60 years of age can undergo compensatory hypertrophy to the same extent as younger patients as early as seven months after surgery [29, 30]. Thus, despite the anatomic changes noted earlier, the senescent kidney possesses some reserve and can still respond to stimuli expected to induce an increase in GFR.

EFFECT OF AGE ON TUBULAR FUNCTION

As noted earlier, because the anatomic changes affecting the glomeruli are paralleled by those in the tubules, glomerular-tubular balance is usually adequately maintained in the elderly [8, 31].

THE RENIN-ANGIOTENSIN-ALDOSTERONE SYSTEM

Plasma renin activity (PRA) and plasma aldosterone (PA) have been measured in different age groups during unrestricted (120 mEq sodium per day) and low sodium (Na) diets (< 10 mEq per day) in the supine and standing positions [32–34]. Both PRA and PA decrease progressively with each decade of life, starting after the fourth decade. The same pattern persists whether subjects are on an unrestricted or a restricted sodium diet, supine or standing. The mechanism(s) responsible for the decrease in renin production is not clear. Since neither the substrate concentration (angiotensinogen) nor the total renin content of the plasma changes with age, a decrease in the ability of the elderly to activate prorenin to renin has been postulated by some as the most likely explanation for the lower PRA [35, 36]. The decreased aldosterone level can be partially explained by a lower active renin level, per se, since the response to corticotrosin administration, which directly stimulates the cells of the zona glomerulosa, is similar in both young and elderly subjects [34].

SODIUM METABOLISM

LOW SODIUM DIET

In the study by Weidman et al [34], in which 12 patients aged 20 to 30 years and seven patients aged 62 to 70 years were placed on a low sodium diet (< 10 mEq per day), overall urinary excretion of Na (measured daily) was similar in the two groups except on day nine, when the older group showed greater Na excretion. Crane and Harris [33] noted that patients older than 50 years of age tend to excrete more Na in the urine when placed on a 10 mEq Na per day diet; however, statistical significance was achieved only in the 70- to 79-year age group. Epstein and Hollenberg [37], rather than measuring daily Na excretion in the older age group on a low Na diet, determined the rate at which balance was achieved. They concluded that cumulative Na balance per se cannot be used as an index because of the widely differing starting points that result from the variable dietary Na intake beforehand. They found that from age 30 to 60 years dietary Na restriction is associated with a constant half-time for renal Na conservation of 23.4 + 1.1 hours compared to 30.9 + 2.8 hours for subjects over 60 years of age.

It appears that age does influence the kidney's capacity to conserve Na [38]. The underlying mechanism for this phenomenon is not clear. During salt restriction, there is experimental evidence that both proximal and distal parts of the nephron participate in the increased reabsorption. Despite a reduction in nephron number and cortical blood flow in the elderly, medullary flow is well preserved [39]. As a result of this disparate blood flow, medullary washout might take place, reducing the efficacy of the countercurrent system and thereby decreasing the amount of Na removed by the ascending limb of deep nephrons. Another factor that might contribute to the inability of the elderly patient to conserve salt normally is the decrease in activity of the autonomic nervous system with age. There is experimental evidence that this system contributes to the increased proximal Na reabsorption noted during salt restriction [40].

VOLUME EXPANSION

As shown by Luft et al [41], subjects older than 40 years excreted a similar saline load more slowly than younger subjects, although the plasma Na was similar in both groups. In this particular study creatinine clearance was not measured. Since GFR decreases with age, one explanation for the blunted natriuresis is a decrease in the filtered load. In a more recent study, Kirkland et al [42] found reduced 24-hour urine Na and potassium excretion in the elderly (mean age 66.5 years) compared with that in younger subjects (mean age 29.2 years). Compared with younger persons, the elderly subjects excreted Na, potassium, and total solutes at a proportionately higher rate at night. The baseline plasma atrial natriuretic peptide (ANP), a substance that participates in the natriuresis associated with volume expansion, increases with age [43–45], in part due to a decrease in its catabolic rate [46]. Since saline loading in the elderly results in a significant rise in ANP [43], the blunted natriuresis cannot be attributed to an inappropriate response.

URINARY ACIDIFICATION

The kidneys play a very important role in acid-base homeostasis by reabsorbing the bulk of filtered bicarbonate and generating new bicarbonate through the titration of buffers, the most important being ammonia and titratable acids (phosphate, sulfate). The latter mechanism depends on the active secretion of hydrogen ion (H^+) by tubular cells. Blood pH and bicarbonate levels do not change significantly with age, and the elderly kidney maintains its ability to acidify the urine maximally in the presence of appropriate stimuli [47].

Unfortunately, bicarbonate reabsorption by the proximal tubule has not been studied under different loads; however, since plasma bicarbonate remains unchanged despite a gradual decrease in GFR with age, it appears that glomerular-tubular balance for this ion is well maintained. Nevertheless, one would expect the elderly to excrete a bicarbonate load more slowly than younger subjects, making them more prone to the development of metabolic alkalosis.

Under normal circumstances the excretion of titratable acid and ammonium is similar among different age groups [47]. However, after a 2 mmol per kg ammonium chloride load, urinary excretion of net acid is significantly lower in elderly subjects. The difference can be accounted for solely by a decrease in ammonium excretion, since titratable acid excretion is no different. This impairment of ammonium excretion represents an intrinsic tubular defect, the mechanism of which is not known.

URINARY CONCENTRATION

Rowe et al [48] noted that after 12 hours of water deprivation the elderly (mean age 68 years) achieved a mean urine osmolality of 882 compared with 1051 in a middle-aged group (mean age 49 years) and 1109 mOsm per kg H_2O in a younger group of subjects (mean age 33). The differences among the three groups were statistically significant. The authors concluded that aging is associated with a decrease in the ability to concentrate the urine maximally. Identical conclusions have been reached by Dontas et al [8].

To achieve maximal urine concentration the following features should prevail:

1. A normally functioning hypothalamic-hypophyseal axis. If anything, it has been shown that there is a significant age-related increase in osmoreceptor sensitivity. For the same osmolar stimulus elderly subjects released twice as much antidiuretic hormone (ADH) as younger subjects [49].
2. Adequate fluid delivery to the distal segment of the nephron. The GFR does decrease with age; however, no significant relationship between creatinine clearance and urine osmolality was found by Rowe and colleagues [48], suggesting that fluid delivery is not a limiting factor.
3. A normally functioning ascending limb of Henle. As mentioned earlier, a state of relative medullary washout exists in the elderly. As a consequence, there is enhanced solute removal from the medullary interstitium that probably contributes to the impaired ability of the elderly to achieve the same maximum urinary concentration as younger subjects.
4. A collecting tubule responsive to ADH. Experimental studies in the aged rat suggest that the concentrating defect is due to a decrease in water permeability along the collecting duct [50]. Miller and Shock [51] have measured the urine-plasma (U/P) inulin concentration ratio in three different age groups in humans following the administration of 0.5 milliunits of pitressin during water diuresis. As can be seen from Figure 1-2, U/P inulin was significantly lower in the elderly compared with that in the younger age groups. These results are compatible with a relative insensitivity of the collecting tubule to ADH.

In summary, it appears that the impaired ability of the elderly kidney to concentrate the urine maximally is a consequence of medullary washout and relative insensitivity of the collecting tubules to ADH.

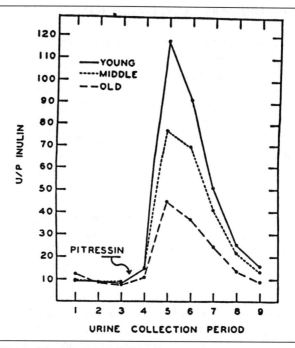

FIGURE 1-2. Mean value of U/P inulin ratio for each of three age groups before and after the intravenous administration of pitressin. Urine collection periods 1 to 9 represent nine consecutive 12-minute periods. Pitressin was administered immediately after the conclusion of period 3. (From Miller JH and Shock NW: Age differences in the renal tubular response to antidiuretic hormone. *J Gerontol* 8:446–450, 1953. By permission of S. Karger AG; Basel.)

TUBULAR REABSORPTION OF GLUCOSE

The effects of age on the minimal rate of renal tubular reabsorption of glucose have been examined by Miller and co-workers [52], who demonstrated a linear decrease with age. Since GFR decreases as well, however, glycosuria at normal plasma levels does not occur.

REFERENCES

1. Westking D, Pushparaj N, and O'Toole K: Morbidity and mortality in the aged. *Hosp Pract* 17:97–109, 1982.
2. Tauchi H, Tsuboi K, and Okutomi J: Age changes in the human kidney of the different races. *Gerontologia* 17:87–97, 1971.

3. Griffiths GJ, et al: Loss of renal tissue in the elderly. *Br J Radiol* 49:111–117, 1976.
4. Moore RA: The total number of glomeruli in the normal human kidney. *Anat Rec* 48:153–168, 1931.
5. Kappel B and Olsen S: Cortical interstitial tissue and sclerosed glomeruli in the normal human kidney, related to age and sex: A quantitative study. *Virchows Arch [A]* 387:271–277, 1980.
6. Kaplan C, et al: Age-related incidence of sclerotic glomeruli in human kidneys. *Am J Pathol* 80:227–234, 1975.
7. Darmady EM, Offer J, and Woodhouse MA: The parameters of the aging kidney. *J Pathol* 109:195–207, 1973.
8. Dontas AS, Marketos SG, and Papanayiotou P: Mechanisms of renal tubular defects in old age. *Postgrad Med J* 48:295–303, 1972.
9. Langeveld JPM, et al: Chemical characterization of glomerular and tubular basement membrane of men of different ages. *Kidney Int* 20:104–114, 1981.
10. Brenner B, Meyer TW, and Hostetter TH: Dietary protein intake and the progressive nature of kidney disease: The role of hemodynamically mediated glomerular injury in the pathogenesis of progressive glomerular sclerosis in aging, renal ablation and intrinsic renal disease. *N Engl J Med* 307:652–659, 1982.
11. Kasiske BL: Relationship between vascular disease and age associated changes in the human kidney. *Kidney Int* 31:1153–1159, 1987.
12. Hollenberg NK, et al: Senescence and the renal vasculature in normal man. *Circ Res* 34:309–316, 1974.
13. McLachlan MSF, et al: Vascular and glomerular changes in the aging kidney. *J Pathol* 121:65–78, 1977.
14. Yamaguchi T, Omae T, and Katsuki S: Quantitative determination of renal vascular changes related to age and hypertension. *Jpn Heart J* 10:248–258, 1969.
15. Davies DF and Shock NW: Age changes in glomerular filtration rate: Effective renal plasma flow and tubular excretory capacity in adult males. *J Clin Invest* 29:496–507, 1950.
16. Rowe JW, et al: The effect of age on creatinine clearance in man: A cross-sectional and longitudinal study. *J Gerontol* 31:155–163, 1976.
17. Lindeman RD, Tobin J, and Shock NW: Longitudinal studies on the rate of decline in renal function with age. *J Am Geriatr Soc* 33:278–285, 1985.
18. Rowe JW, et al: Age-adjusted standards for creatinine clearance. *Ann Intern Med* 84:567–569, 1976.
19. Kampman J, et al: Rapid evaluation of creatinine clearance. *Acta Med Scand* 196:517–520, 1974.
20. Forbes GB and Reina JC: Adult lean body mass declines with age: Some longitudinal observations. *Metabolism* 19:653–663, 1970.
21. Cockcroft DW and Gault MH: Prediction of creatinine clearance from serum creatinine. *Nephron* 16:31–41, 1976.
22. Drusano GL, et al: Commonly used methods of estimating creatinine clearance are inadequate for elderly debilitated nursing home patients. *J Am Geriatr Soc* 36:437–441, 1988.
23. Gral T and Young M: Measured versus estimated creatinine clearance in the elderly as an index of renal function. *J Am Geriatr Soc* 28:492–496, 1980.
24. Durakovic Z: Creatinine clearance in the elderly: A comparison of direct measurement and calculation from serum creatinine. *Nephron* 44:66–69, 1986.
25. Friedman JR, Norman DC, and Yoshikawa TT: Correlation of estimated re-

nal function parameters versus 24-hour creatinine clearance in ambulatory elderly. *J Am Geriatr Soc* 37:1485–1489, 1989.

26. Lindeman RD, Tobin JD, and Shock NW: Association between blood pressure and the rate of decline in renal function with age. *Kidney Int* 26:861–868, 1984.

27. Beukhof HR, et al: Effect of low-dose dopamine on effective renal plasma flow and glomerular filtration rate in 32 patients with IgA glomerulopathy. *Am J Nephrol* 5:267–270, 1985.

28. Bosch JP, et al: Renal functional reserve in humans. Effect of protein intake on glomerular filtration rate. *Am J Med* 75:943–950, 1983.

29. Boner G, Shery J, and Riesebach RE: Hypertrophy of the normal human kidney following contralateral nephrectomy. *Nephron* 9:364–370, 1972.

30. Eklund L and Gothlin J: Compensatory renal enlargement in older patients. *J Roentgenol* 127:713–715, 1976.

31. Dontas AS, et al: The effect of bacteriuria on renal functional patterns in old age. *Clin Sci* 34:73–81, 1968.

32. Flood C, et al: The metabolism and secretion of aldosterone in elderly subjects. *J Clin Invest* 46:960–966, 1967.

33. Crane MG and Harris JJ: Effect of aging on renin activity and aldosterone excretion. *J Lab Clin Med* 87:947–959, 1976.

34. Weidman P, et al: Effect of aging on plasma renin and aldosterone in normal man. *Kidney Int* 8:325–333, 1975.

35. Tsunoda K, et al: Effect of age on the renin-angiotensin-aldosterone system in normal subjects: Simultaneous measurement of active and inactive renin, renin substrate and aldosterone in plasma. *J Clin Endocrinol Metab* 62:384–389, 1986.

36. Higaki J, et al: Effects of aging on human plasma renin: Simultaneous multiple assays of enzyme activity and immunoactivity of plasma renin. *Acta Endocrinol* 120:81–86, 1989.

37. Epstein M and Hollenberg NK: Age as a determinant of renal sodium conservation in normal men. *J Lab Clin Med* 87:411–417, 1976.

38. Macias Nuñea JF, et al: Renal handling of sodium in old people. A functional study. *Age Aging* 7:178–181, 1980.

39. Takazakura E, et al: Intrarenal vascular changes with age and disease. *Kidney Int* 2:224–230, 1972.

40. Gottschalk CW: Renal nerves and sodium excretion. *Ann Rev Physiol* 41:229–240, 1979.

41. Luft FC, et al: Effects of volume expansion and contraction in normotensive whites, blacks and subjects of different ages. *Circulation* 59:643–650, 1979.

42. Kirkland JL, et al: Patterns of urine flow and electrolyte excretion in healthy elderly people. *Br Med J* 287:1665–1667, 1983.

43. Ohashi M, et al: High plasma concentration of human natriuretic polypeptide in aged man. *J Clin Endocrinol Metab* 64:81–85, 1987.

44. Clark BA, Elahi D, and Epstein FH: Age and dose related differences in response to atrial natriuretic peptide in man. *Kidney Int* 35:282A, 1989.

45. Haller BGD, et al: Effects of posture and aging on circulating atrial natriuretic peptide levels in man. *J Hypertension* 5:551–556, 1987.

46. Inscho EW, Wilfinger WW, and Banks RO: Age related differences in the natriuretic and hypotensive properties of rat atrial extracts. *Endocrinology* 121:1662–1670, 1987.

47. Agarwal BN and Cabebe FG: Renal acidification in elderly subjects. *Nephron* 26:291–295, 1980.

48. Rowe JW, Shock NW, and DeFronzo RA: The influence of age on the renal response to water deprivation in man. *Nephron* 17:270–278, 1976.
49. Helderman JH, et al: The response of arginine vasopressin to intravenous ethanol and hypertonic saline in man: The impact of aging. *J Gerontol* 33: 39–47, 1978.
50. Bengele HH, et al: Urinary concentrating defect in the aged rat. *Am J Physiol* 240:F147–150, 1981.
51. Miller JH and Shock NW: Age differences in the renal tubular response to antidiuretic hormone. *J Gerontol* 8:446–450, 1953.
52. Miller JH, McDonald RK, and Shock NW: Age changes in the maximal rate of renal tubular reabsorption of glucose. *J Gerontol* 7:196–200, 1952.

2 DISORDERS OF WATER AND SALT METABOLISM

Normally, plasma osmolality is maintained within a narrow range despite wide daily variations in water intake. More than 90 percent of the osmotic pressure of plasma (and other extracellular fluids) is accounted for by sodium (Na) and its anions, with urea and glucose providing the remainder. The constancy of plasma osmolality is maintained by rapid adjustments in water excretion or intake to oppose any changes in the plasma concentration of Na and its anions.

Changes in osmolality are perceived quite rapidly by neurons located in the anterior hypothalamus, where there is integration and transmission of the neural signals to cells of the supraoptic and paraventricular nuclei responsible for antidiuretic hormone (ADH) synthesis, and to the so-called thirst centers. The secretion of ADH serves to retain water by increasing its reabsorption by the kidneys. Its absence has the opposite effect. The system is sensitive enough to perceive changes in plasma osmolality as small as 1 percent, although the mechanism responsible for such a response is not yet entirely clear [1].

Besides changes in osmolality, nonosmotic variables also independently affect ADH release, including (1) hemodynamic events (hypotension or hypovolemia) mediated primarily by pressure-sensitive receptors located in the left atrium and large arteries of the chest and neck [2]; (2) drugs such as barbiturates, opiates, chlorpropamide, tolbutamide, vinca alkaloids, carbamazepine, and clofibrate; (3) other agents such as catecholamines and acetylcholine [3]; and (4) nausea [4]. The different factors involved in water excretion are summarized in Figure 2-1.

How does this situation apply to the elderly? Both serum osmolality and plasma Na are well maintained in the elderly; however, there are alterations in the physiologic patterns outlined in Figure 2-1 that make the elderly person more susceptible to disorders of water balance:

1. A decrease in thirst with hypodypsia related to a defect in the opioid-associated drinking drive [5] has been found in elderly persons subjected to 24 hours of water deprivation [6].
2. The ADH response to changes in volume-pressure (nonosmotic stimuli) as estimated by orthostasis is blunted in the elderly. This defect appears to be distal to the vasomotor center in the baroreceptor reflex arc, since norepinephrine release is intact [7].

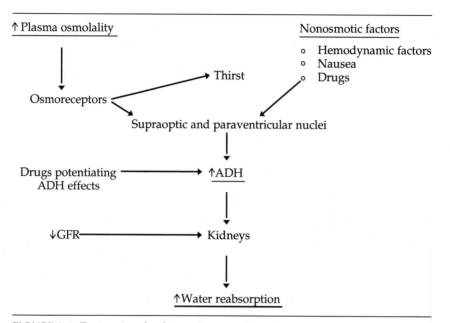

FIGURE 2-1. Factors involved in water excretion.

3. Despite a larger increase in ADH release in the elderly compared with younger subjects when faced with an increase in osmolality, the elderly do not achieve as high a urinary concentration [8].

HYPONATREMIA

INCIDENCE AND PREVALENCE
In a study of all patients hospitalized during a 3-month period in their institution, Baran and Hutchinson [9] found 78 patients with a serum Na less than or equal to 128 mEq per liter. Sixty percent were over the age of 60, with 31 percent aged 61 to 70 years, 24 percent aged 71 to 80 years, and 5 percent over 80 years old. Of 683 patients admitted to an acute geriatric care unit during a 10-month period, 77 (11.3 percent) had a plasma Na concentration below 130 mEq per liter [10]. Kleinfield and associates [11], in a random sampling of plasma Na of 160 patients in a chronic care facility, reported that 36 patients (22.5 percent) had chronic hyponatremia.

It appears from these data that hyponatremia is rather common in the elderly. Indeed, in a prospective study of patients with hyponatremia admitted to the Hospital of the University of Colorado Health Sciences Center, the mean age varied between 57 and 63 years in the different groups studied [12]. Of 22 patients with symptomatic hyponatremia reported by Cogan and colleagues [13], most were elderly.

PATHOGENESIS

Before a diagnosis of hyponatremia is made, pseudohyponatremia due to hyperlipidemia, hyperproteinemia, or hyperglycemia must be eliminated [14]. In the case of hyperlipidemia and hyperproteinemia, serum osmolality is normal in the presence of hyponatremia. In the case of hyperglycemia, for each 100 mg per dl increment in serum glucose, there is a decrement of 1.6 mEq per liter in serum Na [15]. Pseudohyponatremia may also be due to increased serum concentration of osmotically active solutes such as mannitol, ethanol, or ethylene glycol. In such cases the difference between the measured and calculated serum osmolality will be more than 10 mOsm per kg H_2O [16]. Once these conditions are ruled out, the hyponatremic patient can be classified as normovolemic, edematous, or hypovolemic depending on the clinical assessment of the extracellular fluid volume (Table 2-1) [12]. Whereas the diagnosis of edematous hyponatremia can be easily made at the bedside, differentiating between normovolemic and hypovolemic hyponatremia may be difficult on clinical grounds, especially in the elderly, in whom useful signs of hypovolemia such as poor skin turgor or orthostasis may be absent. A low sodium concentration ($<$ 20 mEq per liter) in a spot urine specimen strongly suggests a hypovolemic state, whereas the urine sodium is usually greater than 40 mEq per liter in the normovolemic hyponatremic patient [17].

TABLE 2-1. Classification of hyponatremia

A. Normovolemic
    Syndrome of inappropriate secretion of ADH (SIADH)
    Diuretic-induced
    Postoperative
    Others—hypothyroidism, adrenal insufficiency, acute respiratory
      failure
B. Edematous
    Congestive heart failure
    Liver disease
    Nephrotic syndrome
    Chronic obstructive pulmonary disease
C. Hypovolemic
D. Hypoalbuminemic hyponatremia—a syndrome of variable etiology in
    the elderly

TABLE 2-2. Cause of inappropriate secretion of ADH

Central nervous system disorders: vascular abnormalities, infections

Intrathoracic disorders: tumors, infections

Idiopathic

Drug-induced: chlorpropamide, carbamazepine, vinca alkaloids, phenothiazines, clofibrate

---

Normovolemic Hyponatremia

The syndrome of inappropriate secretion of ADH (SIADH) and diuretic administration constitute the most common causes of normovolemic hyponatremia in the elderly.

SIADH. Several conditions have been associated with this syndrome (Table 2-2). In the series of Sunderam and Mankikar [10], stroke, chest infection, and carcinoma were the most common causes. Of the 13 patients older than 60 years reported by Kleinfeld et al [11], three had a cerebrovascular accident, three were taking pharmacologic agents known to impair water excretion, two had a malignancy, and the remaining five had a variety of disorders. These latter five patients may have had an idiopathic form as recently described by Goldstein and colleagues [18], who reported one patient with SIADH without any associated disease and found nine other previously reported cases. Edward et al [19] subsequently described an 86-year-old patient with the syndrome. In the 11 patients described in these two reports, seven (64 percent) were older than 60 years, which suggests that advanced age predisposes to this form of SIADH. The mechanism for ADH release in these patients is not clear, but in some patients stress might serve as a stimulus [20]. Such patients, however, should be followed carefully, since clinically detectable malignancy has been identified several months after a diagnosis of "idiopathic" SIADH has been made [21, 22].

Several pharmacologic agents have been associated with SIADH including vincristine, vinblastine, phenothiazines, MAO inhibitors, clofibrate, chlorpropamide, and carbamazepine. Among this list, the latter two drugs are commonly used in the elderly for the management of adult-onset diabetes mellitus and tic douloureux (trigeminal neuralgia), respectively. Of the five patients with chlorpropamide hyponatremia studied by Weissman et al [23], four were over the age of 60.

Elevated plasma ADH levels in patients with SIADH have been confirmed by Zerbe et al [24] in 79 patients. They have shown that plasma ADH levels inappropriate for the hypotonicity of body fluids exist (Fig.

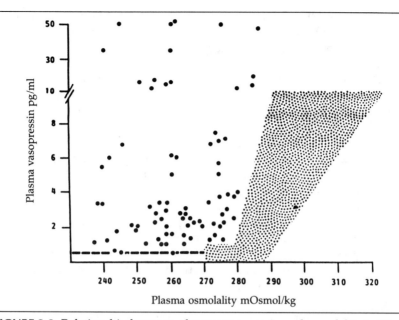

FIGURE 2-2. Relationship between plasma vasopressin and osmolality in 79 patients with clinical features of SIADH (shaded area represents the range of normal values). (From Zerbe R, Stropes L, and Robertson G: Vasopressin function in the syndrome of inappropriate antidiuresis. *Ann Rev Med* 31:315–327, 1980. By permission of Annual Reviews Inc.).

2-2). The changes in serum Na concentration that occur are accounted for primarily by changes in solute and water balance, as shown by Cooke et al [25]. Atrial natriuretic factor is elevated acutely and chronically during SIADH and may be responsible in part for the natriuresis seen early in this syndrome [26]. In some patients with SIADH, salt wasting due to an inability of the distal part of the nephron to reabsorb salt maximally has been reported [27]. Such patients differ markedly from those with the more common "pure" form of SIADH in that volume restriction is associated with an increased loss of sodium in the urine, resulting in severe volume contraction. It is important to recognize such patients because they generally require administration of large doses of mineralocorticoids [28].

Besides hyponatremia, hypouremia has also been encountered frequently in patients with SIADH [29, 30], secondary to both an increase in urinary losses of urea and body fluid dilution [30]. Beck [31] reported a mean serum urate concentration of 2.9 ± 4 mg per dl in patients with SIADH compared with 7.7 ± 0.8 mg per dl in those with other forms of hyponatremia. Hypouricemia has been demonstrated by others and has been attributed both to increased tubular secretion of uric acid and a decrease in the postsecretory reabsorption rate [32, 33].

DIURETIC-INDUCED HYPONATREMIA. The true incidence of diuretic-induced hyponatremia in the elderly is not known. Of 48 episodes of hyponatremia studied retrospectively by Abramow and Cogan [34], 14 instances (29 percent) were explained solely on the basis of diuretic use. Seven of 59 patients with severe hyponatremia (mean Na of 112 mEq per liter) reported by Booker [20] were taking a diuretic. The thiazide group of diuretics and, rarely, the potassium-sparing diuretics such as triamterene or amiloride may be responsible for the syndrome, which is seen most often in elderly women. Seventy-seven percent of reported patients were over 60 years old, and 85 percent of these were women, as reported by Grenfell [35]. In the series of Abramow and Cogan [34], the mean age was 76.5 years, and 11 of the 12 patients (92 percent) were women. The reason why diuretic-induced hyponatremia is more prevalent in elderly women is not clear.

Approximately 60 percent of the patients come to medical attention because of symptomatic hyponatremia, ranging from nausea and vomiting to confusion, seizures, or coma. The mechanisms responsible for the hyponatremia are probably multiple and include urinary Na losses, potassium depletion [36, 37] and an increase in water intake [38]. It should be noted, however, that hypokalemia is not present in all reported patients. The inappropriate release of ADH has also been suggested as a cause of diuretic-induced hyponatremia [39, 40]. Finally, there is experimental evidence that a sulfonamide diuretic can potentiate the effect of ADH on the collecting tubule [41]. In the presence of a submaximal concentration of ADH (2.5 mU per ml), indapamide (a sulfonamide diuretic) significantly increases the hydraulic permeability of the isolated cortical collecting tubule. Figure 2-3 schematically describes how these factors play a role in diuretic-induced hyponatremia.

Another reason why diuretic-induced hyponatremia is seen most commonly with thiazides could be related to their different effect on prostaglandins compared with furosemide. Furosemide increases urinary prostaglandin excretion, which antagonizes the hydro-osmotic effect of ADH, whereas the thiazides have no effect on prostaglandin release [42].

POSTOPERATIVE HYPONATREMIA. In younger individuals postoperative antidiuresis is usually a transient phenomenon secondary to ADH release due to pain, analgesic use, and so on. By contrast, in the elderly this problem may be severe and prolonged. Deutsch and associates [43] reported a group of patients (average age 75 years) in whom

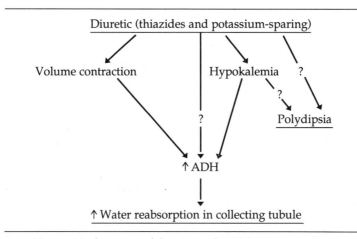

FIGURE 2-3. Mechanisms of diuretic-induced hyponatremia.

symptoms of hyponatremia, including moderate to marked changes in level of consciousness, occurred within the first 5 postoperative days. Likely contributing factors included narcotic use during the pre-, peri-, and postoperative periods and excessive hypotonic fluid administration in the presence of nonosmotic stimulated secretion of ADH [44]. Based on these findings, fluid replacement in the postoperative elderly patient should be carefully planned and should be limited to replacing losses on an hourly basis, if possible. In these patients serum electrolytes should be measured periodically or whenever a change in the level of consciousness is noted.

Hyponatremia has also been reported following transurethral prostatic resection. The true incidence of this problem is not known; however, in a prospective study carried out by Rhymer and co-workers [45], 7 of 100 patients developed significant hyponatremia (range 103–133 mEq per liter). They found a significant correlation between the weight of the resected prostate and the postoperative decrease in serum Na, as well as between the weight of the gland resected and the volume of irrigation fluid (glycine) used. Since the hyponatremia most likely represents reabsorption of electrolyte-free solution by the open prostatic veins [46], the larger the gland and the longer the surgery, the more irrigating solution will be reabsorbed. Another factor contributing to the amount of irrigating solution reabsorbed was the irrigating pressure maintained. It is recommended that the latter be kept below 60 mm Hg during the procedure [47]. Symptoms usually appeared near the end or immediately following surgery and included increasing apprehension, disorientation, blood pressure elevation, bradycardia, irritability, twitching, nausea, vomiting, and convulsions. In general, the prognosis is good, but it depends on the rate at which serum Na is lowered. Six of the seven patients reported by Rhymer and associates [45] recovered within 48 hours. Sunderrajan et al [47] quoted a mortality as high as 50 percent for the group in whom a rapid fall in serum Na occurred. Our own experience is limited to four symptomatic patients; three recovered and one expired after developing a grand mal seizure. All four patients were on a low Na diet in the hospital, and diuretic therapy for hypertension was continued in three, so that preoperative volume contraction with persistent ADH release might have contributed to the postoperative water retention in these patients.

OTHER ASSOCIATED CONDITIONS. Endocrine disorders such as hypothyroidism and adrenal insufficiency may be associated with hyponatremia. It is not known how often this complication is seen in elderly patients with these disorders. In both situations persistent release of ADH, although playing a significant role, does not entirely explain the water retention [48]. It is important to note that transient asymptomatic hyperthyroxinemia can occur during hyponatremia [49] and that hyperthyroidism has been reported to affect as many as 10 percent of elderly patients [50].

Acute respiratory failure has also been associated with hyponatremia. Szatalowitz and colleagues [51] reported 13 patients with acute respiratory failure (average age 59 years) whose ADH levels were significantly elevated. The nonosmotic stimulus for the ADH release in these patients is not clear. The hyponatremia observed was mild (plasma Na 133 ± 1 mEq per liter) and was reversible on correction of the acute problem. It seems prudent to administer hypotonic fluid cautiously to patients with acute respiratory failure to avoid severe hyponatremia.

Edematous Hyponatremia
CONGESTIVE HEART FAILURE. Hyponatremia is not an uncommon finding in patients with congestive heart failure [52, 53]. Dzau and colleagues [54] compared biochemical and hemodynamic parameters in hyponatremic and normonatremic patients with congestive heart failure. Ejection fraction was similar in both groups; however, plasma angiotensin II, renin activity, aldosterone, and prostaglandins (PGE_2 and 6 keto-$PGF_{1\alpha}$) were higher in the hyponatremic group. In patients with congestive heart failure, kidney function is decreased in those with hyponatremia compared with normonatremic patients [55]. Rondeau and co-workers [56] found that plasma ADH levels were higher in 31 elderly patients with heart failure compared with age-matched controls, with plasma Na and osmolality lower in the heart failure group. The nonosmotic stimulation of ADH release in heart failure does not appear to depend on the renin-angiotensin system, since plasma renin activity does not correlate with plasma ADH [57]. The hyponatremia of congestive

heart failure is multifactorial and depends on (1) increased water intake secondary to the dipsogenic effect of increased angiotension II [58]; (2) intrarenal factors; and (3) nonosmotic release of ADH. As a rule, the more severe the heart failure, the higher the plasma ADH level. Since the level of ADH decreases as cardiac function improves, cardiac function may represent the main determinant for the nonosmotic release of the hormone [59]. In patients with milder forms of the disease, control of the heart failure will correct the hyponatremia; however, in more severe states, the combined use of furosemide (daily dose tailored to the patient's diuretic response) and captopril (started at an initial dose of 12.5 mg given every 8 hours and titrated to achieve maximal hemodynamic response) has been found to be very helpful and should be used in such patients [60, 61].

LIVER DISEASE. The hyponatremia of chronic liver disease is also multifactorial. Renal hemodynamics have been found by Lancestremere and associates [62] to play a role. Plasma ADH levels are usually elevated in hyponatremic patients with cirrhosis [63], but diuresis can occur without concomitant suppression of ADH in some patients, suggesting that the hormone may represent a "permissive" rather than a pivotal factor in the impairment of water excretion [64]. A decrease in effective arterial blood volume has been suggested as the nonosmotic stimulus for the ADH release, since the latter can be suppressed by head-out water immersion, a maneuver associated with central blood volume expansion [65, 66]. The importance of ineffective blood volume and catecholamines, which have been thought to play a role in the hyponatremia seen in cirrhosis [67, 68], is still a matter of controversy, however. Recently, urinary PGE_2 was found to be lower in cirrhotic patients with hyponatremia compared with those with normonatremia [69]. As noted, PGE_2 modulates the effect of ADH in the cortical collecting tubule, so that a lower PGE_2 level results in the reabsorption of a larger percentage of the water presented to this site. The reason for the decreased urinary excretion of PGE_2 in these patients is not known.

The management of hyponatremia in the cirrhotic patient consists mainly of water and moderate salt restriction and gentle diuresis. Demeclocycline has been tried, but the incidence of side effects is rather high in this patient population. Oral urea (see Treatment) is worth trying in recalcitrant cases.

NEPHROTIC SYNDROME. Hyponatremia has not been a common occurrence in elderly patients with the nephrotic syndrome (occurring in less than 1 percent). Three (8.3 percent) of the patients of Kleinfeld et al with hyponatremia had nephrotic syndrome [11]. Usberti et al [70] found an inverse correlation between blood volume or plasma volume and the ability to excrete a water load. Expansion of blood volume with 20 percent albumin reduced the plasma level of ADH and promoted a water diuresis. Bichet and Schrier [71] also found a lower glomerular filtration rate (GFR), lower fractional excretion of Na, higher plasma renin activity (PRA), higher plasma aldosterone (PA) and catecholamines, and impaired water excretion in hyponatremic patients with the nephrotic syndrome, suggesting that a decrease in blood volume might be the nonosmotic stimulus for ADH release.

CHRONIC OBSTRUCTIVE PULMONARY DISEASE (COPD). Farber et al [72] have reported a high incidence of hyponatremia in edematous patients with COPD and respiratory failure (mean age 57 ± 7 years). When compared to controls, these patients had a lower effective renal plasma flow and GFR together with elevated PRA and PA levels. Plasma ADH could not be suppressed despite the lower plasma osmolality. It appears that the hyponatremia is a consequence of both intrarenal hemodynamics and persistent ADH release. Again, the cause of nonosmotic release of ADH is not clear. Therefore, one should be cautious about the amount of hypotonic solution infused in such patients. Even in normonatremic patients with COPD, the percentage of a water load excreted may be significantly lower than that in normal subjects.

Hypovolemic Hyponatremia
The hyponatremia that occurs in this group of patients is the result of a release of ADH due to a persistent volume stimulus in a patient with free access to water. The source of volume losses is usually the gastrointestinal tract (severe diarrhea) or the kidneys (osmotic diuresis of hyperglycemia and glycosuria, continued use of a diuretic and a low salt diet in the elderly hypertensive patient hospitalized for other problems, or overdiuresis for congestive heart failure). The diagnosis is not difficult in most patients because physical signs of volume contraction such as weight loss, an orthostatic drop in blood pressure, and poor skin turgor are usually present. However, the signs of hypovolemia may be difficult to detect in the elderly, as noted earlier. In those patients not taking a diuretic, the urine Na concentration is low (< 20 mEq per liter). When renal failure is present, the BUN is usually disproportionately higher than the serum creatinine. Therapy should be directed toward correcting the cause of the fluid losses and expanding the extracellular volume with a saline solution.

Hypoalbuminemic Hyponatremia
Dandona et al [73] have recently described six patients with severe hyponatremia and pronounced hypoalbuminemia. Age was given only for three of the six patients, all of whom were older than 60 years. The explanation for the inability of these patients to excrete water is not clear; however, since the hypo-osmolality could be corrected by plasma al-

bumin infusion, hypovolemia might have been the stimulus for persistent ADH release. We have seen 12 patients (all elderly women) with hypoalbuminemia (range 1.5–2.0 g per dl) and hyponatremia (110–120 mEq per liter). All were patients who were hospitalized for either cerebrovascular disease or advanced dementia (possibly the stimulus for ADH release) and were receiving large volumes of nasogastric feedings low in Na. Three of these patients were edematous with normal PRA and PA levels. These patients responded well to water restriction. After correction of the hyponatremia, NaCl (2 g daily) was added to the tube feedings without any further problems. In another three patients, edema was absent, and PRA and PA levels were both elevated, suggesting volume contraction. The addition of 4 g of NaCl to their feedings resulted in prompt correction of the hyponatremia.

CLINICAL MANIFESTATIONS

Studies done by Arieff et al [74] have demonstrated that symptoms are related to both the magnitude and the rate of development of hyponatremia. Of the 36 patients reported by Kleinfeld et al [11], nine were asymptomatic; in the remaining 27 patients the various symptoms were to a great extent secondary to the underlying disease. The clinical features attributable to hyponatremia are summarized in Table 2-3.

TREATMENT

Asymptomatic Patients

The therapy of hyponatremia depends on the clinical situation. The traditional method in the asymptomatic patient consists of fluid restriction. When a drug is the cause, it should be discontinued. Unfortunately, normonatremia is difficult to maintain with fluid restriction alone, and other therapies may be necessary in patients with chronic hyponatremia as in those with SIADH. Several approaches have been recommended.

LITHIUM. Lithium carbonate can produce a nephrogenic diabetes insipidus; however, its effectiveness is limited to only a minority of patients,

TABLE 2-3. Clinical features attributable to hyponatremia in 77 patients

Clinical feature	No. of patients
weakness	28
confusion	21
postural hypotension	17
falls	13
transient hemiparesis	1
seizures	2

SOURCE: Sunderam SG and Mankikar GD: Hyponatremia in the elderly. *Age Aging* 12:77–80, 1983.

and it is potentially toxic, limiting its usefulness in the elderly, in whom the half-life of the drug is prolonged [75, 76].

DEMECLOCYCLINE. This tetracycline antibiotic inhibits the action of ADH in the cortical collecting tubule. Doses of 600 to 1200 mg per day are generally used. The drug is well tolerated, but its use in patients with pre-existing kidney or liver disease is limited [77–79]. Side effects include nausea, photosensitivity, and extracellular fluid volume contraction [80].

UREA. A dose of 40 to 90 g per day orally has been reported by Decaux et al [81] to be beneficial in the long-term management of patients with SIADH or the hyponatremia associated with liver disease. The drug has both an antinatriuretic and a diuretic effect. According to the passive countercurrent model, the antinatriuretic action is secondary to increased NaCl reabsorption in the thin ascending limb of Henle [82]. Its diuretic effect is due to the osmotic force of unabsorbed urea. Although side effects have been minimal, its use has been limited to a relatively small number of patients [83].

PHENYTOIN. At a dose of 100 mg 3 times daily orally, this drug has been used successfully for up to 8 months in one patient [84]. It acts by inhibiting the release of ADH from the hypophysis [85]. A trial in a large number of patients is necessary before its routine use can be recommended.

FUROSEMIDE. The combination of furosemide and a high salt diet has been used long term by Decaux and associates [86] with good results.

ADH ANALOGUES. The advent of new analogues of ADH with specific antagonist activity against the antidiuretic properties of this hormone allow more specific therapy of SIADH and other chronic hyponatremic states [87].

Symptomatic Patients
The presence of symptoms related to hyponatremia depends on the rapidity with which hypotonicity occurs as well as on the absolute level of the serum Na. When symptoms are present, rapid correction is indicated. To estimate the Na deficit in such patients the following formula has been recommended:

desired Na concentration − observed Na concentration × (0.6 × body weight in kg)

However, based on Table 2-4 it is evident that total body water represents 45 to 50 percent of body weight in the elderly, and therefore the

TABLE 2-4. Body water compartments
throughout life span (as percent of body weight)

Age	Sex	Body weight (kg)	Total body water (%)	Extra-cellular water (%)	Intra-cellular water (%)
0–11 days			76.4	41.6	34.8
11–180 days			72.8	34.9	37.9
6 months–2 years			62.2	27.5	34.7
2–7 years			65.5	25.6	36.9
7–14 years			64.2	17.5	46.7
23–54 years	male	72.5	54.3	23.4	30.9
			±1.4*	±0.6	±0.9
23–51 years	female	59.3	48.6	22.7	25.9
			±1.5	±0.5	±1.0
71–84 years	male	68.1	50.8	25.4	25.4
			±1.6	±1.4	±0.6
61–74 years	female	63.9	43.4	21.4	22.4
			±1.3	±0.5	±1.0

*Standard error of the mean.
SOURCE: Weitzman R and Kleeman CR: Water metabolism and the neurohypophyseal hormones. In Maxwell MH and Kleeman CR (eds): *Clinical Disorders of Fluid and Electrolyte Metabolism*, 3rd ed. New York, McGraw-Hill, 1980, pp. 531–645. With permission.

use of 60 percent will tend to overestimate the Na deficit, as recently discussed by Shankel [88]. This question is of more than academic interest because overcorrection has been associated with central pontine myelinolysis, also called osmotic demyelination syndrome [89, 90]. Clinical manifestations of this syndrome range from minimal to severe neurologic deficits with flaccid quadriplegia and facial weakness. The incidence of this syndrome in the overtreated hyponatremic patient is a matter of controversy, however [91].

Once the decision to treat hyponatremia has been made, some authors have advised rapid correction at rates approaching 2 mEq per liter per hour [92, 93]; however, slower correction usually works as well [94, 95]. Ashouri [96] reported eight symptomatic patients with diuretic-induced hyponatremia who received correction at a rate of 0.78 ± 0.26 mEq per liter per hour, requiring 28.8 ± 6 hours. All the patients recovered with complete resolution of the neurologic symptoms. Recent evidence suggests that an increase in plasma sodium of 20 mEq per liter or less in the initial period of therapy is associated with recovery without sequelae in most patients [97]. Our approach consists of reaching a serum Na of 120 to 125 mEq per liter, corrected at a rate of 0.5 to 0.8 mEq per liter per hour, using hypertonic NaCl alone (512 mM per liter) for the volume-depleted patient. Intermittent doses of intravenous furosemide (1 mg per kg body weight), as recommended by Hantman et al [98], are added for patients with SIADH and edema. In the latter group of patients, diuresis should be initiated with furosemide before any salt is infused. We have used this regimen successfully in 20 elderly patients with symptomatic hyponatremia. Examination of the pons in five of these patients, who died from unrelated conditions long after correction of their hyponatremia, failed to show any evidence of myelinolysis.

MORTALITY IN HYPONATREMIC PATIENTS
In the study of Anderson and colleagues [12], the fatality rate for patients with hyponatremia was 11.2 percent compared with 0.19 percent for the remainder of the patient population examined during the same period of time; however, in other published series as well as our own experience, hyponatremia appears to be a marker for severe underlying disease that generally carries a poorer prognosis.

HYPERNATREMIA

Hypernatremia is less common in the elderly than hyponatremia. For instance, among 14,133 patients over the age of 60 seen during a three-year period in a Veterans Administration hospital, 212, or 1.5 percent, had a serum Na greater than 148 mEq per liter [99]. Of 10 patients seen by us for hypernatremia during a one-year period, eight were elderly.

ETIOLOGY
Hypernatremia is the result of either the addition of a hypertonic Na solution to the extracellular fluid or hypotonic fluid losses. Extracellular hypertonic fluid gain occurs mainly following the infusion of Na bicarbonate during cardiopulmonary resuscitation. Accidental ingestion of salt is rather rare in the elderly. Hypotonic fluid losses through the gastrointestinal tract secondary to diarrhea are the most common cause of hypernatremia in the elderly [99]. In our experience, the most common cause of such diarrhea in the hospital setting is hyperosmolar tube feeding and lactulose administration in the patient with portosystemic encephalopathy [100, 101]. Renal loss of water due to osmotic diuresis associated with glycosuria (mainly in patients with the hyperglycemic hyperosmolar syndrome), mannitol or glycerol infusion, or high-protein tube feeding is the next most common cause of hypernatremia [102].

CLINICAL MANIFESTATIONS
The clinical manifestations associated with hypernatremia are usually those of the underlying disease. In one large series the conditions most often seen were dementia (32 percent), pneumonia (27 percent), sepsis (25 percent), heart failure (20 percent), and stroke (8 percent) [99]. Occa-

sionally an acute confusional state due to the hyperosmolar state brings the patient to medical attention [103]. The sensation of thirst, which is probably present in many of these patients, may not be verbalized, since those affected frequently have a depressed sensorium.

With hypotonic losses from the gastrointestinal tract, evidence of volume contraction will be found on physical examination. It should be noted, however, that changes usually associated with dehydration such as poor skin tone and sunken eye sockets may be seen with aging per se. Urinary Na concentration is usually less than 20 mEq per liter unless the patient has chronic renal failure, develops acute tubular necrosis owing to the accompanying shock, or the hypernatremia is marked [104]. In the patient who has received Na bicarbonate, the history should be helpful, and the urinary Na concentration is usually greater than 60 mEq per liter. The urinary osmolality is generally greater than twice the plasma osmolality unless there is superimposed acute or chronic renal insufficiency. In our experience this combination (hypotonic losses through the GI tract and renal failure) has been the rule rather than the exception in the elderly with severe extracellular fluid volume losses. Hypernatremia secondary to water losses through osmotic diuresis should be suspected in patients receiving either high-protein tube feedings or an osmotic diuretic such as mannitol (e.g., during aortic aneurysm surgery or following a cerebrovascular accident) or in those with severe hyperglycemia and glycosuria. In these situations, the urine Na tends to be above 30 mEq per liter, and the urine osmolality is close to isotonicity.

TREATMENT
Water losses should be estimated before instituting therapy. Several formulas have been described, but we have found the following most helpful:

$$BW_2 = Na_1 \times BW_1/Na_2$$

where BW_2 represents the current body water, Na_1 the normal serum Na (145 mEq per liter), BW_1 the original volume of body water (50 percent of body weight in the elderly), and Na_2 the current serum Na. The water loss is the difference between BW_1 and BW_2. For instance, in a 70-kg man with a serum Na of 165 mEq per liter, $BW_2 = 145 \times 35/165 = 5075/165 = 31$ liters. The water deficit would then be $35 - 31 = 4$ liters.

Type of Solution
Dextrose in water should be given to the patient with hypernatremia secondary to Na excesses, with careful monitoring of the urinary output. If the patient is oliguric, intravenous furosemide can be tried. In

postcardiac arrest patients with acute oliguric renal failure in whom large volumes of sodium bicarbonate have been infused, dialysis should be initiated. For the patient with hypotonic fluid losses and hypotension, rapid expansion of the extracellular fluid can be achieved with a 0.9 percent NaCl infusion. Once normotension has been achieved, one can switch to any of the hypotonic solutions available (we usually base our decision on determination of the urine Na).

Rate of Infusion

It is recommended that calculated losses be repaired within 48 to 72 hours. In the series of Snyder et al [99], the mortality in patients in whom the deficit was replaced within 48 to 72 hours was 31 percent compared with 66 percent in those corrected within 24 hours. The marked difference was attributed to the probable development of cerebral edema. The overall mortality in this series was 42 percent. The severity of the hypernatremia does not appear to contribute directly to the mortality rate (Table 2-5). When other problems such as chronic renal failure, ischemic heart disease, surgery, or pneumonia were present concurrently, the mortality increased, which suggests that hypernatremia in the elderly is often a marker for more serious illness, as with hyponatremia. Of 48 elderly patients with hypernatremic dehydration reported by Himmelstein and associates [105], 24 died (50 percent).

TABLE 2-5. Association of clinical characteristics
with mortality in 162 elderly patients with hypernatremia

Measure of severity of hypernatremia	Survivors	Non-survivors
Serum sodium levels (mEq/liter)		
Peak	154	153
Mean (for entire episode)	151	151
Total body water deficit at time of peak sodium level (%)	10.7	9.5
Duration of episode (days)	2.1	1.9
Age (yr)*	78 ± 9	77 ± 9
Sex (%)		
Women	41	42
Men	59	58
Race (%)		
White	69	72
Black	26	22
Other	5	6

*Value given as mean ± SD
SOURCE: Snyder NA, Feigel DW, and Arieff AI: Hypernatremia in elderly patients. A heterogeneous, morbid, and iatrogenic entity. *Ann Intern Med* 107:309–319, 1987.

DIABETES INSIPIDUS

INCIDENCE
Diabetes insipidus (DI) is rather rare in the elderly. Of 85 adult patients reported in the literature, only three were 60 years or older [106–113].

ETIOLOGY
DI is secondary to either a deficiency in ADH synthesis by the pituitary gland (neurogenic DI) or an inability of the cells of the renal collecting tubule to respond to circulating ADH (nephrogenic DI). The causes of these two varieties of DI are outlined in Table 2-6.

CLINICAL MANIFESTATIONS
DI should be suspected in any elderly patient presenting with polyuria and hypotonic urine. The most important diagnosis to be ruled out is psychogenic polydipsia (compulsive water drinking), a condition more common in this age group than DI. Patients with psychogenic polydipsia are usually women who have a history of psychiatric disease [114]. In some patients (mostly males), the syndrome develops on a background of chronic alcoholism, and in others chronic hiccups is the reason for ex-

TABLE 2-6. Causes of diabetes insipidus

Neurogenic diabetes insipidus
  Hypophysectomy
  Intracranial surgery
  Head trauma
  Intracranial tumors
    Primary—suprasellar or intrasellar
    Metastatic—breast or lung carcinoma, myeloproliferative disorders
  Granulomatous disease
    Tuberculosis
    Sarcoidosis
  Vascular abnormalities—aneurysms
  Infections (viral)
  "Empty sella" syndrome
Nephrogenic diabetes insipidus
  Congenital
  Chronic renal insufficiency
  Electrolyte disorders
    Hypokalemia
    Hypercalcemia
  Drugs
    Lithium
    Demeclocycline
    Other?

cessive drinking [115]. In contrast to DI patients, who are in general normo- or even hypernatremic, patients with compulsive water drinking are hyponatremic, and the condition is at times severe and symptomatic. Laboratory evidence of rhabdomyolysis has been reported in these patients [115], the mechanism of which is not clear. The diagnosis of psychogenic polydipsya can be confirmed by water restriction, which leads to an increase in plasma ADH and urine osmolality (to greater than plasma osmolality) as free water clearance becomes negative. In some patients ADH is released, and urine osmolality increases at a plasma osmolality that is clearly abnormally low, suggesting a resetting of the osmostat. Besides a defect in the secretion of ADH, patients with psychogenic polydipsia exhibit unexplained deficits in urinary dilution and osmoregulation of water intake [116]. In psychotic patients, an increase in water intake tends to occur during exacerbations of the psychiatric problem and improves with therapeutic intervention.

· During water deprivation, patients with neurogenic DI achieve a urine osmolality above that of plasma after ADH administration. A dose of 5 IU of aqueous ADH is used subcutaneously. The plasma ADH concentration and osmolality after administration of hypertonic (5 percent) saline infused at a rate of 0.05 to 0.06 ml per kg body weight per min. will also help to differentiate neurogenic from nephrogenic DI [112]. It is important to remember to correlate plasma ADH levels with plasma osmolality and to interpret the results according to normal values obtained by using the same assay and procedure, as emphasized by Zerbe and Robertson [112]; however, nomograms, similar to those reported by Robertson et al [117], have yet to be published for the elderly. Such data would be valuable because ADH, as noted earlier, increases with age. In older men, basal plasma ADH levels can reach values three times as high as those obtained in 25-year-olds [118].

TREATMENT
The therapy of choice for patients with neurogenic DI consists of intranasal administration of dDAVP. A starting dose of 2.5 mg once daily has been suggested, with gradual increases until polyuria is adequately controlled [111]. Certain patients may require a divided dose. The drug is generally well tolerated, and only an occasional patient develops resistance to the drug. In patients who cannot tolerate dDAVP and in those with congenital nephrogenic DI or chronic renal insufficiency, the urine volume can be significantly decreased by the use of indomethacin, a thiazide diuretic, and salt restriction. Care must be taken to avoid excessive volume contraction with postural hypotension or a further decrease in kidney function. Since nephrogenic DI in the elderly is most likely secondary to other disorders (see Table 2-6), management is that of the underlying problem.

PROGNOSIS AND MORTALITY
Both prognosis and mortality in patients with DI depend primarily on the underlying disease; however, in the elderly, who may not be able to replace water losses because of decreased mentation and an inability to comprehend or respond to thirst or an inability to take liquids because of infirmity and lack of attention, severe volume contraction and even shock may occur, leading to significant morbidity and even mortality.

REFERENCES

1. Robertson GL, et al: Development and clinical application of a new method for the radioimmunoassay of arginine vasopressin in human plasma. *J Clin Invest* 52:2340–2352, 1973.
2. Robertson GL: Osmotic and hemodynamic control of vasopressin: Functional and anatomical relationships. In Takacs L (ed): *Advances in Physiological Sciences*. Vol II: *Kidneys and Body Fluids*. Budapest Akademiai, Kiado, Pergamon, 1981.
3. Sklar AH and Schrier RW: Central nervous system mediators of vasopressin release. *Physiol Rev* 63:1243–1280, 1983.
4. Rowe JW, et al: Influence of the emetic reflex on vasopressin release in man. *Kidney Int* 16:729–735, 1979.
5. Silver AJ and Morley JE: Role of the opioid in hypodipsia of aging. *Clin Res* 37:90A, 1980.
6. Phillips PA, et al: Reduced thirst after water deprivation in healthy elderly men. *N Engl J Med* 311:753–759, 1984.
7. Rowe JW, et al: Age related failure of volume-pressure mediated vasopressin release. *J Clin Endocrinol Metab* 54:661–664, 1982.
8. Helderman JH, et al: The response of arginine vasopressin to intravenous ethanol and hypertonic saline. The impact of aging. *J Gerontol* 33:39–47, 1978.
9. Baran D and Hutchinson TA: The outcome of hyponatremia in a general hospital population. *Clin Nephrol* 22:72–76, 1984.
10. Sunderam SG and Mankikar GD: Hyponatremia in the elderly. *Age Aging* 12:77–80, 1983.
11. Kleinfeld M, Casimir M, and Borra S: Hyponatremia as observed in a chronic disease facility. *J Am Geriatr Soc* 27:156–161, 1979.
12. Anderson RJ, et al: Hyponatremia: A prospective analysis of its epidemiology and the pathogenic role of vasopressin. *Ann Intern Med* 102:164–168, 1985.
13. Cogan E and Abramow M: Transient hyperthyroxinemia in symptomatic hyponatremic patients. *Arch Intern Med* 146:545–547, 1986.
14. Weisberg LS: Pseudohyponatremia: A reappraisal. *Am J Med* 86:313–318, 1989.
15. Katz M: Hyperglycemia-induced hyponatremia. Calculation of expected serum sodium depression. *N Engl J Med* 289:843–844, 1973.
16. Glasser L, et al: Serum osmolality and its applicability to drug overdose. *Am J Clin Pathol* 60:695–699, 1973.
17. Chung HM, et al: Clinical assessment of extracellular fluid volume in hyponatremia. *Am J Med* 83:905–908, 1987.
18. Goldstein CS, Braunstein S, and Goldfarb S: Idiopathic syndrome of inap-

propriate antidiuretic hormone secretion possibly related to advanced age. *Ann Intern Med* 99:185–188, 1983.

19. Edward K, Barken F, and Lovold JA: Age and inappropriate antidiuretic hormone secretion. *Ann Intern Med* 100:766, 1984.
20. Booker JA: Severe symptomatic hyponatremia in elderly outpatients. The role of thiazide therapy and stress. *J Am Geriatr Soc* 32:108–113, 1984.
21. Martinez-Maldonado M: Inappropriate antidiuretic hormone secretion of unknown origin. *Kidney Int* 17:554–567, 1980.
22. Verbalis JG: Tumoral hyponatremia. *Arch Intern Med* 146:1686–1687, 1986.
23. Weissman PN, Shenkman L, and Gregerman RI: Chlorpropamide hyponatremia. *N Engl J Med* 284:65–71, 1971.
24. Zerbe R, Stropes L, and Robertson G: Vasopressin function in the syndrome of inappropriate antidiuresis. *Ann Rev Med* 31:315–327, 1980.
25. Cooke RC, Turin MD, and Walker GW: The syndrome of inappropriate antidiuretic hormone secretion (SIADH): Pathophysiologic mechanisms in solute and volume regulation. *Medicine* 58:240–251, 1979.
26. Cogan E, et al: Natriuresis and atrial natriuretic factor. Secretion during inappropriate anti-diuresis. *Am J Med* 84:409–417, 1988.
27. Al-Mufti H and Arieff AI: Hyponatremia due to central salt-wasting syndrome. Combined cerebral and distal tubular lesion. *Am J Med* 77:740–746, 1984.
28. Ishikawa SE, et al: Hyponatremia responsive to fludrocortisone acetate in elderly patients after head injury. *Ann Intern Med* 146:187–191, 1987.
29. Barter FC and Schwartz WB: The syndrome of inappropriate secretion of antidiuretic hormone. *Am J Med* 42:790–806, 1967.
30. Decaux G, Genette F, and Mockel J: Hypouremia in the syndrome of inappropriate secretion of antidiuretic hormone. *Ann Intern Med* 93:716–717, 1980.
31. Beck LH: Hypouricemia in the syndrome of inappropriate secretion of antidiuretic hormone. *N Engl J Med* 301:528–530, 1979.
32. Shichiri M, et al: Renal handling of urate in the syndrome of inappropriate secretion of antidiuretic hormone. *Arch Intern Med* 145:2045–2047, 1985.
33. Decaux G, et al: Mechanisms of hypouricemia in the syndrome of inappropriate secretion of antidiuretic hormone. *Nephron* 39:164–168, 1985.
34. Abramow M and Cogan E: Clinical aspects and pathophysiology of diuretic-induced hyponatremia. *Adv Nephrol* 13:1–28, 1984.
35. Grenfell RF: Hyponatremia with the administration of diuretics. In Puschett JB and Greenberg A (eds): *Diuretics II. Chemistry, Pharmacology, and Clinical Applications.* New York, Elsevier, 1986.
36. Ashraf N, Locksley R, and Arieff AI: Thiazide-induced hyponatremia associated with death or neurologic damage in outpatients. *Am J Med* 70:1163–1168, 1981.
37. Fichman MP, et al: Diuretic-induced hyponatremia. *Ann Intern Med* 75:853–863, 1971.
38. Friedman E, et al: Thiazide induced hyponatremia. Reproducibility by single dose rechallenge and an analysis of pathogenesis. *Ann Intern Med* 110:24–30, 1989.
39. Hamburger S, et al: Thiazide-induced syndrome of inappropriate secretion of antidiuretic hormone. Time course of resolution. *JAMA* 246:1235–1236, 1981.
40. Sonnenblick M, Algur N, and Rosin A: Thiazide induced hyponatremia and vasopressin release. *Ann Intern Med* 110:751, 1989.
41. Abramow M and Dratwa M: Interaction of vasopressin and diuretics in the isolated collecting tubule. *Eur J Clin Invest* 4:353, 1974.

42. Keischi A, et al: Effect of furosemide on urinary excretion of prostaglandin E in normal volunteers and patients with essential hypertension. *Prostaglandins* 14:513–521, 1977.
43. Deutsch S, Goldberg M, and Dripps RD: Postoperative hyponatremia with the inappropriate release of antidiuretic hormone. *Anesthesiology* 27:250–256, 1966.
44. Chung H-M, et al: Postoperative hyponatremia. A prospective study. *Arch Intern Med* 146:333–336, 1987.
45. Rhymer JC, et al: Hyponatremia following transurethral resection of the prostate. *Br J Urol* 57:450–452, 1985.
46. Griffin M: Toxic symptoms accompanied by hemolysis during transurethral prostatectomy. *J Urol* 59:431–436, 1984.
47. Sunderrajan S, et al: Post-transurethral prostatic resection hyponatremic syndrome. Case report and review of the literature. *Am J Kidney Dis* 4:80–84, 1984.
48. Weiss JM and Robertson GL: Water metabolism in endocrine disorders. *Sem Nephrol* 4:303–315, 1984.
49. Cogan E and Abramow M: Transient hyperthyroxinemia in symptomatic hyponatremic patients. *Arch Intern Med* 146:545–547, 1986.
50. Sawin CT, et al: The aging thyroid: Increased prevalence of elevated serum thyrotropin levels in the elderly. *JAMA* 242:247, 1979.
51. Szatalowitz VL, Goldberg JP, and Anderson RJ: Plasma antidiuretic hormone in acute respiratory failure. *Am J Med* 72:583–587, 1982.
52. Weston RE, et al: The pathogenesis and treatment of hyponatremia in congestive heart failure. *Am J Med* 25:558–572, 1958.
53. Bell NH, Schedl HP, and Bartter FC: An explanation for abnormal water retention and hypoosmolality in congestive heart failure. *Am J Med* 36:351–360, 1964.
54. Dzau VJ, et al: Prostaglandins in severe congestive heart failure. Relation to activation of the renin-angiotensin system and hyponatremia. *N Engl J Med* 310:347–352, 1984.
55. Szatalowitz VL, et al: Radioimmunoassay of plasma arginine vasopressin in hyponatremic patients with congestive heart failure. *N Engl J Med* 305:263–266, 1981.
56. Rondeau E, et al: High plasma antidiuretic hormone in patients with cardiac failure: Influence of age. *Min Electr Metab* 8:267–274, 1982.
57. Korfas C, et al: Non-osmotic stimulation of vasopressin (ADH) is independent of the renin-angiotensin (RAS) in severe congestive heart failure (CHF) in man. *Am Soc Nephrol* 18th Annual Meeting 44A, 1985.
58. Johnson AK, et al: Plasma angiotensin II concentration and experimentally induced thirst. *Am J Physiol* 240:R229–R234, 1981.
59. Bichet DG, et al: Modulation of plasma and platelet vasopressin by cardiac function in patients with heart failure. *Kidney Int* 29:1188–1196, 1986.
60. Dzau VJ and Hollenberg NK: Renal response to captopril in severe heart failure: Role of furosemide in natriuresis and reversal of hyponatremia. *Ann Intern Med* 100:772–782, 1984.
61. Packer M, Medina N, and Yushak M: Correction of dilutional hyponatremia in severe chronic heart failure by converting enzyme inhibition. *Ann Intern Med* 100:782–789, 1984.
62. Lancestremere RG, et al: Renal failure in Laennec's cirrhosis: III. Diuretic response to administered water. *J Lab Clin Med* 60:967–975, 1962.
63. Bichet D, et al: Role of vasopressin in abnormal water excretion in cirrhotic humans. *Ann Intern Med* 96:413–416, 1982.

64. Epstein M, et al: Relationship between plasma arginine vasopressin and renal water handling in decompensated cirrhosis. *Min Electr Metab* 10:155–165, 1984.

65. Bichet DG, Groves BM, and Schrier RW: Mechanisms of improvement of water and sodium excretion by immersion in decompensated cirrhotic patients. *Kidney Int* 24:788–794, 1983.

66. Shapiro MD, et al: Interrelationship between cardiac output and vascular resistance as determinants of effective arterial blood volume in cirrhotic patients. *Kidney Int* 26:206–211, 1985.

67. Bichet DG, Van Patten VJ, and Schrier RW: Potential role of increased sympathetic activity in impaired sodium and water excretion in cirrhosis. *N Engl J Med* 307:1552–1557, 1982.

68. Epstein M, Larios O, and Johnson O: Effects of water immersion on plasma catecholamines in decompensated cirrhosis. Implications for deranged sodium and water homeostasis. *Min Electr Metab* 11:25–34, 1985.

69. Perez-Ayuso RM, et al: Evidence that renal prostaglandins are involved in renal water metabolism in cirrhosis. *Kidney Int* 26:72–80, 1984.

70. Usberti M, et al: Role of plasma vasopressin in the impairment of water excretion in nephrotic syndrome. *Kidney Int* 25:422–429, 1984.

71. Bichet DG and Schrier RW: Water metabolism in edematous disorders. *Sem Nephrol* 4:325–333, 1984.

72. Farber MO, et al: Abnormalities of sodium and water handling in chronic obstructive lung disease. *Arch Intern Med* 142:1326–1330, 1982.

73. Dandona P, Fanseca V, and Baron DN: Hypoalbuminemic hyponatremia: A new syndrome? *Br Med J* 291:1253–1255, 1985.

74. Arieff A, Llack F, and Massry S: Neurologic manifestations and morbidity of hyponatremia: Correlation with brain water and electrolytes. *Medicine* 55:121–129, 1976.

75. Forrest JN, et al: Superiority of demeclocycline over lithium in the treatment of chronic syndrome of inappropriate antidiuretic hormone. *N Engl J Med* 298:173–177, 1978.

76. Chapron DJ, Cameron IR, and White LD: Observations on lithium disposition in the elderly. *J Am Geriatr Soc* 30:651–655, 1982.

77. DeTroyer A: Demeclocycline treatment for the syndrome of inappropriate antidiuretic hormone secretion. *JAMA* 237:2723–2726, 1977.

78. Miller PD, Linas SL, and Schrier RW: Plasma demeclocycline levels and nephrotoxicity. Correlation in hyponatremic cirrhotic patients. *JAMA* 243:2513–2515, 1980.

79. Geheb M and Cox M: Renal effects of demeclocycline. *JAMA* 243:2519–2520, 1980.

80. Danovitch G, LeRoith D, and Glick S: Renal function during treatment of inappropriate secretion of antidiuretic hormone with demeclocycline. *Isr J Med Sci* 14:852–857, 1978.

81. Decaux G, Unger J, and Mockel J: Urea therapy for inappropriate antidiuretic hormone secretion from tuberculosis meningitis. *JAMA* 244:589–590, 1980.

82. Decaux G, et al: Treatment of hyponatremic cirrhotic with ascites resistant to diuretics by urea. *Nephron* 44:337–343, 1986.

83. Decaux G, et al: Treatment of the syndrome of inappropriate secretion of antidiuretic hormone by urea. *Am J Med* 69:99–106, 1980.

84. Taney A, et al: Long-term treatment of the syndrome of inappropriate antidiuretic hormone secretion with phenytoin. *Ann Intern Med* 90:50–52, 1979.

85. Fichman MP, Bethune JE, and Kleeman CR: Inhibition of antidiuretic hormone by diphenylhydantoin (abstract). *Clin Res* 15:141, 1967.
86. Decaux G, et al: Treatment of the syndrome of inappropriate secretion of antidiuretic hormone with furosemide. *N Engl J Med* 304:329–330, 1981.
87. Lazlo FA, Csatis S, and Balaspiri L: Prevention of hyponatremia and cerebral edema by the vasopressin antagonist D/CH$_2$/Tyr/ET/VAVP in rats treated with pitressin tannate. *Acta Endocrinol* 116:56–60, 1984.
88. Shankel SW: A new formula for correction of hyponatremia. *Am Soc Nephrol* 19th Ann Meeting 59A, 1986.
89. Sterns RH, Riggs JE, and Schochet SS Jr: Osmotic demyelination syndrome following correction of hyponatremia. *N Engl J Med* 314:1535–1542, 1986.
90. Ayus JC: Diuretic-induced hyponatremia. *Arch Intern Med* 146:1295–1296, 1986.
91. Norenberg MD: Treatment of hyponatremia: The case for a more conservative approach. Dubois GD, Arieff AI: Treatment of hyponatremia: The case for rapid correction. In Norins RG (ed): *Controversies in Nephrology and Hypertension*. New York, Churchill-Livingstone, 1984.
92. Ayus JC, Olivero JJ, and Frommer JP: Rapid correction of severe hyponatremia with intravenous hypertonic saline solution. *Am J Med* 72:43–48, 1982.
93. Ayus JC, Krothapalli RK, and Arieff AI: Changing concepts in treatment of severe symptomatic hyponatremia: Rapid correction and possible relation to central pontine myelinolysis. *Am J Med* 78:897–902, 1985.
94. Stern RH: Severe symptomatic hyponatremia: Treatment and outcome. A study of 64 cases. *Ann Intern Med* 107:656–664, 1987.
95. Sterns R: The prognosis of severe symptomatic hyponatremia. *Am Soc Nephrol* 19th Annual Meeting 56A, 1986.
96. Ashouri OS: Severe diuretic-induced hyponatremia in the elderly. A series of eight patients. *Arch Intern Med* 146:1355–1357, 1986.
97. Ayus JC, Krothapolli RK, and Arieff AI: Treatment of symptomatic hyponatremia and its relation to brain damage: A prospective study. *N Engl J Med* 317:1190–1195, 1987.
98. Hantman D, et al: Rapid correction of hyponatremia in the syndrome of inappropriate secretion of antidiuretic hormone. An alternative treatment to hypertonic saline. *Ann Intern Med* 78:870–875, 1973.
99. Snyder NA, Feigal DW, and Arieff AI: Hypernatremia in elderly patients. A heterogeneous, morbid and iatrogenic entity. *Ann Intern Med* 107:309–319, 1987.
100. Nelson DC, McGrew WRG Jr, and Hoyumpa AM Jr: Hypernatremia and lactulose therapy. *JAMA* 249:1295–1298, 1983.
101. Warren SE, Mitas JA II, and Swerdlin AHR: Hypernatremia in hepatic failure. *JAMA* 243:1257–1261, 1980.
102. Gault MH, et al: Hypernatremia, azotemia and dehydration due to high-protein tube feeding. *Ann Intern Med* 68:778–791, 1968.
103. Jana DK and Romano-Jana L: Hypernatremic psychosis in the elderly. Case reports. *J Am Geriatr Soc* 21:473–477, 1973.
104. Ross EJ and Christie SBM: Hypernatremia. *Medicine* 48:441–467, 1969.
105. Himmelstein DV, Jones AA, and Woolhandler S: Hypernatremic dehydration in nursing home patients: An indicator of neglect. *J Am Geriatr Soc* 31:466–471, 1983.
106. Vavra I, et al: Effect of a synthetic analogue of vasopressin in animals and in patients with diabetic insipidus. *Lancet* 1:948–952, 1968.

107. Andersson KE and Arner B: Effects of DDAVP, a synthetic analogue of vasopressin in patients with cranial diabetes insipidus. *Acta Med Scand* 192: 21–27, 1972.

108. Edwards CRW, et al: Vasopressin analogue DDAVP in diabetes insipidus: Clinical and laboratory studies. *Br Med J* 3:375–378, 1973.

109. Ward MK and Fraser TR: DDAVP in treatment of vasopressin-sensitive diabetes insipidus. *Br Med J* 3:86–89, 1974.

110. Robinson AG: DDAVP in the treatment of central diabetes insipidus. *N Engl J Med* 294:507–511, 1976.

111. Cobb WE, Spare S, and Reichlin S: Neurogenic diabetes insipidus: Management with dDavp (1-desamino-8-D-arginine vasopressin). *Ann Intern Med* 88:131–188, 1978.

112. Zerbe RL and Robertson GL: A comparison of plasma vasopressin measurements with a standard indirect test in the differential diagnosis of polyuria. *N Engl J Med* 305:1539–1546, 1981.

113. Milles JL, Spruce B, and Baylis PH: A comparison of diagnostic methods to differentiate diabetes insipidus from primary polydipsia, a review of 21 patients. *Acta Endocrinol* 104:410–416, 1983.

114. Hariprasad MK, Eisinger RP, and Nadler IM: Hyponatremia in psychogenic polydipsia. *Arch Intern Med* 140:1639–1642, 1980.

115. Cronin RE: Psychogenic polydipsia with hyponatremia: Report of eleven cases. *Am J Kidney Dis* 9:410–416, 1987.

116. Goldman MB, Luchins DJ, and Robertson GL: Mechanisms of altered water metabolism in psychotic patients with polydipsia and hyponatremia. *N Engl J Med* 318:397–403, 1988.

117. Robertson GL, et al: Development and clinical application of a new method for the radioimmunoassay arginine vasopressin in human plasma. *J Clin Invest* 52:2340–2352, 1973.

118. Os I, et al: Evidence of age-related variation in plasma vasopressin in normotensive man. *Scand J Clin Lab Invest* 45:263–268, 1985.

3 DISORDERS OF POTASSIUM METABOLISM

NORMAL PHYSIOLOGY

Serum potassium (K) in the normal individual is maintained within the narrow range of 3.5 to 5.5 mEq per liter despite wide fluctuations in intake. Both extrarenal and renal mechanisms are involved in K homeostasis. During the first few hours after a K load, it is estimated that 50 percent of the load will be disposed of by extrarenal mechanisms and the remainder by the kidney.

EXTRARENAL MECHANISMS OF K HOMEOSTASIS

Gastrointestinal Tract
In response to K loading the colonic surface mucosal cells undergo structural changes leading to increased excretion. The basolateral membrane Na-K-ATPase may increase as much as 40 percent in such circumstances, with serum aldosterone and plasma K concentration constituting the two main regulators [1, 2].

Insulin
This hormone exerts its effect by shifting K from the extracellular to the intracellular space, mainly in hepatocytes (which account for 70 perecnt of the insulin effect), with other peripheral tissues such as muscle and fat accounting for the remainder. Insulin acts directly on plasma membranes, resulting in an increase in Na-K-ATPase–dependent pumps [3].

Adrenergic Nervous System
The effector organ of the adrenergic nervous system seems to be muscle cells, with the membrane beta-2 adrenergic receptor primarily involved [4]. This effect requires activation of membrane-bound adenylate cyclase and stimulation of Na-K-ATPase–dependent pumps, leading to K entry into the cell. The alpha-adrenergic system has been found to have the opposite effect [5].

Mineralocorticoids
In addition to its effect on the colon, aldosterone participates in extrarenal K homeostasis [6] through mechanisms yet to be completely elucidated [7].

Glucagon

Glucagon has been found to induce a transient mobilization of K from the splanchnic region [8]. The contribution of glucagon and the gluco-corticoids in the day-to-day maintenance of K homeostasis is not entirely clear, however.

RENAL MECHANISM OF K HOMEOSTASIS

Since virtually all of the filtered K is reabsorbed in the proximal portion of the nephron, urinary K excretion reflects the secretion of K in the distal nephron. In experimental animals the principal cells of the cortical collecting tubules have been shown to undergo surface density changes in the basolateral membrane under varying K loads [9]. Potassium present in the surrounding plasma and interstitial fluid is actively transported by these cells through an ATP-driven Na-K exchange pump across the basolateral membrane, whereas K diffuses passively across the luminal membrane. Also, during adaptation to K loading, the cells of the papillary collecting duct undergo an increase in luminal membrane surface area with no change in the basolateral surface. It appears that there is a pump that moves K from the cell to the luminal fluid in these cells [10].

Several factors are involved in the regulation of K secretion by the distal nephron.

Plasma Factors

SERUM POTASSIUM. The higher the plasma K level, the greater the K secretion.

ALDOSTERONE. Aldosterone, by increasing sodium reabsorption in the cortical collecting tubule, induces a depolarization of the luminal membrane, thereby amplifying the electrochemical driving force for K movement from cell to lumen.

ACID-BASE STATUS. During metabolic acidosis K moves out of the cell as hydrogen ions move intracellularly. This occurs in renal as well as in extrarenal cells. Furthermore, a low systemic pH could decrease K conductance per se. The opposite action occurs in alkalosis [11].

ANTIDIURETIC HORMONE. This hormone has been found to increase K secretion by the distal nephron in the rat [12].

Luminal Factors

FLOW RATE. Increasing tubular flow rate has been shown to stimulate K secretion in the rat [13].

CHANGES IN TRANSEPITHELIAL VOLTAGE. The presence of a large concentration of either endogenous (bicarbonate) or exogenous (e.g., carbenicillin) unreabsorbable anions will increase K secretion by making the luminal fluid more negative [14].

LUMINAL CHLORIDE CONCENTRATION. Potassium secretion is stimulated in the presence of a low luminal chloride concentration [15].

POTASSIUM RECYCLING. It has been shown in the rat that the pars recta or the descending limb of Henle can secrete K [16]. The magnitude of K secreted varies with the K status of the animal [17, 18].

CHANGES IN K METABOLISM WITH AGE

Total body potassium decreases as muscle mass decreases with age. Table 3-1 summarizes the average total body K according to age as described by Novak [19]. Serum K in the healthy elderly is maintained within the same narrow range of 3.5 to 5.5 mEq per liter found in younger individuals despite the progressive decrease in glomerular filtration rate seen with advancing age. Therefore, both extrarenal and renal mechanisms involved in K homeostasis must remain intact to adapt to the progressive nephron loss.

HYPOKALEMIA

INCIDENCE AND PREVALENCE
In a survey of 3,684 hospitalized patients, Morgan and Young [20] found 70 (1.9 percent) with hypokalemia. The incidence was 1.4 percent among newly admitted cases. The mean age was 61 years, with 57 percent older than 65 years at a time when 41 percent of the inpatient population was over 65 years. McCarthy [21] reported that 1.1 percent of 50 geriatric pa-

TABLE 3-1. Average total body potassium in different age groups

	Body potassium (mEq)	
Age (yr)	Male (±50)	Female (±50)
45–55	3775 (425)	2575 (291)
55–65	3607 (433)	2403 (287)
65–85	3168 (234)	2351 (200)

SOURCE: Novak LP: Aging, total body potassium fat-free mass and cell mass in males and females between ages 18 and 85 years. J Gerontol 27:438–443, 1972.

tients hospitalized for acute conditions were hypokalemic. The incidence of hypokalemia in the outpatient elderly is not known; however, given the frequency of hypertension and heart failure, and the use of diuretics in this age group, it must be relatively common.

ETIOLOGY
There is very little specific information available on the distribution of etiologic factors causing hypokalemia in elderly inpatients. In 40 elderly patients seen at our hospital the causes of hypokalemia (serum K < 3.0 mEq per liter) were renal losses in 62 percent, gastrointestinal tract losses in 15 percent, and mixed losses in 13 percent; mixed losses were more common in patients with severe hypokalemia (serum K < 1.5 mEq per liter). Potassium redistribution from the extracellular to the intracellular fluid occurred in 10 percent (Table 3-2). Other causes included injury, acute transient hypokalemia, and hypokalemia with no obvious cause.

PATHOGENESIS
Diuretics (thiazides and loop diuretics) induce hypokalemia by increasing tubular flow and sodium delivery to the distal convoluted tubule and also by producing chloride depletion. There is also some experimental evidence suggesting that furosemide might directly stimulate renal tubular K secretion [22]. Acetazolamide increases K loss owing to its effect on proximal tubular bicarbonate and the increased delivery of this anion to the distal tubule. Some of our patients were receiving acetazolamide and large doses of intravenous bicarbonate to alkalinize the urine to manage uric acid stones. In such patients, the presence of bicarbonate in the distal nephron and the increased urinary volume serve as stimuli for increased K secretion. In diuretic-induced hypokalemia the urinary K is usually greater than 30 to 40 mEq per liter while the patient is still taking the drug. If a history of diuretic use is not elicited, the clinical picture might suggest Bartter's syndrome. This entity is, however, initially diagnosed earlier in life [23, 24]. In patients in whom the diuretic has been recently discontinued, urinary K may be low (< 10 mEq per liter).

The hypokalemia associated with sodium carbenicillin is due to the carbenicillin, which is a nonreabsorbable anion that induces a favorable electrical gradient for K secretion in the distal nephron.

The causes of hypokalemia associated with hypomagnesemia are not entirely clear but probably include both proximal and distal (aldosterone) tubular mechanisms (see Chap. 5).

The presence of hypokalemic metabolic alkalosis with high urinary chloride and urinary K concentrations in a normotensive elderly person should lead to a suspicion of mineralocorticoid excess, frequently due to licorice ingestion [25]. Our patients were usually women who generally did not volunteer the information unless specifically asked.

TABLE 3-2. Etiology of hypokalemia

Potassium losses through the kidneys (25 patients)
  Diuretic use: thiazides, furosemide, Diamox (14)
  Other drugs: carbenicillin, bicarbonate (5)
  Magnesium deficiency: due to diarrhea or aminoglycosides (4)
  Mineralocorticoid excess (2)
Potassium losses through the gastrointestinal tract (6 patients)
  Diarrhea (6)
Potassium losses through both kidneys and gastrointestinal tract (5 patients)
Potassium redistribution from the extracellular to the intracellular fluid
    (4 patients)
  Respiratory alkalosis (3)
  Hyperalimentation (1)

Patients lose K through the gastrointestinal tract usually due to severe diarrhea. Significant hyperchloremic metabolic acidosis with evidence of volume contraction is generally present. The urinary K in such patients tends to be low, less than 20 mEq per liter.

Patients with intestinal obstruction that requires prolonged nasogastric suction develop hypokalemia associated with both gastrointestinal and urinary K losses. These patients have a metabolic alkalosis and a low urinary chloride level (< 10 mEq per liter), and most of the K is lost during the initiation phase of the alkalosis when there is significant bicarbonaturia.

Hypokalemia related to transcellular shifts occurs in patients with respiratory alkalosis or those receiving hypertonic glucose and insulin during hyperalimentation.

The postulated mechanism for the so-called acute transient hypokalemia is an intracellular shift of K, most likely secondary to an increase in catecholamine secretion, which may be expected in acutely ill patients [4, 20]. In some, however, prior thiazide therapy may play a role, since it has been shown that this diuretic can increase catecholamine-induced hypokalemia [26]. Indeed, a similar mechanism could also be at work in the hypokalemia which develops in patients with acute myocardial infarction [27–29].

CLINICAL MANIFESTATIONS
Moderate to severe K deficiency may have important effects on cardiac, skeletal, and smooth muscle, intermediary metabolism (carbohydrate and protein), and the kidney's ability to concentrate the urine maximally [30, 31]. Severe manifestations of hypokalemia are, fortunately, uncommon in the elderly in our experience. Furthermore, because most of our patients were acutely ill, the overwhelming clinical manifestations were mainly those of the underlying disease.

The elderly ambulatory patient with hypokalemia is usually asymptomatic, although a small minority have ill-defined complaints of musculoskeletal origin, which are reversible on K replacement.

THERAPY AND PROGNOSIS

Since most of the total body K is stored in muscle, direct muscle K measurement represents the most accurate way of assessing deficits. This is, however, impractical in clinical practice. Sterns et al [32], by analyzing pure K depletion in humans, concluded that a decrease in plasma K of 0.3 mEq per liter is, in general, associated with an average total body deficit of 100 mEq. These data are compatible with studies in which muscle K was measured in patients on diuretic therapy [33–35].

Patients with acute transient hypokalemia can be watched for several days if there are no specific symptoms because most will become normokalemic within a week. In the absence of spontaneous correction, oral or parenteral K supplementation may be required.

Patients with acute myocardial infarction and hypokalemia present a more difficult problem because the incidence of ventricular fibrillation in this group appears to be significantly higher than in those with normal serum K [27, 29, 36]. It is not clear whether the hypokalemia serves as a marker or is etiologically responsible for the ventricular arrhythmia, since the latter is not necessarily prevented by K supplementation. Intravenous administration of a nonselective beta blocker has been recommended and has been used with some success in such patients [37].

Parenteral administration of potassium chloride (KCl) is frequently necessary in hospitalized patients with increased losses through the kidneys or gastrointestinal tract. In patients with associated renal insufficiency (acute or chronic), careful monitoring of the serum K is mandatory to avoid hyperkalemia. In most patients, normokalemia, once achieved, is maintained except in those with associated hypomagnesemia, in whom long-term oral therapy may be required.

In elderly ambulatory patients on diuretics hypokalemia is usually well tolerated, although controversy exists as to whether the incidence of ventricular arrhythmia is increased [38, 39]. Some authors recommend K supplementation for every patient taking a diuretic in view of the fact that the cellular concentration of K may be significantly decreased even in the presence of a normal serum K [40]. Furthermore, it has been shown in a short-term study that the addition of KCl to the diuretic regimen of a hypertensive patient may induce a significant fall in blood pressure [41]. We recommend treatment for preventing hypokalemia only in those elderly patients taking a diuretic who have heart disease, a history of previous arrhythmias, or are taking digitalis.

Hypokalemia can be prevented or treated in these patients with the use of one of the several KCl preparations available or with K-sparing agents such as aldactone, triamterene, or amiloride. In the elderly patient on such therapy the K level should be monitored, particularly if a drug known to interfere with K metabolism such as a converting enzyme inhibitor, beta blocker, or nonsteroidal anti-inflammatory agent is used concurrently or if the patient has diabetes mellitus or renal insufficiency.

The amount of KCl required to achieve normokalemia in a diuretic-treated patient is quite variable. In one study of a small group of patients, 60 mEq per day of KCl effectively corrected hypokalemia in 80 percent of the patients [42]. In another study, a dose as high as 96 mEq per day was required [43]. Our practice is to start with 20 mEq twice a day and gradually increase the dose until normokalemia is achieved. Gastrointestinal upset has been the most common side effect encountered. A slow release tablet containing 8 mEq of KCl is available, which has the advantage of producing a lower incidence of ulcerative lesions of the gastrointestinal tract. The price and the large number of tablets required to correct hypokalemia with this preparation constitute major drawbacks for the elderly, however.

Spironolactone acts by binding competitively to the aldosterone receptor site, thereby preventing its action. The most common side effect associated with its use is hyperkalemia, which occurs in 10 percent of patients [44]. At greatest risk for this complication are patients with renal insufficiency and those concurrently taking either KCl supplements or other drugs known to produce an increase in serum K. The required dose is 25 to 150 mg per day. Therapy should be initiated with the smallest dose, since a significant elevation of plasma K may be seen even with the daily ingestion of 25 mg. The drug is relatively expensive [45].

Triamterene and amiloride both act by blocking the entry of Na into the renal tubular cell. This leads to a decrease in the amount of Na extruded across the basolateral cell membrane with a concomitant decrease in K uptake by the cell [46]. In addition, both drugs decrease the electrochemical driving force for cell-to-lumen efflux of K by making the cell interior more electrically negative [46]. The recommended dose for triamterene is 100 to 300 mg per day in divided doses. Elevation of serum creatinine, acute renal failure (when combined with indomethacin), and nephrolithiasis are reported side effects [47, 48]. The amiloride dose is 5 to 20 mg per day, given as a single dose. Hyperkalemia is the most common side effect, particularly in diabetic patients. Either drug will add a substantial burden to the already limited budget of many elderly patients. It is estimated that the elderly patient fills an average of 12 prescriptions per year [49], so that one alternative to treating diuretic-induced hypokalemia is to use one of the available K-sparing agents combined with the diuretic. Spironolactone-hydrochlorothiazide and triamterene-hydrochlorothiazide have been tried in the elderly and found to be relatively well tolerated [50]. An amiloride-hydrochlorothiazide combination is also available and may be preferable in patients for whom maintenance of glomerular filtration rate is prostaglandin dependent (such as those with heart failure or liver cirrhosis). Urinary prostaglandin E_2 (PGE_2) excretion was found to increase in patients receiving amiloride-hydrochlorothiazide, whereas in the group receiving triamterene-hydrochlorothiazide urinary PGE_2 may decrease [51]. The required dose should be established by individual titration of each component before switching to the combination. Again, it cannot be emphasized enough that KCl supplementation should not be used together with a K-sparing agent in the elderly because of the possibility of fatal hyperkalemia. In patients in whom correction of the hypokalemia is difficult, mainly those who are hospitalized, are taking diuretics, or who have diarrhea, the serum magnesium should be measured, since normokalemia can be achieved only after the former has been adequately corrected if found to be low [52].

HYPERKALEMIA

INCIDENCE AND PREVALENCE
The true incidence of hyperkalemia in the geriatric population is not known; however, the frequency of this complication does increase with age. Significant hyperkalemia was found in 406 (1.4 percent) out of 29,063 hospitalized patients in a Scottish hospital [53]. The average age of these patients was 58 ± 1.6 years, significantly older than 1,218 randomly selected controls. Of 4,921 patients receiving potassium chloride, hyperkalemia developed in 179 (3.6 percent). The age distribution of these hyperkalemic patients, summarized in Table 3-3, shows a disproportionate number 60 years or older. Similarly, the patients with hyperkalemia reported by Shemer et al [54] were also significantly older than the control group (66.8 ± 13.7 versus 56.0 ± 19.1 years). The reason for the susceptibility of the elderly patient to hyperkalemia is not clear but probably is related to the existence in a single individual of several risk factors such as renal insufficiency and multiple drug interactions, as suggested by Shemer et al [54].

ETIOLOGY AND PATHOGENESIS
The etiology of hyperkalemia in the elderly is similar to that in younger patients. Pseudohyperkalemia related to hemolysis, leukocytosis, or thrombocytosis should be ruled out first in every patient with an elevated serum K. The etiology of hyperkalemia in 50 consecutive elderly patients seen by us is summarized in Table 3-4.

Drug-Induced Hyperkalemia
Drug ingestion was the most common cause of hyperkalemia in our series, with KCl replacement the cause in 50 percent. Normal humans can

TABLE 3-3. Frequency of hyperkalemia according to age

Age (yr)	Hyperkalemia (%)
<50	0.8
50–59	4.2
60–69	4.3
70–79	4.6
80+	6.0

SOURCE: Lawson DH: Adverse reactions to potassium chloride. *Q J Med* 171:433–440, 1974.

TABLE 3-4. Etiology of hyperkalemia

Drug-induced (20 patients)
    KCl replacement (10)
    K-sparing diuretic (3)
    Nonsteroidal anti-inflammatory agents (3)
    Converting enzyme inhibitors (2)
    Beta blockers (1)
    Heparin (1)
Renal tubular hyperkalemia (16 patients)
Renal failure (9 patients)
    Acute (7)
    Chronic (2)
Disturbed intracellular-extracellular gradient (5)
    Hyperglycemia (3)
    Acid-base disturbances (2)

handle diets containing as much as 300 mEqK per day without developing hyperkalemia [55]. A shift in sodium reabsorption from a proximal to a distal nephron site as well as an elevated aldosterone level are key factors in the adaptation to the high K diet [55]. In the elderly, however, decreased aldosterone levels and an associated blunted aldosterone response to various stimuli most likely contribute to their susceptibility to KCl-induced hyperkalemia. In addition, the BUN tends to be higher in elderly persons on KCl replacement with hyperkalemia than in those who are normokalemic, suggesting that renal insufficiency may also play a role.

Potassium-sparing diuretics produce hyperkalemia by interfering with K secretion in the distal part of the nephron, as discussed earlier.

Nonsteroidal anti-inflammatory drugs (NSAIDs) are commonly used in the elderly. Hyperkalemia has been one of the reported complications and for some reason is found mainly with the use of indomethacin, although occasionally piroxicam and ibuprofen have been implicated as well [56–59]. The frequency of this problem is not known; however, in one reported prospective study of 50 patients on indomethacin, the serum K concentration exceeded 5.0 mEq per liter in 23 patients (46 percent) [60]. Older age and mild pre-existing kidney disease were significant risk factors for those developing hyperkalemia. Of 22 patients reported in the literature, 15 (68 percent) were over 60 years old, further suggesting a higher prevalence of this complication in the elderly [56–59, 61–67]. Mild elevation in BUN and serum creatinine was present in the majority of the patients prior to starting the NSAID. Hyperkalemia may develop at any time after starting the drug (average 3–4 days), and dose did not appear to play a role. In addition to hyperkalemia, worsening of kidney function with oliguric renal failure and hyperchloremic metabolic acidosis is also quite common following NSAID ingestion [56, 59, 64, 66, 67]. The fact that the hyperkalemia and renal failure are easily reversible on discontinuing the offending agent favors a functional mechanism rather than a structural alteration. Indeed, it has been shown that indomethacin, by decreasing renal PGE_2 production, induces a hyporenin-hypoaldosterone state that can explain the hyperkalemia [62, 63]. McCarthy and associates [68] have suggested a possible direct role of these agents in inhibiting excretion as well as cellular uptake of K. Inhibition of renal prostaglandin synthesis could also explain the renal failure, since under conditions of circulatory stress prostaglandins appear to play a major role in the maintenance of glomerular filtration rate. Thus, it appears to be a good practice to monitor serum K and kidney function in any elderly patient taking a NSAID. If one of these agents is necessary, sulindac is apparently the safest [69]. It should be noted, however, that the risk of acute renal failure, particularly in patients with concomitant cardiovascular and renal problems, is still increased [70].

Hyperkalemia associated with the use of a converting-enzyme inhibitor has been seen in three patients. All three had pre-existing impairment of kidney function, in keeping with the experience of others [71]. Therefore, care should be taken in using these drugs in elderly patients with renal insufficiency. Age per se, however, does not constitute a risk factor. It should be noted that concomitant use of a beta blocker will substantially increase the likelihood of hyperkalemia in the presence of renal impairment.

Isolated beta blocker–induced hyperkalemia is rare. We have seen it in only one elderly patient with severe renal insufficiency (creatinine 4.2 mg per dl). Normokalemia followed withdrawal of the drug, and hyperkalemia reappeared after the drug was inadvertently reinstituted. A similar problem was reported by Swenson [72] in an elderly man treated for glaucoma with timolol maleate. In general, elderly patients with severe renal insufficiency are at risk for developing hyperkalemia secondary to beta blockers [73]. The rise in serum K most likely represents the inhibition of its translocation from the extracellular to the intracellular fluid compartment.

Parenteral or subcutaneous administration of heparin causes hypoaldosteronism by inhibiting the conversion of cortisone to 18-hydroxycorticosterone [74, 75]. The development of hyperkalemia, however, is rather rare with this agent. Patients with chronic renal insufficiency or uncontrolled diabetes mellitus are particularly at risk and deserve to have their serum K monitored regularly while receiving heparin [76, 77]. Hyperkalemia may be noted as early as 5 days and up to months after initiation of therapy. Hyperchloremic metabolic acidosis is a frequently associated abnormality, probably a consequence of the elevated K concentration (see the following section).

Renal Tubular Hyperkalemia

A defect in the tubular secretion of K occurs in 32 percent of elderly patients with hyperkalemia [78] (see Table 3-4). Seventy-four percent of patients reported in the literature were over age 60 [79–87]. Patients are usually asymptomatic with mild to moderate hyperkalemia (5.6–6.0 mEq per liter). Renal insufficiency (creatinine 2.0–5.0 mg per dl) is universally present. Diabetic nephropathy or tubulointerstitial nephropathy of various etiologies is usually responsible for the renal insufficiency. Obstructive uropathy should be ruled out in these patients, particularly if the etiology of the renal failure is obscure [88]. Hyperchloremic metabolic acidosis is found in 50 percent of the patients. The acidosis is explained in part by a decrease in ammonia production and delivery to the loop of Henle, with a subsequent lowering of the concentration gradient between the loop and the inner medullary collecting duct [89, 90]. The rate of H^+ secretion in the medullary collecting duct is also decreased owing to a decrease in distal sodium delivery as well as a decrease in pump activity, a direct effect of aldosterone deficiency [89, 91]. The underlying defect responsible for the syndrome may be an abnormality in the production of renin, aldosterone, or both. Some patients, however, have a normal renin-angiotensin-aldosterone axis but an isolated defect in tubular K secretion. In others, both these factors might be at play, as summarized in Table 3-5.

This syndrome may be due to a variety of structural or physiologic problems including (1) sclerosis of the juxtaglomerular apparatus due to the underlying kidney disease [92]; (2) defective conversion of inactive renin to active renin [93, 94]; (3) an abnormality in the synthesis of prostaglandin E_2 and kallikrein [95]; (4) a deficiency in prostacyclin [96]; (5) suppression of renin production (and aldosterone) by volume expansion, resulting from the renal insufficiency found in practically all these patients, and associated with an increase in atrial natriuretic peptide [97]; and (6) the "chloride shunt" [98]. In this last form of renal tubular

TABLE 3-5. PRA, PA, and urinary pH in the three forms of renal tubular hyperkalemia

Defect	PRA (ng/ml/hr)			PA (ng/ml/hr)			Urine pH
	Baseline	*After stimulation*		*Baseline*	*After stimulation*		
		Posture	*Furosemide*		*ACTH*	*AII*	
Renin production	low	—	—	low/normal	↑	↑	can reach 5.5 or less
Aldosterone synthesis	low/normal	↑	↑	low	—	—	as above
Tubular defect in K secretion	normal	↑	↑	normal	↑	↑	>6.0

PRA = plasma renin activity; PA = plasma aldosterone; ACTH = adrenocorticotropic hormone; AII = angiotensin II.

hyperkalemia the distal tubule has a higher than usual rate of chloride reabsorption. As a consequence, volume expansion ensues with subsequent suppression of the renin-aldosterone axis. In fact, following furosemide administration plasma renin increases out of the "range" found in normals. In this group, the glomerular filtration rate is normal, and hypertension is frequently present (70 percent). This problem must be rather rare in the elderly, because none of the 28 patients reported in the literature and reviewed by Gordon [99] was over 60 years of age, and only three were in their sixth decade of life.

None of our patients had Addison's disease; however, this problem should be kept in mind when evaluating a hyperkalemic patient, particularly if marked volume contraction exists.

A tubular defect in K secretion occurs less commonly than hyporenin-hypoaldosteronism [100]. In patients with this defect, urinary pH remains above 6.0 in the presence of acidosis compared with those with hyporenin-hypoaldosteronism, in whom the urine pH may be 5.5 or less [101]. Whereas patients with hyporenin-hypoaldosteronism increase their fractional excretion of K after administration of a mineralocorticoid or sodium sulfate, those with a defect in tubular secretion are unresponsive. Because of its similarity to the effect of amiloride, this form of hyperkalemic acidosis has been labeled a voltage-dependent type of renal tubular acidosis [102].

Renal Failure

Seven patients had acute oliguric renal failure of diverse etiology. In three of these patients, hemolysis and increased tissue breakdown (rhabdomyolysis) were probably contributing factors owing to the associated increased K load. Two patients had advanced chronic renal insufficiency (creatinine 5.0 mg per dl and 6.2 mg per dl, respectively), and one might have been ingesting a salt substitute (the K content of these substitutes varies between 10 and 13 mEq per g).

Disturbed Intracellular-Extracellular Gradient

HYPERGLYCEMIA. If a 50-g dose of glucose is given to an insulin-dependent diabetic, plasma K increases by an average of 1.3 mEq per liter, peaking 30 to 60 minutes following the load [103, 104]. If such a diabetic patient has superimposed hypoaldosteronism or renal insufficiency, one might expect the serum K to rise even more. Our three patients had renal insufficiency (serum creatinine ranging from 1.8 to 2.1 mg per dl). We did not measure the plasma aldosterone concentration, but it has been found to be decreased in such patients. Because the hyperkalemia may be quite severe at times, care should be exercised in administering glucose to a comatose diabetic patient [105–108].

ACID-BASE DISTURBANCES. Hyperkalemia was a complication of acute metabolic acidosis in two patients. When H^+ is added to the extracellular fluid it undergoes buffering by intracellular proteins, leaving free K to be redistributed from the intracellular to the extracellular fluid. The extent of K movement depends on the quantity of acid buffered rather than the arterial pH. In general, the rise in serum K associated with acidosis due to an increase in organic acids (such as lactate) tends to be less than that with acidosis related to mineral acids (such as chloride) [109]. Since organic anions tend to accumulate in the cell with subsequent cell swelling, some K will remain in the intracellular fluid [110]. Hyperkalemia can also occur with respiratory acidosis.

CLINICAL MANIFESTATIONS
The clinical manifestations of hyperkalemia are related primarily to interference with the electrophysiologic events underlying muscle contraction. Even though all muscle groups may be involved, cardiac tissue is exceptionally vulnerable to hyperkalemia. The magnitude of the hyperkalemia as well as the rate at which it develops determines cardiotoxicity. Since it is very difficult to predict progression to fatal cardiotoxicity, the presence of any electrocardiographic abnormality is an indication for immediate therapy. The earliest ECG change is symmetric peaking of the T wave, followed by widening of the QRS complex and prolongation of the PR interval. Heart block, atrial standstill, and a sine wave configuration (due to the merging of QRS complex with the T wave) are late events often followed by ventricular fibrillation or asystole.

TREATMENT

General Measures
Several measures are available for the management of cardiotoxicity in the hyperkalemic patient. These fall into three broad categories and may be undertaken simultaneously to maximize the chances of full recovery.

CALCIUM. The infusion of calcium restores a more normal differential between the threshold and resting transmembrane potential. The usual approach is to infuse 10 to 30 ml of 10 percent calcium gluconate under constant ECG monitoring. This form of therapy does not change the serum K but can rapidly reverse the ECG changes.

SODIUM BICARBONATE. One or two ampules (44 mEq per 50 ml) infused over a 10-minute period may be used initially. Additional amounts should be administered depending on the presence and severity of acidosis.

GLUCOSE AND INSULIN. The usual approach is to administer 50 ml of 50 percent glucose followed by a continuous infusion of 10 percent glucose until the K level normalizes. Insulin can be added to the glucose infusion at the rate of 10 to 20 units of regular insulin for each 100 g of glucose. This form of therapy constitutes the most efficient way to lower the serum K rapidly in the patient with end-stage kidney disease pending the initiation of hemodialysis [111].

The latter two forms of therapy act by redistributing K from the extracellular to the intracellular compartment. By so doing, they increase the transmembrane potential toward normal. Nebulized albuterol at a dose of 10 to 20 mg has also been used successfully in such patients [112]. This approach, however, may not be very helpful in the elderly, given the reduced sensitivity of their beta receptors to the beta agonists [113].

In addition to the above methods, which act relatively rapidly, measures to remove excess K from the body can be initiated. These include the use of sodium polystyrene sulfonate (a K-exchange resin), 15 to 30 g of which is usually administered in a liquid suspension given orally, or 50 to 100 g in 200 ml of water given as a retention enema. Hemodialysis or peritoneal dialysis may be necessary in patients with significant renal insufficiency.

Specific Therapies

Once the serum K has been brought down to a normal level, more specific measures should be undertaken for the long-term management of the patient. In patients with drug-induced hyperkalemia, the offending agent should be discontinued. For those with renal failure, dialytic therapy may be necessary. On occasion, patients on maintenance hemodialysis will require interdialytic administration of alkali (for those who tend to maintain a serum bicarbonate below 15 mEq per liter) or sodium polystyrene sulfonate (15–30 g bid). Oral sodium bicarbonate can be used; however, compliance, in our experience, is generally poor because of gastric complaints.

Once the diagnosis of hyporenin-hypoaldosteronism has been made, correction of systemic acidosis and hyperkalemia can be sustained by administration of fludrocortisone in daily doses of 0.1 to 0.3 mg [86]. Side effects, such as extracellular fluid retention and hypertension, may limit the use of this drug, however. Other alternatives, which can also be used for the patient with the voltage-dependent tubular acidosis and hyperkalemia, include (1) administration of alkali (1.5–2.0 mEq of sodium bicarbonate per kg per day) combined with dietary K restriction (2 g K daily); (2) potassium-binding resins (see preceding section on glucose and insulin for dose); and (3) furosemide administration, the dose depending on the level of kidney function [114]. Since the aciduric response to furosemide is somewhat attenuated by aldosterone deficiency, in those patients with both voltage-dependent hyperkalemia and hypoaldosteronism hyperkalemia, furosemide in combination with fludrocortisone may be useful as long as no contraindication to the use of the mineralocorticoid exists [115].

PROGNOSIS

In patients with acute hyperkalemia, the prognosis depends on how rapidly the cardiotoxicity is reversed. Otherwise, mortality depends mainly on the underlying disease. None of our 50 patients died as a direct result of hyperkalemia.

REFERENCES

1. Hirsch DJ and Hayslett JP: Adaptation to potassium. *News in Physiological Sciences* 1:54–57, 1986.
2. Sweiry JC and Binder HJ: Characterization of aldosterone-induced potassium secretion in rat distal colon. *J Clin Invest* 83:844–851, 1989.
3. Gavryck WA, Moore RD, and Thompson RC: Effect of insulin upon membrane-bound $(NA^+ + K^+)$-ATPase extracted from frog skeletal muscle. *J Physiol* 252:43–58, 1975.
4. Brown MJ, Brown DC, and Murphy MB. Hypokalemia from β_2-receptor stimulation by circulating epinephrine. *N Engl J Med* 309:1414–1419, 1983.
5. Williams ME, et al: Impairment of extrarenal potassium disposal by α-adrenergic stimulation. *N Engl J Med* 311:145–149, 1984.
6. Bia MJ and DeFronzo RA: Extrarenal potassium homeostasis. *Am J Physiol* 240:F257–F268, 1981.
7. Cox M, Sterns RH, and Singer I: The defense against hyperkalemia: The roles of insulin and aldosterone. *N Engl J Med* 299:525–532, 1978.
8. Massara F, et al: Pathophysiological doses of glucagon cause a transient increase of the hepatic vein potassium concentration in man. *Min Electrol Metab* 12:142–146, 1986.
9. Stanton BA, et al: Structural and functional study of the rat distal nephron: Effects of potassium adaptation and depletion. *Kidney Int* 19:36–48, 1981.
10. Rastegar A, et al: Changes in membrane surfaces of collecting duct cells in potassium adaptation. *Kidney Int* 18:293–301, 1980.
11. Sterns RH and Spital A: Disorders of internal potassium balance. *Semin Nephrol* 7:206–222, 1987.
12. Field MJ, Stanton BA, and Giebisch GH: Influence of ADH on renal potassium handling: A micropuncture and microperfusion study. *Kidney Int* 25:502–511, 1984.
13. Good DW and Wright FS: Luminal influences of K secretion: Sodium concentration and fluid flow rate. *Am J Physiol* 236:F192–F205, 1979.
14. Sullivan LP: Effect of Na and impermanent anions on renal K transport during stopped flow. *Am J Physiol* 201:774–780, 1961.
15. Velazquez H, Wright FS, and Good DW: Luminal influences on potassium secretion: Chloride replacement with sulfate. *Am J Physiol* 242:F46–F55, 1982.

16. Jamison RL, et al: Potassium secretion by the descending limb of pars recta of the juxtamedullary nephron in vivo. *Kidney Int* 9:323–332, 1976.
17. Battilana CA, et al: Effect of chronic potassium loading on potassium secretion by the pars recta or descending limb of the juxtamedullary nephron in the rat. *J Clin Invest* 62:1093–1103, 1978.
18. Arrascue JF, Dobyan DC, and Jamison RL: Potassium recycling in the renal medulla: Effects of acute potassium chloride administration to rats fed a potassium-free diet. *Kidney Int* 20:348–352, 1981.
19. Novak LP: Aging, total body potassium, fat free mass and cell mass in males and females between ages 18 and 85 years. *J Gerontol* 27:438–443, 1972.
20. Morgan DB and Young RM: Acute transient hypokalemia: New interpretation of a common event. *Lancet* 2:751–752, 1982.
21. McCarthy ST: Body fluid, electrolytes and diuretics. *Curr Med Res Opin* 7:87–95, 1982.
22. Tannen RL and Gerrits L: Response of the renal K conserving mechanism to a kaliuretic stimuli: Evidence for a direct kaliuretic effect of furosemide. *Clin Res* 31:752A, 1983.
23. Tannen RL: Potassium metabolism. In Gonick HC (ed): *Current Nephrology*, Vol 6. New York, Wiley, 1983.
24. Jamison RL, et al: Surreptitious diuretic ingestion and pseudo-Bartter's syndrome. *Am J Med* 73:142–147, 1982.
25. Conn JW, Rovner DR, and Cohen EL: Licorice-induced pseudoaldosteronism. *JAMA* 205:492–496, 1968.
26. Struthers AD, Whitesmith R, and Reid JL: Prior thiazide diuretic treatment increases adrenaline-induced hypokalaemia. *Lancet* 1:1358–1361, 1983.
27. Solomon RJ: Ventricular arrhythmias in patients with myocardial infarctions and ischemia. Relationship to serum potassium and magnesium. *Drugs* (Suppl 1) 28:66–76, 1984.
28. Nordrehang JE, Johannessen KA, and Von der Lippe G: Serum potassium concentrations as a risk factor of ventricular arrhythmias early in acute myocardial infarction. *Circulation* 71:645–649, 1985.
29. Reuben SR and Thomas RD: The relationship between serum potassium and cardiac arrhythmias following cardiac infarction in patients aged over 65 years. *Curr Med Res Bull* 7: (Suppl 1) 79–82, 1982.
30. Knochel JP: Hypokalemia. *Adv Intern Med* 30:317–335, 1984.
31. Halevy J, Gunsherowitz M, and Rosenfeld JB: Life-threatening hyperkalemia in hospitalized patients. *Min Electrol Metab* 14:163–167, 1988.
32. Sterns RM, et al: Internal potassium balance and the control of the plasma potassium concentration. *Medicine* 60:339–354, 1981.
33. Villamil MF, et al: Effect of long term treatment with hydrochlorothiazide on water and electrolytes of muscle in hypertensive subjects. *Am Heart J* 65:294–302, 1963.
34. Bergstrom J and Hultman E: The effect of thiazides, chlorthalidone and furosemide on muscle electrolytes and muscle glycogen in normal subjects. *Acta Med Scand* 180:363–376, 1966.
35. Morgan DB and Davidson C: Hypokalemia and diuretics: An analysis of publications. *Br Med J* 280:905–908, 1980.
36. Nordrehang JE and Von der Lippe G: Hypokalemia and ventricular fibrillation in acute myocardial infarction. *Br Heart J* 50:525–529, 1983.
37. Norris RM, et al: Prevention of ventricular fibrillation during acute myocardial infarction by intravenous propranolol. *Lancet* 2:883–886, 1984.

38. Kassirer JP and Harrington JT: Fending off the potassium pushers. *N Engl J Med* 312:785–787, 1985.
39. Kaplan NM: Our appropriate concern about hypokalemia. *Am J Med* 77:1–4, 1984.
40. Abraham AS, et al: Intra-cellular cations and diuretic therapy following acute myocardial infarction. *Arch Intern Med* 146:1301–1303, 1986.
41. Kaplan NM, et al: Potassium supplementation in hypertensive patients with diuretic-induced hypokalemia. *N Eng J Med* 312:746–749, 1985.
42. Schwartz AB and Swartz CD: Dosage of potassium chloride elixir to correct thiazide-induced hypokalemia. *JAMA* 230:702–704, 1974.
43. Papademetrion V, et al: Effectiveness of potassium chloride or triamterene in thiazide hypokalemia. *Arch Intern Med* 145:1986–1990, 1985.
44. Greenblat DJ and Koch-Weser J: Adverse reactions to spironolactone. A report from the Boston Collaborative Drug Surveillance Program. *JAMA* 225:40–43, 1973.
45. Ramsay LE, et al: Amiloride spironolactone and potassium chloride in thiazide-treated hypertensive patients. *Clin Pharmacol Ther* 27:533–543, 1980.
46. Cannon-Babb ML and Schwartz AB: Drug-induced hyperkalemia. *Hosp Pract* 21:99–127, 1986.
47. Sica DA and Gehr TWB: Triamterene and the kidney. *Nephron* 51:454–461, 1989.
48. Weinberg MS, et al: Anuric renal failure precipitated by indocin and triamterene. *Nephron* 40:216–218, 1985.
49. Williams P and Rush DR: Geriatric polypharmacy. *Hosp Pract* 6:104–120, 1986.
50. Finnegan TP, Spence JD, and Cape RD: Potassium-sparing diuretics: Interaction with digoxin in elderly men. *J Am Geriatr Soc* 32:129–131, 1984.
51. Zawada ET Jr: Antihypertensive therapy with triamterene-hydrochlorothiazide vs. amiloride-hydrochlorothiazide. *Arch Intern Med* 146:1312–1314, 1986.
52. Whang R, et al: Magnesium depletion as a cause of refractory potassium depletion. *Arch Intern Med* 145:1686–1688, 1985.
53. Paice B, et al: Hyperkalemia in patients in hospital. *Br Med J* 286:1189–1192, 1983.
54. Shemer J, et al: Incidence of hyperkalemia in hospitalized patients. *Isr J Med Sci* 19:659–661, 1983.
55. Hen RJ, et al: Adaptation to chronic potassium loading in normal man. *Min Electrol Metab* 12:165–172, 1986.
56. Frais MA, Burgers ED, and Mitchell LB: Piroxicam-induced renal failure and hyperkalemia. *Ann Intern Med* 99:129, 1980.
57. Grossman LA and Moss S: Piroxicam and hyperkalemic acidosis. *Ann Intern Med* 99:282, 1983.
58. Miller KP, Lazar EJ, and Fotino S: Severe hyperkalemia during piroxicam therapy. *Arch Intern Med* 144:2414–2415, 1984.
59. Corwin HL and Bonventre JV: Renal insufficiency associated with non-steroidal anti-inflammatory agents. *Am J Kidney Dis* 4:147–152, 1984.
60. Aimran A, et al: Incidence of hyperkalemia induced by indomethacin in a hospital population. *Br Med J* 291:107–108, 1985.
61. Findling JW, et al: Indomethacin-induced hyperkalemia in three patients with gouty arthritis. *JAMA* 244:1127–1128, 1980.
62. Tan SY, et al: Indomethacin-induced prostaglandin inhibition with hyperkalemia. *Ann Intern Med* 90:783–785, 1979.

63. Beroniade V, Corneille L, and Haraoui B: Indomethacin-induced inhibition of prostaglandin with hyperkalemia. *Ann Intern Med* 91:499–500, 1979.
64. Kimberly RP, et al: Reduction of renal function by newer nonsteroidal anti-inflammatory drugs. *Am J Med* 64:804–807, 1978.
65. Meier DE, et al: Indomethacin-associated hyperkalemia in the elderly. *J Am Geriatr Soc* 31:371–373, 1983.
66. Geller M, Folkert VW, and Schlondorff D: Reversible acute renal insufficiency and hyperkalemia following indomethacin therapy. *JAMA* 246:154–155, 1981.
67. Goldszer RC, et al: Hyperkalemia associated with indomethacin. *Arch Intern Med* 141:802, 1981.
68. McCarthy EP, Frost GW, and Stokes GS: Indomethacin-induced hyperkalemia. *Med J Austr* 1:550, 1979.
69. Swainson CP and Griffiths P: Acute and chronic effects of sulindac on renal function in chronic renal disease. *Clin Pharmacol Ther* 37:298–300, 1985.
70. Nesher G, Zimran A, and Hershkoc C: Reduced incidence of hyperkalemia and azotemia in patient's receiving sulindac compared with indomethacin. *Nephron* 48:291–295, 1988.
71. Textor SC, et al: Hyperkalemia in azotemic patients during angiotensin-converting enzyme inhibition and aldosterone reduction with captopril. *Am J Med* 73:719–725, 1982.
72. Swenson ER: Severe hyperkalemia as a complication of timolol, a topically applied β-adrenergic antagonist. *Arch Intern Med* 146:1220–1221, 1986.
73. Yang WC, et al: Beta adrenergic-mediated extrarenal potassium disposal in patients with end-stage renal disease: Effect of propranolol. *Min Electrol Metab* 12:186–193, 1986.
74. Coun JW, et al: Inhibition of heparinoid of aldosterone biosynthesis in man. *J Clin Endocrinal Metab* 26:527–532, 1966.
75. Sherman RA and Ruddy MC: Suppression of aldosterone production by low-dose heparin. *Am J Nephrol* 6:165–168, 1986.
76. Leehy D, Gantt C, and Lim V: Heparin-induced hypoaldosternism. *JAMA* 246:2189–2190, 1981.
77. Edes TE and Sunderrajan EV: Heparin-induced hyperkalemia. *Arch Intern Med* 145:1070–1072, 1985.
78. Perez GO, Pelleys R, and Oster JR: Renal-tubular hyperkalemia. *Am J Nephrol* 2:109–114, 1982.
79. Gerstein AR, et al: Aldosterone deficiency in chronic renal failure. *Nephron* 5:90–105, 1968.
80. McGiff JC, et al: Interrelationships of renin and aldosterone in a patient with hypoaldosteronism *Am J Med* 48:247–253, 1970.
81. Perez G, Siegel L, and Schreiner GE: Selective hypoaldosteronism with hyperkalemia. *Ann Intern Med* 76:757–763, 1972.
82. Gossain VV, et al: Impaired renin responsiveness with secondary hyperaldosteronism. *Arch Intern Med* 132:885–890, 1973.
83. Weidmann P, et al: Syndrome of hyporeninemic hypoaldosteronism in renal disease. *J Clin Endocrinol Metab* 36:965–977, 1973.
84. Oh MS, et al: A mechanism for hyporeninemic hypoaldosteronism in chronic renal disease. *Metabolism* 23:1157–1166, 1974.
85. DeLeiva A, et al: Big renin and biosynthetic defect of aldosterone in diabetes mellitus. *N Engl J Med* 295:639–643, 1976.
86. Sebastian A, et al: Amelioration of metabolic acidosis with fludrocortisone therapy in hyporeninemic hypoaldosteronism. *N Engl J Med* 297:576–583, 1977.

87. Schambelan M, Sebastian A, and Biglieri EG: Prevalence, pathogenesis and functional significance of aldosterone deficiency in hyperkalemic patients with chronic renal insufficiency. *Kidney Int* 17:89–101, 1980.

88. Battle DC, Arruda JAL, and Kurtzman NA: Hyperkalemic distal renal tubular acidosis associated with obstructive uropathy. *N Engl J Med* 304:373–380, 1981.

89. Dubose TD and Caflisch CR: Effect of selective aldosterone deficiency on acidification in nephron segments of the rat inner medulla. *J Clin Invest* 82:1624–1632, 1988.

90. Szylman P, et al: Role of hyperkalemia in the metabolic acidosis of isolated hyperaldosteronism. *N Engl J Med* 294:361–365, 1976.

91. Sebastian A, et al: Effect of mineralocorticoid replacement therapy in renal acid-base homeostasis in adrenalectomized patients. *Kidney Int* 18:767–769, 1980.

92. Phelps KRR, et al: Pathophysiology of the syndrome of hyporeninemic hypoaldosteronism. *Metabolism* 29:186–199, 1980.

93. Tan SY, Antonipillae I, and Mulrow PJ: Inactive renin and prostaglandin E_2 production in hyporeninemic hypoaldosteronism. *J Clin Endocrinol Metab* 51:849–853, 1980.

94. Tuck ML and Mayes DM: Mineralocorticoid biosynthesis in patients with hyporeninemic hypoaldosteronism. *J Clin Endocrinol Metab* 50:341–347, 1980.

95. Kaufman JS, et al: Isolated hypoaldosteronism and abnormalities in renin, kallikrein and prostaglandin. *Nephron* 43:203–210, 1986.

96. Nadler JL, et al: Evidence of prostacyclin deficiency in the syndrome of hyporeninemic hypoaldosteronism. *N Engl J Med* 314:1015–1020, 1986.

97. Williams GH: Hyporeninemic hypoaldosteronism. *N Engl J Med* 314:1041–1042, 1986.

98. Schambelan M, Sebastian A, and Rector F: Mineralocorticoid resistant renal hyperkalemia without salt wasting (type II pseudohypoaldosteronism): Role of increased renal chloride reabsorption. *Kidney Int* 19:716–727, 1981.

99. Gordon RD: Syndrome of hypertension and hyperkalemia with normal glomerular filtration rate. *Hypertension* 8:93–102, 1986.

100. Arruda JAL, et al: Hyperkalemia and renal insufficiency: Role of selective aldosterone deficiency and tubular unresponsiveness to aldosterone. *Am J Nephrol* 1:160–167, 1981.

101. Battle DC: Hyperkalemic hyperchloremic metabolic acidosis associated with selective aldosterone deficiency and distal renal tubular acidosis. *Semin Nephrol* 1:260–274, 1981.

102. Arruda JAL, et al: Voltage-dependent distal acidification defect induced by amiloride. *J Lab Clin Med* 95:407–416, 1980.

103. Viberti GC: Glucose-induced hyperkalemia: A hazard for diabetics? *Lancet* 1:690–691, 1978.

104. Nicolio GL, et al: Glucose-induced hyperkalemia in diabetic subjects. *Arch Intern Med* 141:49–53, 1981.

105. Goldfarb S, et al: Paradoxical glucose-induced hyperkalemia. *Am J Med* 59:744–750, 1975.

106. Goldfarb S, et al: Acute hyperkalemia induced by hyperglycemia: Hormonal mechanisms. *Ann Intern Med* 84:426–432, 1976.

107. Ammon RA, May SW, and Nightingale SD: Glucose-induced hyperkalemia with normal aldosterone levels. *Ann Intern Med* 89:349–351, 1978.

108. Montolin J and Revert L: Lethal hyperkalemia associated with severe hyperglycemia in diabetic patients with renal failure. *Am J Kidney Dis* 1:47–48, 1985.

109. Adrogue HJ and Madias NE: Changes in plasma potassium concentration during acute acid-base disturbances. *Am J Med* 71:456–467, 1981.
110. Oster JR, et al: Plasma potassium response to acute metabolic acidosis induced by mineral and non-mineral acids. *Min Electrol Metab* 4:28–36, 1980.
111. Blumberg A, et al: Effect of various therapeutic approaches on plasma potassium and major regulating factors in terminal renal failure. *Am J Med* 85:507–512, 1988.
112. Allon M, Dunlay R, and Copkney C: Nebulized albuterol for acute hyperkalemia in patients on hemodialysis. *Ann Intern Med* 110:426–429, 1989.
113. Vestral RE, Wood AJJ, and Shand DG: Reduced beta-adrenoreceptor sensitivity in the elderly. *Clin Pharmacol Ther* 26:181–186, 1979.
114. Rastogi SP, et al: Effect of furosemide on urinary acidification in distal renal tubular acidosis. *J Lab Clin Med* 104:271–282, 1984.
115. Sebastian A, Schambelan M, and Sutton JM: Amelioration of hyperchloremic acidosis with furosemide therapy in patients with chronic renal insufficiency and type 4 renal tubular acidosis. *Am J Nephrol* 4:287–300, 1984.

4 ACID-BASE DISORDERS

NORMAL ACID-BASE BALANCE

The maintenance of normal acid-base balance in humans depends on the balance between hydrogen ion (H) production and excretion. H, primarily a consequence of cellular metabolism, is present in the blood in two forms: carbonic acid (H_2CO_3) and fixed acids. The former is excreted by the lungs as CO_2 and the latter by the kidney. Under normal circumstances net daily fixed acid production is 50 to 100 mM (1 mM per kg). In addition to cellular metabolism, dietary foodstuffs (protein, fat, carbohydrate), absorption by the gut of available base equivalents, and buffering by bone also contribute to net acid production [1]. The kidneys participate in the excretion of fixed acids through their regulation of bicarbonate (a major extracellular buffer) absorption and excretion, NH_3 production, and titrable acid excretion.

RENAL BICARBONATE REGULATION

Bicarbonate (HCO_3) is freely filtered through the glomerular capillary wall at a rate related to the plasma HCO_3 concentration and the glomerular filtration rate (GFR). In the proximal tubule, HCO_3 reabsorption is linked to the luminal secretion of H, as shown by the following reaction:

$$H^+ + HCO_3 \rightleftharpoons H_2CO_3 \rightleftharpoons H_2O + CO_2$$

The dissociation of H_2CO_3 to $H_2O + CO_2$ is almost immediate owing to the presence of carbonic anhydrase (CA) in the proximal tubule brush border. The CO_2 produced diffuses back into the cell to participate in the formation of HCO_3, which then diffuses into the peritubular interstitial space, and H, which will be secreted into the lumen, completing the cycle:

$$_{Ca}CO_2 + H_2O \overset{CA}{\rightleftharpoons} H_2CO_3 \rightleftharpoons HCO_3 + H^+$$

Eighty to eighty-five percent of the filtered HCO_3 is absorbed by this method in the early segments of the proximal tubule. An increase in luminal HCO_3 concentration, luminal flow rate, or arterial pCO_2 stimulates proximal HCO_3 reabsorption. Renal nerve stimulation and angiotensin II also increase HCO_3 reabsorption. On the other hand, an increase in peritubular HCO_3 concentration inhibits HCO_3 reabsorption [2].

Both the medullary and cortical segments of the thick ascending limb of Henle participate in HCO_3 reabsorption through an active process that requires CA. The process can be stimulated by metabolic acidosis or an increase in dietary sodium and is inhibited by metabolic alkalosis, low sodium diet, vasopressin, and medullary hypertonicity [3]. A large part of the HCO_3 that escapes proximal tubular reabsorption is reabsorbed in this segment.

Both the inner and the outer medullary collecting ducts also participate in HCO_3 absorption [4, 5], which can be modulated by mineralocorticoids and various peptide hormones through cyclic AMP [6].

AMMONIA PRODUCTION
The regeneration of HCO_3 and the adaptation to changes in acid-base status occur mainly through variations in the synthesis of ammonia (NH_3) from amino acids (chiefly glutamine) by the cells of the early proximal tubular segment. NH_3 excretion increases during metabolic acidosis and decreases during metabolic alkalosis. Besides changes in peritubular H concentration, luminal flow rate and K concentration are important regulators of NH_3 synthesis.

The synthesis of NH_3 from glutamine also results in the formation of HCO_3. The latter is preferentially transported across the basolateral membrane of the proximal tubule into the systemic blood, whereas the NH_3 formed is secreted into the tubular fluid, much of which is reabsorbed in the thick ascending limb, leading to its accumulation in the medulla by countercurrent multiplication. From the medullary interstitium, NH_3 is passively secreted across the collecting duct epithelium, where it combines with H, secreted actively, resulting in the formation of ammonium (NH_4), which is excreted in the final urine [7].

TITRABLE ACID EXCRETION
The titrable acids (TA) consist of all the filtered buffers present in the urine (with the exception of NH_3) combined with H. These buffers are usually organic acids such as phosphate, creatinine, and beta-hydroxybutyrate. Phosphate accounts for the bulk of TA and is generated mainly in the proximal tubule through the conversion of Na_2HPO_4 to NaH_2PO_4. Under ordinary circumstances, 33 to 50 percent of the total H load is excreted as TA [8]. Factors known to affect the rate of formation and excretion of TA include the degree of acidosis and the concentration and pK

of the filtered buffers. In summary, net acid excretion (NAE) is the sum of the NH_3 and TA excreted minus any HCO_3 loss:

$$NAE = NH_4 + TA - HCO_3$$

EFFECTS OF AGE ON ACID-BASE METABOLISM

Blood pH and plasma HCO_3 do not change with age [9]. Therefore, the aging kidney is able to maintain acid-base homeostasis under basal conditions; however, when subjected to an acute acid load, the elderly do not increase NAE to the same degree as younger patients (see Chap. 1). This phenomenon is secondary to a lower NH_4 excretion, which cannot be accounted for solely by the progressive decrease in GFR seen with age. Additional factors not yet elucidated must be responsible for this impairment.

ACID-BASE DISORDERS

Judging from our own experience, acid-base disorders are rather common in the elderly. The true incidence, however, is not known. In 7,433 abnormal blood gas measurements obtained from patients of various ages by Hodgkins and colleagues [10], metabolic alkalosis was present in 36 percent, respiratory alkalosis in 21 percent, mixed abnormality in 19 percent, respiratory acidosis in 16 percent, and metabolic acidosis in 8 percent. No breakdown according to age was available in this study. We retrospectively analyzed 130 consecutive abnormal arterial blood gas determinations obtained from elderly hospitalized patients. Metabolic acidosis was present in 30 percent, mixed abnormalities in 23 percent, respiratory acidosis in 18 percent, metabolic alkalosis in 17 percent, and respiratory alkalosis in 12 percent, suggesting differences in acid-base metabolism in the elderly and/or different medical problems associated with these metabolic disturbances compared with those in the general population. Most of the data presented in this section are drawn from this experience, since there are relatively few data in the literature that specifically address acid-base disturbances in the elderly.

METABOLIC ACIDOSIS

Etiology

The etiology of metabolic acidosis is dependent on the type of acidosis present, which is classified in the elderly like that in younger patients: (1) increased anion gap acidosis, which is due (in decreasing order of frequency) to severe chronic renal insufficiency, lactic acidosis, ketoacidosis, drugs, or poisons, and (2) nonanion gap acidosis, which is due to mild or moderate chronic renal insufficiency with or without tubular hyperkalemia, HCO_3 losses through the gastrointestinal tract, drugs, renal tubular acidosis, or diabetes mellitus.

Clinical Manifestations and Pathogenesis

In general, the clinical manifestations in patients with metabolic acidosis are those of the associated disease state. The conscious patient may complain of shortness of breath. On physical examination, Kussmaul breathing may be present as well as asterixis, particularly if the acidosis is severe.

The pathogenesis of the acidosis (both anion gap and nonanion gap varieties) associated with renal insufficiency (which is responsible for more than 30 percent of cases of metabolic acidosis in elderly patients) is discussed in Chaps. 3 and 11.

Lactic acidosis is generally found in states of poor tissue perfusion (e.g., septic or cardiogenic shock) and results from an imbalance between production (by the poorly perfused organs) and utilization (by an ischemic liver and other tissues) [11]. It may be present in a pure form or associated with other anion or nonanion gap acidosis. An increase in the blood lactate level with acidosis has also been reported in elderly patients with certain types of malignancy such as lymphomas and carcinoma of the breast, lung, and bowel [12]. The exact mechanism responsible for the increase in lactate production in these patients has not been completely elucidated [13]. Lactic acidosis may also be associated with a number of other conditions such as seizures, short bowel syndrome, and hereditary defects [14], but their occurrence in the elderly is rather rare. In the appropriate setting, the diagnosis of lactic acidosis is confirmed by a plasma lactate level ≥ 5 mmol per liter.

Ketoacidosis occurs in diabetes mellitus, starvation, and alcoholism. The inorganic acids generated endogenously are beta-hydroxybutyric (from incompletely burned body fat) and acetoacetic. Of the various drugs and chemicals (salicylate, methanol, ethylene glycol, paraldehyde, acetaminophen) capable of causing an anion-gap acidosis [15–18] when ingested either accidentally or in a suicidal attempt, salicylate poisoning is the only one of significant clinical importance in the elderly. In the absence of a definite history of salicylate ingestion, the clinical picture can be easily confused with other clinical states seen in the elderly such as a primary central nervous system event, alcoholic intoxication, or sepsis [19]. The presence of a mixed acid-base picture (respiratory alkalosis and metabolic acidosis) should raise the suspicion of this diagnosis, which is confirmed by measuring the plasma salicylate level. A level of 40 to 60 mg per dl is associated with mild toxicity, 60 to 100 mg per dl with moderate intoxication, and greater than 100 mg per dl with severe intoxication. The acidosis is secondary to the accumulation of ketones and lactate in the extracellular fluid, resulting from the disturbed carbohydrate metabolism, which is a consequence of uncoupling of mitochondrial oxidative phosphorylation by salicylates. In addition, the salicylate itself contributes to the increase in the anion gap [20, 21].

Gastrointestinal losses of HCO_3 secondary to diarrhea constitute the second most common cause of nonanion gap acidosis in the elderly (mild to moderate renal insufficiency being the most common). At the time of diagnosis, renal failure (acute or chronic), severe volume contraction, hypophosphatemia, and hypophosphaturia were usually present in our patients. Since renal failure decreases NH_3 availability, a low distal Na delivery associated with volume contraction interferes with H secretion, and hypophosphaturia limits urinary TA, the kidneys undoubtedly contribute to the acidosis in many of these patients.

Hyperchloremic acidosis of varying severity occurs in 55 percent of elderly patients treated with carbonic anhydrase inhibitors (e.g., acetazolamide) for glaucoma [22, 23]. This high incidence in the elderly may be due in part to a higher blood concentration of the drug at the commonly prescribed doses than that seen in younger patients [23]. Since these drugs act by inhibiting tubular HCO_3 secretion, the urine pH during the early phase of therapy is greater than 7. During more chronic administration, however, a lower pH (5–6) may be found. Other drugs such as amiloride, spironolactone, and the converting-enzyme inhibitors can also produce a nonanion gap acidosis, although in our experience it has been rare.

Defective urinary acidification occurring in either the proximal or the distal portion of the nephron is classified as renal tubular acidosis (RTA). In proximal RTA (type II), massive urinary HCO_3 losses lead to a steady-state metabolic acidosis in association with a normal NAE. The pH in a first morning urine sample in these patients is characteristically less than 6.0 and can be as low as 5.3 following an acid load. In addition to HCO_3, other solutes usually absorbed in the proximal tubule such as glucose, phosphate, uric acid, and amino acids may also be lost. In patients with distal RTA (type I), the first morning urine pH is usually greater than 6.0 and will remain greater than 5.3 following an acid load. Hypercalciuria and hypocitruria associated with nephrolithiasis are common in these patients. In both forms of RTA, hypokalemia is common. Hyperkalemic distal RTA, also referred to as type IV RTA, is a common entity in the elderly as discussed in Chap. 3, but pure type I RTA is rare in this age group. In one recent review of 40 adults with type I RTA, only two (5 percent) were over the age of 60 [24]. Type I RTA in the elderly is almost always secondary to other diseases such as amyloidosis, multiple myeloma, rheumatoid arthritis, or Sjögren's syndrome.

Hyperchloremic metabolic acidosis may be seen in the patient with uncontrolled diabetes at the time of presentation to the hospital or following treatment for ketoacidosis [25]. Because these patients are usually not severely volume depleted, the continued excretion of keto-anions will exceed the capacity of the kidneys to regenerate alkali and also lead to a loss of HCO_3 precursors, resulting in a hyperchloremic state [26].

It is possible to use a variety of guidelines and formulas to diagnose a pure metabolic acidosis. During steady-state metabolic acidosis the ventilatory response is usually quite predictable and can be calculated from the formula $pCO_2 = 1.54 \times$ serum $HCO_3 + 8.36$, or derived from the fact that for each 1 mEq per liter decrease in serum HCO_3 there is a 1.3 mm Hg decrease in pCO_2. If the measured pCO_2 is 2 mm Hg or greater over the calculated pCO_2, there is probably an accompanying respiratory acidosis, whereas if it is 2 mm Hg or more below the pCO_2, a primary respiratory alkalosis is probably present.

Treatment

$NaHCO_3$ administration remains the mainstay of treatment for metabolic acidosis. The distribution space of HCO_3 is estimated to be 50 percent of total body weight for a serum HCO_3 above 5 mEq per liter and 80 to 100 percent for values below this range. In patients with severe, acute acidosis, we usually attempt to increase the serum HCO_3 concentration to 10 to 12 mEq per liter. The amount required for a given patient should be infused as an isotonic or hypotonic solution rather than as "bolus pushes," which are hypertonic. Since this regimen requires the administration of a significant amount of fluid, volume overload may be a danger, and furosemide may be given in conjunction with the $NaHCO_3$. Dialysis may be necessary in patients with associated severe renal or heart failure.

Treatment of the metabolic acidosis of chronic renal failure is discussed in Chap. 11.

The use of HCO_3 therapy in patients with lactic acidosis is controversial [27, 28]. In patients with malignancy-related acidosis, alkali therapy will normalize the serum HCO_3 concentration in patients in whom the tumors either respond to chemotherapy or are surgically removed [12]. In patients with lactic acidosis due to tissue anoxia, the primary effort should be directed at correcting the underlying problem (improving cardiac function, reversing hypotension, treating sepsis, and so on). Even though raising the plasma pH and HCO_3 does not lead to any change in systemic hemodynamics or in mortality [29], we agree with Narins and Cohen [28] that in patients with severe acidemia (pH < 7.2, $HCO_3 < 8$ mEq per liter) alkali therapy is indicated to bring the serum HCO_3 to 10 mEq per liter to buy sufficient time to eliminate the cause of the acidosis. Dichloroacetate 50 mg per kg body weight, given intravenously as a bolus at 2-hour intervals, has been shown to lower the serum lactate level in a small number of elderly patients. The effect of this drug on the long-term survival of patients with lactic acidosis remains to be determined, however [30].

The acidosis associated with alcoholic and starvation ketosis is generally mild and responds to dextrose administration. In diabetic ketoacidosis, alkali therapy is indicated only initially and when the acidosis is severe [31].

We use the same guidelines outlined earlier (see Chap. 2) to manage acidotic elderly patients with gastrointestinal losses of alkali, since these patients are generally hypernatremic and severely volume contracted. Volume expansion should be accomplished with a solution containing both HCO_3 and chloride.

Drug intoxications (ethylene glycol or methanol) are best treated by ethanol infusion and HCO_3 hemodialysis. Patients with RTA should be treated with oral alkali as outlined in Chap. 11.

RESPIRATORY ACIDOSIS

Etiology
Respiratory acidosis was the third most common variety of acid-base abnormality seen in our elderly patients and was usually secondary to either chronic obstructive pulmonary disease (COPD) or chest wall deformity such as kyphoscoliosis. Central nervous system depression related to drug ingestion as well as other disease states such as Guillain-Barré syndrome, polymyositis, obesity, and hypoventilation syndrome were rare causes in this age group.

Clinical Manifestations and Pathogenesis
Dyspnea, cough, and a respiratory tract infection are the most common clinical manifestations in these patients. On physical examination, cyanosis, tachypnea, use of the accessory respiratory muscles, increased anteroposterior diameter of the thoracic cage, severe chest deformity (in the kyphoscoliotic patient), and clubbing of the fingers may be found. The retention of CO_2 is responsible for the acidemia through generation of H_2CO_3, which dissociates to $H + HCO_3$. The H enters the cell in exchange for potassium (K) and sodium (Na) and is buffered by cellular proteins. The HCO_3 remains in the extracellular fluid (ECF). In addition, some of the CO_2 enters the red blood cell and undergoes hydration in the presence of CA. The H thus formed is buffered by hemoglobin, whereas the HCO_3 moves into the ECF in exchange for chloride (Cl). These changes occur acutely, and the HCO_3 gain by the ECF by this mechanism is rather modest, approximately 4 to 5 mEq per liter. During respiratory acidosis the kidneys are primarily responsible for the

more significant elevation of the plasma HCO_3 concentration than that seen during the acute phase by generation of new HCO_3 and increasing proximal tubule and collecting duct HCO_3 reabsorption [32, 33].

Clinical observations in humans with acute or chronic respiratory acidosis have shown a highly predictable relationship between the degree of hypercapnia and the HCO_3 level following the physiologic adaptations described above. In acute respiratory acidosis, HCO_3 increases 1 mEq per liter for every 10 mm Hg increase in pCO_2. In chronic respiratory acidosis, HCO_3 increase 3.5 mEq per liter for every 10 mm Hg increase in pCO_2. A deviation from these predictable patterns of response should suggest the presence of an additional acid-base disturbance.

Treatment
During acute exacerbations of acid-base disorders treatment is directed toward maintaining adequate oxygenation while correcting or controlling the precipitating event (infection, heart failure, drugs). The total management of the patient with COPD is beyond the scope of this discussion.

METABOLIC ALKALOSIS

Etiology
Based on the urinary Cl concentration, metabolic alkalosis is usually classified as Cl-responsive (urinary Cl < 10 mEq per liter) and Cl-resistant (urinary Cl > 20 mEq per liter). The former, by far more common in the elderly, is associated with gastric fluid losses, diuretic therapy, and posthypercapnic states. The latter occurs in hyperglucocorticoidism, following the use of mineralocorticoidlike agents (licorice, carbenoxolone), and in patients with primary aldosteronism.

Clinical Manifestations and Pathogenesis
The clinical manifestations of metabolic alkalosis are usually those of the underlying problem, although severe alkalemia (pH > 7.55) may cause mental confusion, muscle cramps, or cardiac arrhythmias (both supraventricular and ventricular), particularly in patients requiring ventilatory support. Independent of origin, the development of metabolic alkalosis can be divided into a generation phase and a maintenance phase [34].

CHLORIDE-RESPONSIVE ALKALOSIS. The generation of metabolic alkalosis during vomiting is related to HCl losses that result in an ECF gain of HCO_3. The latter obligates renal excretion of Na as well as K as accompanying cations (see Chap. 3). If the renal Na and gastric Cl losses are not replaced, volume contraction ensues.

With diuretics such as furosemide, bumetanide, and chlorothiazide, which act by blocking NaCl reabsorption in the thick ascending limb of

Henle or distal convoluted tubule, alkalosis is a consequence of the increased delivery of Na to the cortical collecting tubule, where it is partially reabsorbed, associated with an increased secretion of H and K leading to the enhancement of NAE and kaliuresis. Since the capacity of this nephron segment to reabsorb Na is limited, ECF volume contraction will also develop.

The compensatory increase in serum HCO_3 that occurs during respiratory acidosis is also accompanied by a transient increase in NAE and Cl losses. Once the pCO_2 has returned to normal, the excess HCO_3 will be excreted if Cl is available. If the patient has a deficit of NaCl, however, the elevated serum HCO_3 will persist, leading to metabolic alkalosis.

The maintenance of metabolic alkalosis is a consequence of the inability of the kidneys to excrete HCO_3. Several mechanisms are responsible: (1) a decrease in the filtered load of HCO_3 due to a lower GFR as a result of volume contraction, hypokalemia, or activation of tubuloglomerular feedback; (2) K depletion, which stimulates HCO_3 reabsorption in the proximal tubule; (3) an increase in NAE, since K depletion increases NH_3 synthesis and produces intracellular acidosis. The hyperaldosteronism associated with volume contraction might also participate in the increase in NAE.

CHLORIDE-RESISTANT ALKALOSIS. The generation and maintenance of metabolic alkalosis in the Cl-resistant form depends on the persistence of a mineralocorticoid excess despite ECF volume expansion. As a consequence, distal H secretion increases, resulting in an increase in NAE. The mineralocorticoid excess also stimulates K secretion with ensuing hypokalemia. Hypokalemia then contributes to the increase in NAE and proximal HCO_3 reabsorption.

The respiratory compensatory pattern seen in patients with pure metabolic alkalosis is erratic. In general, the PCO_2 increases 0.6 mm Hg for each mEq per liter increase in serum HCO_3; however, a lesser degree of compensation has also been suggested with $PCO_2 = 0.9 (HCO_3) + 9$ [37]. Significant deviations from these relationships suggest a mixed acid-base disturbance.

Treatment
In Cl-responsive metabolic alkalosis, both Cl and potassium should be replaced. The rate of replacement will depend on the severity of the ECF depletion. In the presence of hypotension and tachycardia, 0.9 percent NaCl is the solution of choice. Once the hemodynamics stabilize, the switch can be made to either 0.45 percent or 0.33 percent NaCl with added K. In patients who are on nasogastric suction, the daily losses should be replaced. We also add an H_2-receptor antagonist (either cimetidine or ranitidine) in an effort to attentuate gastric HCl losses [35].

For treatment of Cl-resistant alkalosis see Chaps. 3 and 12. In patients receiving a saline infusion and pharmacologic doses of glucocorticoid, management should include salt restriction and K replacement.

A significant number of our elderly patients with metabolic alkalosis also had associated acute renal failure. Since volume contraction was responsible for the renal failure in most of these patients, recovery was rapid following volume expansion. For patients with acute renal failure who do not respond to fluids, dialysis (preferably continuous arteriovenous hemofiltration dialysis using NaCl as the replacement solution) may be necessary, since renal failure impairs renal HCO_3 excretion.

In intractable cases (which we have not seen in the elderly) 0.15 normal HCl can be infused into a central vein as an isotonic solution, not to exceed 2 liters per day. The amount required should be calculated from the HCO_3 space (50 percent of body weight) [36].

RESPIRATORY ALKALOSIS
Respiratory alkalosis was diagnosed in 12 percent of our patients. This figure probably represents an underestimate because a large number of hospitalized patients with this abnormality go unnoticed (since a blood gas determination is not routinely performed).

Etiology
Respiratory alkalosis can occur in any situation in which the depth or rate of respiration increases. The hyperventilation in our elderly patients was caused by hypoxia associated with pulmonary or heart disease, sepsis, liver disease, or fever or artificially by overbreathing through respirators. Anxiety, analeptic overdoses, and hyperthyroidism may also be associated with hyperventilation.

Clinical Manifestations and Pathogenesis
Patients with metabolic alkalosis may complain of lightheadedness, perioral numbness, and paresthesias of the extremities, presumably due to a decrease in ionized calcium, the altered pH, and perhaps to the vasoconstrictive effect of a low pCO_2 on the cerebral vasculature. The mechanisms responsible for the hyperventilation associated with sepsis and fever are not completely understood but could represent stimulation of the respiratory center both directly and through peripheral baroreceptors. With drugs such as salicylates, the stimulation is direct. The metabolic alkalosis of liver disease may be related to changes in hormonal balance (estrogen and progesterone).

Diagnosis of pure acute respiratory alkalosis should be made when there is a 2 mEq per liter decrease in HCO_3 for each 10 mm Hg decrease in pCO_2. In the chronic form, HCO_3 decreases 5 mEq per liter for each 10 mm Hg fall in pCO_2. In the early phase, approximately two-thirds of the decrease in plasma HCO_3 is due to tissue buffering and one-third to blood buffering. When the process extends beyond 24 hours, the kidneys respond by decreasing NAE, which leads to the greater decrease in HCO_3.

Treatment
The treatment for respiratory alkalosis is that of the underlying clinical problem.

MIXED ACID-BASE DISORDERS
Mixed acid-base disorders were present in 23 percent of our elderly patients in whom arterial blood gas determinations were performed. The abnormalities encountered were metabolic acidosis/respiratory alkalosis, respiratory and metabolic acidosis, metabolic alkalosis/respiratory acidosis, and respiratory and metabolic alkalosis. A deviation from the expected respiratory compensation for simple metabolic acid-base disturbance (see appropriate section) or disproportionate changes in the anion gap and the HCO_3 level should lead one to suspect the presence of a mixed acid-base disorder [37, 38]. For example, if the ratio between the change in anion gap to the change in serum HCO_3 is less than 0.7, a mixed metabolic acidosis and respiratory alkalosis should be suspected, whereas a value greater than 1.2 suggests a mixed metabolic and respiratory acidosis or a metabolic acidosis and alkalosis. It should be cautioned, however, that these guidelines should be used only as added information to the history and physical examination in assessing the elderly patient in whom a mixed acid-base problem is suspected [39].

A mixed metabolic acidosis and respiratory alkalosis was seen with septic shock, pulmonary edema, and tissue hypoxia related to low cardiac output, severe liver failure, and drug intoxication (salicylate). Most of the patients were in the intesive care unit with multiple organ failure. Mortality in these patients was close to 100 percent.

Mixed respiratory and metabolic acidosis was found in patients with COPD admitted with sepsis (generally secondary to pulmonary infection) or with congestive heart failure. In some patients, renal insufficiency was also present. The mortality in this group was also extremely high.

Mixed metabolic alkalosis and respiratory acidosis was noted in patients who had COPD with associated heart disease or hypertension and who were on salt restriction in the hospital and continued on a diuretic. Two of our patients had COPD and developed metabolic alkalosis following volume expansion with saline while receiving large doses of steroids and cancer chemotherapeutic drugs.

Mixed respiratory and metabolic alkalosis was found in patients who had undergone abdominal surgery and required nasogastric suction while receiving excessive mechanical ventilation or who had sepsis, severe pain, or sustained neurologic damage.

The management of elderly patients with these mixed disorders requires a therapeutic approach that attempts to treat both acid-base abnormalities simultaneously (see appropriate sections).

REFERENCES

1. Toto RD: Metabolic acid-base disorders. In Kokko JP and Tannen RL (eds): *Fluids and Electrolytes*, Vol. 5. Philadelphia: Saunders, 1986, pp. 229–304.
2. Cogan MG: Regulation and control of bicarbonate absorption in the proximal tubule. *Semin Nephrol* 10:115–121, 1990.
3. Good DW: Bicarbonate absorption by the thick ascending limb of Henle's loop. *Semin Nephrol* 10:132–138, 1990.
4. Schuster VL: Bicarbonate reabsorption, and secretion in the cortical and outer medullary collecting duct. *Semin Nephrol* 10:139–147, 1990.
5. Wall SM and Knepper MA: Acid-base transport in the inner medullary collecting duct. *Semin Nephrol* 10:148–158, 1990.
6. Paillard M and Bichara M: Peptide hormone control of urinary acidification and acid-base balance: PTH, ADH and glucagon. *Am J Physiol* 256:F973–F985, 1989.
7. Knepper MA, Packer R, and Good DW: Ammonium transport in the kidney. *Physiol Rev* 69:179–249, 1989.
8. Simpson DP: Control of hydrogen ion homeostasis and renal acidosis. *Medicine* 50:503–541, 1971.
9. Garry PJ, et al: Clinical chemistry reference intervals for healthy elderly subjects. *Am J Clin Nutr* 50:1219–1230, 1989.
10. Hodgkins JE, Soeprono FF, and Chan DM: Incidence of metabolic alkalemia in hospitalized patients. *Crit Care Med* 8:725–728, 1980.
11. Arieff AI and Graf H: Pathophysiology of type A hypoxic lactic acidosis in dogs. *Am J Physiol* 253:E271–E276, 1987.
12. Doolittle GC, et al: Malignancy-induced lactic acidosis. *South Med J* 81:533–536, 1988.
13. Kreisberg RA: Pathogenesis and management of lactic acidosis. *Ann Rev Med* 35:181–193, 1984.
14. Hood VL and Tannen RL: Lactic acidosis. *Kidney* 22:1–6, 1989.
15. Sejersted OM, et al: Formate concentrations in plasma from patients poisoned with methanol. *Acta Med Scand* 213:105–110, 1983.
16. Jacobson D, Ostby N, and Bredesen JE: Studies on ethylene glycol poisoning. *Acta Med Scand* 212:11–15, 1982.
17. Brier LS, Pitts WH, and Gonick HC: Metabolic acidosis occurring during paraldehyde intoxication. *Ann Intern Med* 58:155–158, 1963.
18. Gray TA, Buckley BM, and Vale JA: Hyperlactataemia and metabolic acidosis following paracetanol overdose. *Q J Med* 65:811–821, 1987.
19. Paul BN: Salicylate poisoning in the elderly: diagnostic pitfalls. *J Am Geriatr Soc* 20:387–390, 1972.
20. Hill JB: Salicylate intoxication. *N Engl J Med* 288:1110–1113, 1973.
21. Brenner BE and Simon RR: Management of salicylate intoxication. *Drugs* 24:335–340, 1982.
22. Heller I, et al: Significant metabolic acidosis induced by acetazolamide. Not a rare complication. *Arch Intern Med* 145:1815–1817, 1985.
23. Chapron DJ, Gomolin JH, and Sweeney KR: Azetazolamide blood concentrations are excessive in the elderly: Propensity for acidosis and relationship to renal function. *J Clin Pharmacol* 29:348–353, 1989.

24. Caruana RJ and Buckalew VM Jr: The syndrome of distal (type I) renal tubular acidosis. Clinical and laboratory findings in 58 cases. *Medicine* 67:84–99, 1988.

25. Adrogué HJ, et al: Plasma acid-base patterns in diabetic ketoacidosis. *N Engl J Med* 307:1603–1610, 1982.

26. Oh MS, Carroll HJ, and Uribarri J: Mechanisms of normochloremic and hyperchloremic acidosis in diabetic ketoacidosis. *Nephron* 54:1–6, 1990.

27. Stackpoole PW: Lactic acidosis: The case against bicarbonate therapy. *Ann Intern Med* 105:276–279, 1986.

28. Narins RG and Cohen JJ: Bicarbonate therapy for organic acidosis: the case for its continued use. *Ann Intern Med* 106:615–618, 1987.

29. Cooper JD, et al: Bicarbonate does not improve hemodynamics in critically ill patients who have lactic acidosis. *Ann Intern Med* 112:492–498, 1990.

30. Stackpoole PW, et al: Dichloroacetate in the treatment of lactic acidosis. *Ann Intern Med* 108:58–63, 1988.

31. Hale PJ, Crase J, and Nattrass M: Metabolic effects of bicarbonate in the treatment of diabetic ketoacidosis. *Br Med J* 289:1035–1038, 1984.

32. Cogan M: Chronic hypercapnia stimulates proximal bicarbonate reabsorption in the rat. *J Clin Invest* 74:1942–1947, 1984.

33. McKinney TD and Davidson KK: Effects of respiratory acidosis on HCO_3 transport by rabbit collecting tubules. *Am J Physiol* 255:F656–F665, 1988.

34. Galla JH and Luke RG: Pathophysiology of metabolic alkalosis. *Hosp Pract* 24:123–145, 1987.

35. Barton CH, et al: Cimetidine in the management of metabolic alkalosis induced by nasogastric drainage. *Arch Surg* 114:70–74, 1979.

36. Williams DB and Lyons JH Jr: Treatment of severe metabolic alkalosis with intravenous infusion of hydrochloric acid. *Surg Gynecol Obstet* 150:315–321, 1980.

37. Narins RG and Emmett M: Simple and mixed acid-base disorders: A practical approach. *Medicine* 59:161–187, 1980.

38. Oster JR, Perez GO, and Materson BJ: Use of the anion gap in clinical medicine. *South Med J* 81:225–237, 1988.

39. DiNubile MJ: The increment in the anion gap: Overextension of a concept. *Lancet* 2:951–953, 1988.

5 DISORDERS OF CALCIUM, PHOSPHORUS, AND MAGNESIUM METABOLISM

CALCIUM METABOLISM

NORMAL PHYSIOLOGY

The serum calcium is maintained in the narrow range of 8.5 to 10.5 mg per dl owing to the interaction of several hormonal systems, including parathyroid hormone (PTH), calcitonin, and the D vitamins. The routinely measured total calcium consists of three fractions: an ionized fraction, which constitutes 47 percent of the total and is the physiologically active one; a protein-bound (albumin and globulin) fraction (39 percent); and a complexed fraction (14 percent), bound to multiple organic and inorganic anions [1]. Physiologically significant changes in the level of ionized calcium can occur without corresponding changes in total serum calcium; for example, a rapid increase in pH can decrease and PTH can increase the ionized calcium with only a modest or no change in total calcium. Since changes in serum phosphate can affect serum calcium by binding with free calcium, these two elements should always be measured concurrently.

The concentration of ionized calcium in the blood is the most important factor responsible for the regulation of PTH secretion, since its release is stimulated directly by hypocalcemia and suppressed by hypercalcemia [2–4]. In addition to the extracellular calcium concentration, vitamin D, beta-adrenergic agonists, and histamine (H_2 receptors) have been shown to modulate PTH release [5, 6]. With the exception of vitamin D, however, their physiologic importance remains to be determined.

The synthesis of PTH starts as preproPTH in polyribosomes located within the parathyroid cell matrix. The preproPTH is converted to proPTH by enzymatic activity in or near the reticular membrane. ProPTH is converted to PTH in the Golgi apparatus. The intact hormone, which contains 84 amino acids, gains access to the extracellular fluid by exocytosis. It is metabolized by the liver (and to a lesser extent by the kidneys) into an amino and a carboxy fragment. The amino terminal fragment constitutes the biologically active segment with a half-life in the circulation of less than 5 minutes. The carboxy-terminal fragment has a half-life on the order of 30 to 40 minutes. The latter is significantly increased in patients with renal insufficiency because filtration and excretion by the kidney are the only routes of removal of this fragment from the circulation. To a lesser extent, the amino-terminal fragment is also removed by the kidney, by both glomerular filtration and tubular uptake and secretion. The principal action of PTH is to raise extracellular fluid calcium by increasing renal tubular reabsorption of calcium, mobilizing calcium from bone and increasing intestinal calcium absorption [7].

PTH enhances calcium reabsorption in the cortical thick ascending limb of Henle's loop as well as in the distal tubule by binding to receptors located in the basal membranes of cells in these nephron segments and stimulating adenylate cyclase activity [8]. PTH, through its amino fragment, can activate the osteocytes, osteoblasts, and their precursors [9]. It can have either an anabolic (at low concentration) or a catabolic effect (at high concentration). These functions are also initiated through the activation of cyclic AMP. In the current view of calcium homeostasis in the normal adult, bone has a minimal role in the normal maintenance of plasma calcium. The latter is determined primarily by the relationship between the rate of calcium absorption from the gut (vitamin D–dependent phenomenon) and the renal threshold for calcium (a largely PTH-dependent phenomenon) [10].

Besides its direct action on the renal tubule and bone, PTH participates through vitamin D activation in calcium absorption by the gut. Vitamin D is made available through the diet (D_2, D_3), with absorption taking place in the upper part of the small intestine. It then enters the circulation mainly through the thoracic duct in the chylomicron fraction [11]. Vitamin D is also made available through photosynthesis (ultraviolet light) in the skin, where previtamin D_3 is formed from 7-dehydrocholesterol. The previtamin D_3 so formed undergoes isomerization, resulting in vitamin D_3 formation. The latter is subsequently transferred to the circulation [12].

Vitamin D_3, through carrier proteins, is transported to the liver and undergoes 25-hydroxylation, a reaction catalyzed by both mitochondrial and microsomal enzymes collectively designated vitamin D_3-25 hydroxylase. The synthesis of 25-hydroxyvitamin D_3 (25[OH]D_3) can be inhibited by 1,25-dihydroxyvitamin D_3 (1,25[OH]$_2D_3$) through an increase in hepatocyte cytosolic calcium [13, 14]. In the kidney, 25(OH)D_3 undergoes further hydroxylation by mitochondrial enzymes, 25-hydroxyvitamin D_3-1 hydroxylase to form 1,25(OH)$_2D_3$ and 25-hydroxyvitamin D_3-24 hydroxylase to form 24,25(OH)$_2D_3$. This process takes place in cells in the proximal tubule. 1,25(OH)$_2D_3$ affects active calcium transport throughout the intestinal tract, the ileum being the major site that adapts to changes in dietary calcium [15]. In the enterocyte, the effect of $1,25(OH)_2D_3$ depends on its binding to a protein receptor, located predominantly in the nucleus, resulting in an increased synthesis of messenger RNA for a calcium-binding protein within the intestinal cell. In addition, $1,25(OH)_2D_3$ increases the uptake of calcium at the brush border of the intestinal cell, facilitating its movement into the cell [16]. $1,25(OH)_2D_3$ is also involved in the mobilization of calcium in bone, an action dependent in part on the presence of PTH [17]. Finally, $1,25(OH)_2$-D_3, through receptors located on parathyroid cells [18], exerts a direct inhibitory effect on PTH synthesis, probably by inhibiting PTH gene transcription [19].

Calcitonin (CT) is a 32 amino acid hormone derived from a larger polypeptide. The hormone is synthesized by the C cells located throughout the thyroid gland. Its action results from binding to specific membrane receptors of target cells (osteoblasts, osteocytes perhaps) with subsequent stimulation of cyclic AMP. CT synthesis correlates positively with changes in plasma calcium [20]. Male subjects usually have a greater secretory capacity for CT than females. No change in CT levels occurs with age [21]. The physiologic importance of CT as a plasma calcium regulator in humans remains to be defined.

CHANGES IN THE CALCIUM-PTH-VITAMIN D_3 AXIS WITH AGE

Serum calcium (total and ionized fractions) does not generally change with age. In some studies, however, younger patients were found to have a significantly higher total serum calcium than their older counterparts [22, 23]. This might be due to the fact that the serum albumin level decreases with age [24].

PTH increases gradually with age, and in subjects past the age of 60 it may reach values 2 times the level observed in younger adults [22, 23, 25-27]. As can be seen in Figure 5-1 the variation among patients is rather wide, however. The gradual decrease in GFR seen with age may explain in part the elevated PTH, since in most studies in which creatinine clearance was measured, an inverse correlation could be demonstrated between those two parameters [23, 26]. Besides the lower GFR, the decrease in intestinal calcium absorption seen with increasing age may also play a role [28], since after the oral administration of pharmacologic doses of $25(OH)D_3$, PTH decreases significantly [29]. The reason for the decrease in calcium absorption in the elderly is not fully understood but is of clinical importance because an increase in intestinal calcium absorption constitutes the principal mechanism that prevents a negative calcium balance when dietary calcium intake is decreased [30]. This adaptation is impaired in the elderly [31], which explains why the amount of calcium required to prevent negative calcium balance increases

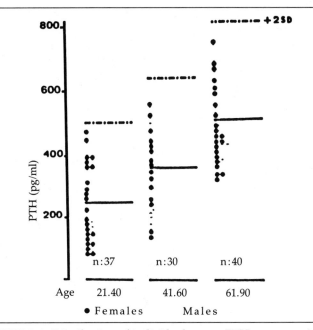

FIGURE 5-1. Distribution of individual serum PTH concentrations in 107 normal subjects aged 21 to 90 years. One normal subject, 75 years old, with the highest PTH value (1700 pg/ml) was omitted in the scattergram. (From Chapuy MC, Durr F, and Chapuy P: Age-related changes in parathyroid hormone and 25-hydroxy-cholecalciferol levels. *J Gerontol* 38:19–22, 1983.)

with age [32]. A possible explanation for the decreased calcium absorption in the elderly is a decrease in plasma $1,25(OH)_2D_3$ levels found by most authors, as seen in Figure 5-2 [28, 33–35]. Indeed, calcium absorption and $1,25(OH)_2D_3$ levels do increase in these patients after administration of a pharmacologic dose of $25(OH)D_3$ [29]. It should be emphasized, however, that the decreased $1,25(OH)_2D_3$ has not been a universal finding [26]. Moreover, in one study the change in calcium absorption did not correlate with the change in plasma $1,25(OH)_2D_3$ [29]. In those elderly with low $1,25(OH)_2D_3$, factors such as a decrease in the sensitivity of the enzyme 1 alpha-hydroxylase to PTH or an increase in the catabolic rate of $1,25(OH)_2D_3$ might be operative [28, 36–39].

The plasma $25(OH)D_3$ level is frequently low in the elderly [40]. This finding is more common in European countries than in the United States, in housebound and institutionalized elderly [41, 42], and during the winter months [34]. In parts of the world where sunlight is more available and where milk is routinely fortified with vitamin D this ten-

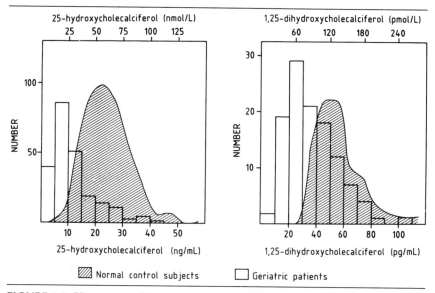

FIGURE 5-2. Histogram of the concentration of 25-hydroxycholecalciferol and 1,25-dihydroxycholecalciferol in elderly patients. Conversion of SI to traditional units: for 25-hydroxycholecalciferol, 1 nmol/liter ≈ 0.4 ng/ml; for 1,25-di-hydroxycholecalciferol, 1 pmol/liter ≈ 0.4 pg/ml. (From Bouillon RA, Subverx JH, Lissens WD, and Pelemans WK: Vitamin D status in the elderly: Seasonal substrate deficiency causes 1,25-dihydroxycholecalciferol deficiency. *Am J Clin Nutr* 45:755–763, 1987. By permission of the American Society for Clinical Nutrition.)

dency is less common [43]. The problem is also compounded by the fact that the skin in the elderly has a greatly diminished capacity to produce previtamin D_3 [44].

A summary of the interactions among serum calcium, PTH, and vitamin D is provided in Figure 5-3.

HYPERCALCEMIA

INCIDENCE AND PREVALENCE
In a screening of 15,903 subjects, Christensson and colleagues [45] found 95 (0.60 percent) with hypercalcemia, 28 of whom (29 percent) were over the age of 60. A marked female preponderance (25:3) was noted. Two to three percent of elderly patients admitted to long-term facilities were found to be hypercalcemic, 60 percent of whom were females [46, 47]. We found hypercalcemia in 5 (2.5 percent, four females, one male) of 200

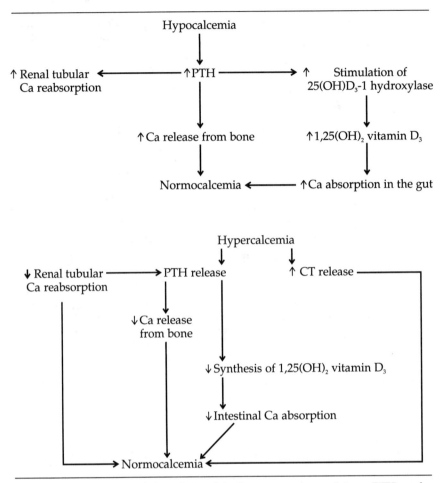

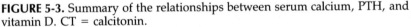

FIGURE 5-3. Summary of the relationships between serum calcium, PTH, and vitamin D. CT = calcitonin.

consecutive elderly patients admitted to our hospital for a variety of reasons in whom a serum calcium determination was done.

ETIOLOGY

The most common causes of hypercalcemia in the elderly are similar to those noted in younger age groups, with primary hyperparathyroidism, malignancy, and drug toxicity (thiazides, D vitamin) accounting for well over 80 percent of the cases. Other etiologies include increased production or sensitivity to $1,25(OH)_2D_3$, benign familial hypercalcemia, adrenal insufficiency, hyperthyroidism, and patients in the recovery phase of acute renal failure secondary to rhabdomyolysis.

TABLE 5-1. Clinical manifestations
reported in association with hypercalcemia

Central nervous system (very common in the elderly)
  Headache
  Impaired concentration
  Memory defects
  Personality changes
  Confusion
  Lethargy
Renal
  Polyuria
  Nephrocalcinosis
  Acute or chronic renal failure
Gastrointestinal
  Anorexia, nausea
  Changes in bowel motility: constipation
  Pancreatitis
Cardiovascular
  Cardiac arrhythmias, heart block
  Hypertension
  Vascular calcification
Musculoskeletal
  Muscle weakness
  Acute arthritis, arthralgia
Ocular
  Conjunctival calcification
  Band keratopathy

CLINICAL MANIFESTATIONS AND PATHOGENESIS

Since calcium plays an important role in the metabolism of every cell, it is not surprising that symptoms produced by hypercalcemia are related to practically every organ. Some of the common symptoms are outlined in Table 5-1. These symptoms can occur in any combination with no specific pattern for a specific etiology. In general, the severity of symptoms is proportionate to the level and rate of rise of the serum calcium.

Primary Hyperparathyroidism

Primary hyperparathyroidism is the single most common cause of hypercalcemia in the elderly. The incidence increases steadily with age, reaching 92 per year per 100,000 elderly males and 188 per year per 100,000 elderly females over the age of 60 in Rochester, Minn. (Fig. 5-4) [48]. An even higher incidence of 250 per year per 100,000 for women over 65 was found by Marx [49]. As noted, the disease is more common in females, with a 7:3 female-to-male ratio. The estimated prevalence has been placed between 1 and 10 percent in one study involving a rela-

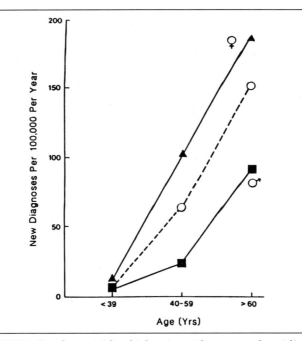

FIGURE 5-4. Incidence with which primary hyperparathyroidism is discovered in subjects of various ages in Rochester, Minnesota. The disease is very rare in subjects below age 40 but grows increasingly common thereafter. Dashed line equals average incidence. (From Mallette LE: Review: Primary hyperparathyroidism, an update: Incidence, etiology, diagnosis and treatment. *Am J Med Sci* 293:239–249, 1987.)

tively small number of elderly males in the United States [50]. Evaluating a larger number of patients, Tibblin and colleagues [51] found a prevalence of 1.5 percent in Sweden. A single adenoma was responsible for hyperparathyroidism in approximately 90 percent of the elderly; multiple adenomas were rarely found [52]. Hyperplasia accounts for the remaining 10 percent. Hyperparathyroidism associated with one of the multiple endocrine neoplasias is usually diagnosed at a younger age.

Carcinoma of the parathyroids can also be associated with an elevated parathyroid hormone level and hypercalcemia. It is not clear how often this entity occurs in the elderly. In two reviews comprising a total of 66 patients reported prior to 1970, only two patients (3 percent) were over the age of 60 [53, 54]. In a more recent review, 14 of 62 patients (23 percent) were elderly [55]. This trend might be due to the greater number of elderly patients with hypercalcemia undergoing extensive clinical evaluation and surgery rather than a true change in incidence.

The etiology of parathyroid adenomas is not known, but it is clear that changes in serum calcium can still influence PTH secretion in most patients, except that the calcium inhibitory set point, defined as the calcium level required to inhibit 50 percent of PTH release, is shifted toward higher calcium values [56, 57]. A lack of complete maximum suppressibility can, however, be found in some adenomas. It has also been shown that the abnormal control of PTH secretion may be related to alterations in calcium transport across the plasma membrane of adenomatous cells [58], perhaps as a consequence of decreased sensitivity of the parathyroid cell receptor to extracellular calcium [59, 60]. Once the new set point is achieved in the individual patient, there is then a higher blood-bone calcium equilibrium [61].

For most patients with primary hyperparathyroidism bone volume is maintained, since the high bone turnover rate results from a parallel increase in both osteoclastic and osteoblastic activity [62]. Calcium losses from bone, therefore, play a relatively minor role in the hypercalcemia of hyperparathyroidism. Rather, the hypercalcemia is maintained primarily by an increase in gut absorption and renal distal tubular reabsorption of calcium. In a small number of patients the hypercalcemia may be due to an alteration in the balance between osteoclastic and osteoblastic activity, which also results in overt bone disease (osteitis fibrosa cystica or bone fractures). Interestingly enough, the plasma $1,25(OH)_2D_3$ level and creatinine clearance have been found to be significantly lower in this group compared to the group in "equilibrium" [35].

The clinical manifestations associated with primary hyperparathyroidism do not differ in the elderly from those found in younger patients. The frequency with which they occur in each group varies somewhat, however. As seen in Table 5-2, neuromuscular complaints (changes in mentation, muscle weakness, asthenia, and fatigue) constitute the most common clinical manifestation of hyperparathyroidism in the elderly, occurring in 29 percent compared to 16 percent in younger patients, in whom renal problems predominate [51, 63, 64]. The prevalance of hyperparathyroidism in a psychogeriatric clinic was found to be approximately 5 percent, mainly among those with newly diagnosed organic brain syndrome [65]. The reason for the increased incidence of central nervous dysfunction, which does not necessarily relate to the severity of the hypercalcemia [66], in the elderly is not clear but may reflect the presence of an already compromised blood supply in the aged. Physical examination in patients complaining of weakness and easy fatigability may demonstrate proximal muscle weakness, more common in the lower extremities. Muscle atrophy, hyperactive deep tendon reflexes, and tongue fasciculations have been reported. A neck mass may be palpable, particularly if carcinoma is present. Serum aspartate aminotransferase

TABLE 5-2. Presenting symptoms in surgically
verified hyperparathyroidism at different ages

Symptoms and signs	<60 Years of age (%) (n = 74)	>60 Years of age (%) (n = 112)	≥70 Years of age (%) (n = 61)
Neuromuscular	16	31	44
Renal	41	19	10
Hypercalcemic crisis	4	4	3
Gastrointestinal	1	1	2
Skeletal abnormalities	2	1	—
Miscellaneous	3	—	2
Incidental finding of elevated serum Ca	31	42	39

SOURCE: Tibblin S, Palsson N, and Rydberg J: Hyperparathyroidism in the elderly. *Ann Surg* 197:135–138, 1983.

(AST), creatinine phosphokinase (CPK), and aldolase levels are, in general, within the normal range [67].

Nephrolithiasis and renal insufficiency (due to nephrocalcinosis or dehydration) are the most common renal manifestations of hyperparathyroidism. Patients with a marked elevation of $1,25(OH)_2D_3$, hypercalciuria, and intestinal hyperabsorption when submitted to a 1,000 mg calcium load, are more prone to these renal complications [68]. The incidence of nephrocalcinosis and nephrolithiasis is lower in the elderly hyperparathyroid patient compared to younger patients and may be explained by the decreased filtered load of calcium due to a decrease in glomerular filtration rate (GFR) and decreased levels of $1,25(OH)_2D_3$. It should be noted, however, that the metabolic profile alone does not always distinguish stone-forming from nonstone-forming patients with primary hyperparathyroidism [69]. Therefore, other still unidentified factors are probably playing a role.

As can be seen in Figure 5-5, hypertension is more common in the elderly with primary hyperparathyroidism than in younger patients when compared with an age-matched control group [70]. The hypertension may be corrected after parathyroidectomy [71]. The mechanisms by which an elevated PTH level and hypercalcemia raise the blood pressure have not been studied in great detail [72]. Plasma renin and aldosterone are usually in the normal range [73, 74]. Plasma catecholamine levels can be either normal [73] or elevated [75]; however, hypertensive hyperparathyroid patients have a more marked response to norepinephrine infusion compared to controls [75]. Other investigators [76] have found an inverse relationship between blood pressure and serum phosphate level.

Gastrointestinal complaints (peptic ulcer, gastritis, chronic constipation) may be the initial problem that brings the patient to medical atten-

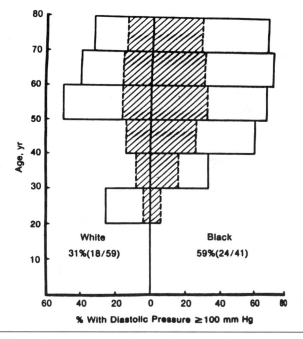

FIGURE 5-5. Percentage of patients with proved hyperparathyroidism for each decade of life. Those with diastolic pressures of 95 mm Hg or more reported by Stamler et al are shown in cross-hatched areas. (From Lafferty FW: Primary hyperparathyroidism: Changing clinical spectrum, prevalence of hypertension and discriminant analysis of laboratory tests. *Arch Intern Med* 141:1761–1766, 1981. By permission of the American Medical Association.)

tion. These symptoms most likely reflect the effect of calcium on stomach acid secretion and on smooth muscle contractility.

Hypercalcemic crisis occurs in the elderly (usually in those with some degree of pre-existing mild renal insufficiency) who develop a rapid rise in serum calcium, occasionally as high as 20 mg per dl [77–79]. Volume contraction, due either to poor intake due to intercurrent illness (e.g., infection) or to increased losses (diarrhea, diuretics, urine concentrating defect), constitutes the triggering factor in the majority of cases. Such patients have central nervous system symptoms including confusion, stupor, and unresponsiveness. These symptoms, although reversible with volume expansion, tend to persist beyond the fall in serum calcium. PTH levels are usually very high (20-fold increase) in these patients.

The diagnosis of primary hyperparathyroidism should be confirmed by the measurement of PTH by immunoassay. One of the major problems encountered in the past had to do with wide interassay variations

[80], forcing clinicians to develop several kinds of discriminant analyses using parameters such as serum calcium, phosphorus, chloride, and albumin to improve diagnostic accuracy in patients in whom primary hyperparathyroidism was suspected [70, 81]. Fortunately, in most recent analyses comparing several commercially available PTH assays, degrees of sensitivity and specificity of 93 to 100 percent have been found in different laboratories using the midregion and C-terminal assays [82, 83]. It is, therefore, recommended that the clinician become familiar with the degree of sensitivity and specificity of the assay being performed by a given laboratory. The midregion assay measures biologically inactive fragments secreted by the parathyroids and those formed catabolically in the liver from the whole PTH molecule, in addition to the biologically active hormone [84]. Since both fragments are normally cleared by the kidney and begin to accumulate when creatinine clearance falls below 40 ml per minute, falsely high values will occur in patients with renal insufficiency. As a general rule, in patients with serum creatinine between 2 and 5 mg per dl and nonparathyroid hypercalcemia, the PTH increase tends to be less than fourfold, whereas in those with primary hyperparathyroidism the increase is significantly greater. Patients with more severe kidney disease (creatinine greater than 5 mg per dl) and hypercalcemia due to "tertiary" hyperparathyroidism may have a 600-fold increase, whereas in similar patients with hypercalcemia due to a nonparathyroid cause, a more moderate increase is usually found (2- to 20-fold).

In a small number of patients with hypercalcemia (5 to 7 percent) the PTH value is normal despite the presence of hyperparathyroidism. In this situation it may be helpful to measure urinary cyclic AMP (expressed as a function of GFR, as long as the latter is above 25 ml per minute), which is elevated in patients with primary hyperparathyroidism [85]. Unfortunately, high levels may also be found in patients with hypercalcemia of malignancy or sarcoidosis, decreasing its diagnostic value substantially [86, 87]. Other approaches include a variety of noninvasive methods for gland localization such as high-resolution real-time ultrasonography. This imaging technique can detect abnormal glands in 78 to 86 percent of cases [88, 89]. There is a 4 to 9 percent false-positive and a 6 to 11 percent false-negative rate. Tumors less than 1 mm in size and those located intrathoracically are usually not detected with this technique. Computed tomography (CT) scanning can identify normal parathyroid glands in 19 to 80 percent of patients. It is particularly helpful for identifying ectopically sited glands. It has a false-positive rate of 14 percent and a false-negative rate of 44 percent [90–92]. The accuracy for both studies combined (ultrasonography and CT) is estimated to be 91 percent [93].

Double tracer subtraction imaging using technetium-99m pertechnetate and thallium chloride-201 has been found to be quite sensitive in detecting single parathyroid adenomas larger than 5 mm in diameter [94]. Its value is somewhat limited in patients with hyperplasia and in those with tumors located low in the mediastinum. The technique can also be of help in locating glands in patients requiring re-exploration of the neck [95].

Magnetic resonance imaging has also been used. False positives (18 percent) do occur, and one major drawback with this technique is its limited availability [96]. This diagnostic procedure, however, might turn out to be the best available for detecting parathyroid glands in patients with recurring disease [97].

Primary hyperparathyroidism and nonparathyroid malignancy may be simultaneously present in an elderly patient with hypercalcemia [98, 99]. If such a patient has superimposed renal insufficiency (as is commonly the case), reaching a definitive diagnosis presents some difficulty. Ljunghall et al [100, 101] attempted to differentiate between these two possibilities by measuring serum calcium and PTH prior to and approximately 8 hours after a single intramuscular injection of 100 IU calcitonin. This dose of calcitonin is usually associated with a 3 to 5 percent drop in serum calcium. This change in serum calcium results in a 10 percent or greater rise in serum PTH in patients with hyperparathyroidism (positive response). No significant change in PTH is seen in patients with nonparathyroid hypercalcemia (negative response). A negative response, however, does not necessarily rule out hyperparathyroidism [102]. Furthermore, the diagnostic value of this test in the patient with hypercalcemia and advanced renal insufficiency (serum creatinine > 5 mg per dl) remains to be determined. In these patients a careful interpretation of all the tests described earlier will be necessary [103].

"NORMOCALCEMIC" HYPERPARATHYROIDISM. A small number of elderly patients have persistently normal to high-normal serum calcium levels despite the presence of hyperparathyroidism. The diagnosis of hyperparathyroidism is usually uncovered in these patients during the investigation for hypophosphatemia. In such patients, the PTH is elevated, and the tubular reabsorption of phosphorus is low. $1,25(OH)_2D_3$ is usually normal, as is the urinary calcium excretion. A resistance to the PTH effect on tubular calcium reabsorption has been postulated as a probable mechanism for the normocalcemia [104].

Malignancy
Malignancy is the most common cause of hypercalcemia in the hospitalized elderly, and both our own experience and the literature suggest that it occurs in 8.5 to 10 percent of adult patients with cancer [105, 106]. The pathogenesis of hypercalcemia in malignancy may differ depending

TABLE 5-3. Hypercalcemia associated with metastatic carcinoma

Primary tumor site	No. patients (%)	Patients with known metastatic disease at diagnosis of hypercalcemia (%)
Lungs	11 (29.7)	8 (72.7)
Breasts	8 (21.6)	7 (87.5)
Head/neck	6 (16.2)	4 (66.7)
Kidney	5 (13.5)	5 (100.0)
Others	7 (19.0)	4 (57.1)
(Thyroid, 2)		
(Colon, 2)		
(Genitalia, 3)		

SOURCE: Adapted from Ray AK and Rao DB: Hypercalcemia and malignant disease in the elderly: Magnesium sulfate therapy. *J Am Geriatr Soc* 22:413–415, 1974; and our own experience.

on the type of tumor. Mundy and Martin [107] have described three tumor categories: (1) solid tumors with metastasis (most common); (2) solid tumors without metastasis (least common); and (3) hematologic malignancies.

SOLID TUMORS WITH METASTASIS. The type of tumor associated with hypercalcemia due primarily to metastases in the elderly is summarized in Table 5-3, which is derived from our own experience combined with that of Ray and Rao [108]. Approximately three-quarters of these patients were known to have bone metastases when hypercalcemia was first noted; however, it should be emphasized that the presence of bone metastases does not necessarily imply a causal relationship between the metastases and the hypercalcemia, since only a small percentage (less than 30 percent) of patients with bone metastases develop hypercalcemia [109]. Furthermore, an inverse rather than a direct correlation has been found in one study between the number of bone metastases and serum calcium levels in patients with cancer-related hypercalcemia [110]. Hypercalcemia in this group is primarily the result of increased bone resorption by the tumor through one or more of the following mechanisms: (1) pressure atrophy with subsequent infarction of surrounding bone and calcium release into the extracellular fluid [109]; (2) release of proteolytic enzymes [111]; (3) stimulation of osteoclastic activity by tumor-produced prostaglandins or other factors such as osteoclastic-activating factor from tumor-derived activated lymphocytes [112].

In 70 percent of the patients we examined, a decrease in GFR was present. The low GFR may contribute to the hypercalcemia by decreasing the filtered calcium load. In the majority of patients, volume contrac-

tion due to poor oral intake and the polyuria that frequently
accompanies hypercalcemia [113] were responsible for the decrease in
GFR, since the BUN and serum creatinine returned to normal after volume expansion and lowering of the serum calcium. Figure 5-6 diagrams
the many ways by which hypercalcemia can alter the renal concentrating
mechanism. In the remaining patients, renal insufficiency was secondary either to a direct effect of the elevated calcium on the glomerulus
[114], obstructive uropathy, or acute tubular necrosis. PTH, nephrogenic

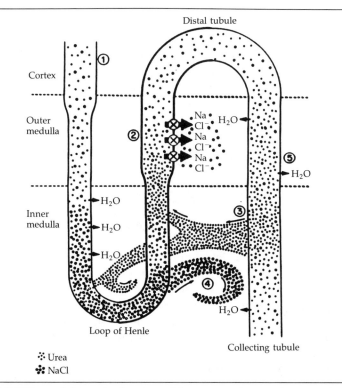

FIGURE 5-6. Schematic drawing of the potential sites of action of
calcium that alter function of the renal concentrating mechanism.
Site 1 = delivery of water and solute to the medulla; site 2 = active
sodium chloride transport across the thick ascending limb of Henle;
site 3 = urea transport across the medullary collecting duct; site
4 = sodium chloride abstraction across the thin ascending limb of
Henle; site 5 = hydro-osmotic transfer of water across collecting
duct epithelium under the influence of antidiuretic hormone
(ADH). (From Goldfarb S and Agus ZS: Mechanism of the polyuria
of hypercalcemia. *Am J Nephrol* 4:69–76, 1984; and modified from
Kokko JP: Renal concentrating and diluting mechanisms. *Hosp Pract*
14:110–116, 1979. By permission of S. Karger AG, Basel.)

cyclic AMP, and $1,25(OH)_2D_3$ are either low or normal in these patients, so that increased renal or intestinal absorption of calcium does not contribute to the hypercalcemia [115].

SOLID TUMORS WITHOUT METASTASES. Table 5-4 summarizes the types of tumors and their relative distribution in 76 elderly hypercalcemic subjects with solid tumors without metastases, also called "humoral hypercalcemia" [116]. Increased bone resorption resulting in skeletal calcium loss through humoral mediators synthesized by the malignant cell is primarily responsible for the hypercalcemia [62]. In some patients, besides volume contraction and a direct lowering effect of growth factors on the GFR [117, 118], there may also be an increase in tubular calcium reabsorption [119, 120]. Both the site and the mechanism of this increased reabsorption remain to be elucidated. Gut calcium absorption is decreased in this group [121, 122]. The specific humoral mediators involved in producing this type of hypercalcemia are described in Table 5-5 [123] and include tranforming growth factors that can stimulate osteoclastic bone resorption and a PTH-related factor. The latter is a protein with a significant sequence homology in the NH_2-terminal region of PTH that has recently been isolated [124, 125] and has been found to be elevated in 55 percent of hypercalcemic patients with an associated malignancy [126]. This protein has been shown to enhance osteoclastic bone resorption in vitro, and its hypercalcemic effect can be averted by using an antisera capable of neutralizing its activity [127]. Concurrent other factors present in the cancer patient such as tumor growth factor alpha, interleukin-1, and tumor necrosis factor most likely play a modifying role as far as the hypercalcemic response to this PTH-related factor is concerned [128].

Multiple myeloma is responsible for most cases of hypercalcemia associated with hematologic malignancies. These patients have increased bone resorption, the result of locally produced cytokines (lymphotoxin) secreted by the malignant cells [129]. Other bone-resorbing factors such as interleukin-1 found in monocytic malignancy [130] and $1,25(OH)_2D_3$ have been reported in some patients with lymphomas [131, 132] (see Table 5-5). In addition to the release of Ca from bone in patients with multiple myeloma, hypercalcemia is frequently augmented by the presence of a decreased GFR [133]. Several factors may be responsible for the renal insufficiency associated with multiple myeloma: (1) direct effects of the tumor including myeloma kidney, amyloidosis, light chain nephropathy, and hyperviscosity; (2) nephrotoxicity due to antibiotic treatment or radiographic contrast media; (3) hypercalcemia and hyperuricemia (rare); (4) severe volume contraction; and (5) sepsis.

In addition to the clinical manifestations of hypercalcemia described earlier, in patients with hypercalcemia and bone involvement, bone pain

TABLE 5-4. Humoral hypercalcemia

Primary tumor site	No. patients (%)
Lungs	22 (28.9)
Kidneys	15 (19.7)
Urogenital	15 (19.7)
Gastrointestinal (including liver)	15 (19.7)
Breasts	7 (9.2)
Head/neck	2 (2.8)
Total	76 (100)

SOURCE: Skrabanck P, McPartlin J, and Powell D: Tumor hypercalcemia and "ectopic hyperparathyroidism." *Medicine* 59:262–282, 1980. Copyright Williams & Wilkins.

(due to direct bone lysis or pathologic fracture) may be the primary reason a patient seeks medical attention. Finally, other potentially reversible causes of hypercalcemia must also be considered when evaluating patients with hypercalcemia.

Thiazides

In our experience, thiazide diuretics constitute the most common cause of drug-induced hypercalcemia. In a minority of patients the increase is mild (serum calcium 10.5–10.8 mg per dl), and since the ionized calcium is normal, the hypercalcemia represents an increase in the fraction bound to the elevated serum albumin secondary to volume contraction. In most patients, however, the ionized calcium is increased [134]. Since the normal negative correlation between ionized calcium and PTH is well maintained, the drug appears to exert its effect directly on calcium metabolism. Indeed, thiazides enhance distal tubular calcium reabsorption [135], but this effect is not essential for the development of hypercalcemia in patients with end-stage renal disease [136]. It has been shown that thiazides directly stimulate calcium release from bone [137].

Patients with thiazide-induced hypercalcemia are usually elderly asymptomatic females taking the drug for hypertension. The hypercalcemia may be seen early or up to 15 years after the institution of therapy. Since this complication occurs most frequently in elderly women, at an age when primary hyperparathyroidism is also most prevalent, this entity should be ruled out, particularly if hypercalcemia persists despite discontinuing the diuretic [138].

Excess of vitamins A and D can produce hypercalcemia. It is not clear how often hypercalcemia due to vitamin A intoxication occurs in the elderly. In general, reported patients have been younger [139]. The diagnosis can be confirmed by the history and measurement of the serum vitamin A level. In recent years many elderly people add calcium or vi-

TABLE 5-5. Pathogenetic classification of the hypercalcemia of cancer

Clinical group	Types of tumors	Bone histologic studies	Bone studies	Radiologic features	Other factors implicated	Local or systemic
Hematologic cancers	Myeloma, lymphosarcoma, Burkitt's lymphoma, adult T-cell lymphoma	Increase in osteoclastic bone resorption adjacent to neoplastic cells	Mainly osteolytic lesions; occasionally diffuse osteopenia		Osteoclast-activating factor; 1,25-dihydroxyvitamin D Lymphotoxin*	Local
Solid tumors with bone metastases	Breast, lung, pancreatic	Increase in local osteoclastic bone resorption; variable osteoblastic response	Discrete lytic lesions; variable sclerotic response		Prostaglandins: direct erosion by tumor cells	Local
Solid tumors without metastases	Lung, kidney, pancreatic, ovarian	Increased osteoclastic bone resorption; decreased bone formation	No abnormality	Increase in fractional excretion of phosphate; increase in nephrogenous cyclic AMP; decrease in immunoreactive PTH	1. PTH 2. Prostaglandins 3. Transforming growth factors 4. Factors that interact with PTH† receptor 5. Colony-stimulating activity	Systemic

*Added by authors of this book.

†PTH = parathyroid hormone.

SOURCE: Mundy GR, et al. The hypercalcemia of cancer: Clinical implications and pathogenic mechanisms. *N Engl J Med* 310:1718–1727, 1984. Reprinted with permission.

tamin D supplements to their diet to treat osteoporosis despite the fact that it probably does not help [140] and may even be harmful [141]. Hypercalcemia may develop in patients taking large doses of vitamin D, over 20,000 units per day. A greater than 10-fold increase in $25(OH)D_3$ is seen in these patients; $1,25(OH)_2D_3$ may also be increased. The hypercalcemia probably represents a direct effect of the high levels of $25(OH)D_3$ on $1,25(OH)_2D_3$ receptors [142]. There may be an additional effect of the 1,25 analog itself, when it is elevated.

Hypercalcemia Due to Increased Production or Sensitivity to $1,25(OH)_2D_3$

This group comprises patients with granulomatous disorders such as sarcoidosis, tuberculosis, fungal diseases, leprosy, and berylliosis. Clinical manifestations are usually those of the underlying disease, but an occasional patient presents with urolithiasis secondary to hypercalciuria (particularly with sarcoidosis). $1,25(OH)_2D_3$ has been found to be increased in these hypercalcemic patients, most likely as a consequence of increased hydroxylation of available $25(OH)D_3$ by 1-alpha-hydroxylase produced by the granulomatous macrophages [143]. An increase in both bone resorption and intestinal calcium absorption due to elevated $1,25(OH)_2D_3$ is probably responsible for the hypercalcemia [144].

Benign Familial Hypercalcemia

A small number of patients (7 to 10 percent) with benign familial hypercalcemia are 60 years or older at the time hypercalcemia is discovered [145]. Complaints similar to those found in patients with hyperparathyroidism such as fatigue, weakness, and mental changes are more frequently reported in this group. Chondrocalcinosis is common. A positive family history, a tendency toward hypermagnesemia, hypocalciuria (calcium-creatinine clearance ratio < 0.018), and an absence of parathyroid gland enlargement on high-resolution parathyroid ultrasonography and other imaging techniques helps to differentiate this syndrome from hyperparathyroidism [146, 147]. Since the pattern of dysfunction in familial hypercalcemia suggests an insensitivity to extracellular calcium by both the kidney tubules and the parathyroid cells, diffuse hyperplasia of the parathyroid glands with elevated PTH levels may be seen in some patients [148]. The hypercalcemia in patients with this syndrome persists despite parathyroid surgery.

Other Causes of Hypercalcemia

Hypercalcemia may be seen in association with pheochromocytoma (due to parathyroid hyperplasia), or it may be present as part of the multiple endocrine neoplasia syndromes, which, as noted earlier, are rarely initially diagnosed in the elderly. In patients with adrenal insufficiency, hypercalcemia is not uncommon and is, for the most part, secondary to hemoconcentration. The hypercalcemia seen with hyperthyroidism is generally mild. It results from a direct effect of thyroid hormone on bone mobilization. Serum PTH and $1,25(OH)_2D_3$ are suppressed, and serum phosphate is elevated [149]. The urinary excretion of hydroxyproline and calcium is increased [150].

TREATMENT OF HYPERCALCEMIA IN THE ELDERLY
The therapy of hypercalcemia can be divided into two stages: emergency therapy and specific therapy.

Emergency Therapy
Since in general no correlation exists between the severity of the symptomatology and the level of hypercalcemia, every symptomatic patient, regardless of the calcium level, and any patient with a serum calcium level greater than 13 mg per dl should receive emergency treatment.

FLUIDS. As noted earlier, patients with hypercalcemia very often have a poor fluid intake, which, when associated with a urinary concentration defect, is a perfect set-up for profound dehydration. We usually start fluid replacement with an infusion of normal saline, 200 ml per hour, with constant monitoring of urinary output, particularly in patients with an elevated serum creatinine. Naturally, signs of fluid overload should be looked for. Since calcium reabsorption in the proximal tubule is significantly linked to sodium reabsorption, the natriuresis accompanying volume expansion will also induce a calciuresis. Attention should be paid to the loss of other electrolytes such as magnesium (Mg) and potassium (K).

LOOP DIURETICS. Intravenous furosemide (100 mg every 2 hours) has been used with volume expansion to treat hypercalcemia [151]. By abolishing the lumen-positive charge in the thick ascending limb, furosemide indirectly interferes with calcium reabsorption, which potentiates the effect of saline expansion [152]. This combination requires even more careful fluid monitoring, since larger urinary losses than those accompanying saline expansion alone must be replaced.

CALCITONIN. This agent lowers the serum calcium by inhibiting bone resorption and decreasing renal tubular reabsorption [153]. The resulting hypercalciuria can occur as early as 30 minutes after administration of the drug and lasts up to 3 hours [154]. The exact tubular site of action has not yet been identified. Calcitonin can be used either intramuscularly or intravenously at 4 to 8 IU per kg per day, administered every 12 hours. A decrease in serum calcium is usually noted within 6 to 8 hours. Bone resorption can be inhibited for up to 72 hours by calcitonin but returns to pretreatment status despite continuous administration of the drug because of down-regulation of calcitonin receptors on bone cells [155]. This "escape" phenomenon can be delayed by concomitant administration of the equivalent of 100 mg of hydrocortisone every 6 hours, with gradual tapering [156]. The mechanism of action of glucocorticoids in lowering serum calcium is not well understood [157].

ETIDRONATE DISODIUM. This drug and other diphosphonates act by decreasing bone resorption, the exact mechanism for which is not known. The number of osteoclasts found in active bone turnover sites decreases substantially after administration of the drug, which is administered intravenously at a dose of 7.5 mg per kg of body weight [158]. It is recommended that the drug be diluted in 250 ml of normal saline and administered over a minimum of 2 hours daily for 3 to 5 days [159]. Etidronate disodium is very effective in treating the hypercalcemia of malignancy. Since its excretory route is mainly renal, it should not be used in patients with a serum creatinine above 3 mg per dl.

MITHRAMYCIN. This drug is not recommended for the emergency treatment of hypercalcemia because it does not produce a decline in serum calcium for 24 to 36 hours. Moreover, it should not be used in patients with renal insufficiency. This drug acts by reducing bone resorption and renal tubular calcium reabsorption [160, 161].

Phosphates and sulfates have also been used in the emergency treatment of hypercalcemia. They are not in wide use in the United States at the present time.

Specific Therapy
After the serum calcium has been lowered quickly, strategies for more chronic or definitive therapy can be planned.

HYPERCALCEMIA OF MALIGNANCY. In addition to administering specific chemotherapeutic agents aimed at controlling the primary tumor, the patient should be encouraged to eat a regular salt diet (unless contraindicated) and to take adequate fluids to maintain adequate hydration. Radiation therapy should be tried if bone pain and localized lesions are present. Several oral agents that lower serum calcium are available and can be added to the patient's therapeutic regimen if necessary. Oral phosphate, 1 to 3 g daily in three divided doses, can be prescribed for patients with normal kidney function. Magnesium sulfate, 15 g twice a day, has proved effective in one study involving a small number of elderly patients. Diarrhea is the most common side effect. The serum Mg level should be monitored in patients with renal insufficiency [108].

Prednisone, 20 to 40 mg per day, is helpful in patients with hypercalcemia associated with lymphoproliferative disorders (myeloma, lymphomas producing 1,25[OH]$_2$D$_3$). Etidronate disodium, 20 mg per kg per day, by mouth is also available; long-term studies of its efficacy are, however, lacking [162, 163].

HYPERCALCEMIA OF HYPERPARATHYROIDISM. The surgical excision of the adenomatous gland constitutes the approach of choice for the treatment of hyperparathyroidism, with normocalcemia achieved in over 90 percent of patients. Persistent hypercalcemia in the remaining patients can be attributed to an inexperienced surgeon, abnormal localization of the tumor, or multiglandular disease [164]. Patients who remain hypercalcemic require further localization studies prior to re-exploration of the neck. Besides the noninvasive procedures described earlier, selective angiography with venous sampling for parathyroid hormone is available and has a high yield of positive results. It is our belief that this procedure should be performed only in experienced centers [90, 96]. In patients with multiple hyperplastic glands, an intraoperative decrease of urinary cyclic AMP to normal has been shown to be helpful in determining the amount of parathyroid tissue to be removed [165]. Postoperative hypocalcemia is the most commonly encountered problem. Its duration depends primarily on the extent of bone disease present at the time. This transient complication can be corrected early with intravenous administration of calcium and regular monitoring of serum calcium. The addition of oral 1,25(OH)$_2$D$_3$ probably does not shorten the time required to correct the hypocalcemia [166].

In 7 percent of patients, hypertension persists after surgery [167]. In 14 percent of those with pre-existing renal insufficiency, kidney function may actually become worse. In the remaining 86 percent GFR either remains stable or improves [167]. The rate of stone formation has been found to decrease from 0.36 before to 0.02 per patient per year after surgery [168].

Carcinoma is found in a small number of elderly patients with primary hyperparathyroidism. Evidence of local invasion of contiguous structures such as the thyroid, neck muscles, or esophagus is usually present. The characteristic histopathologic picture is that of fibrous trabeculae, mitotic figures, and capsular or vascular invasion. More than 5 years of disease-free survival following surgery for parathyroid carcinoma is possible in 30 percent of elderly patients. Local recurrence or distant metastases (liver, lung, bone) occurs in the remaining 70 percent [53–55, 169, 170].

Although most clinicians agree that the presence of complications related to the hypercalcemic state such as urolithiasis, nephrocalcinosis, bone disease (osteopenia, osteitis fibrosa), peptic ulcer disease, or a serum Ca greater than 11 mg per dl is an indication for surgery, controversy exists about the best way of approaching the patient with mild asymptomatic hypercalcemia (serum calcium less than 11 mg per dl) or normocalcemia [171–178]. No specific criteria are available to predict which asymptomatic patient will subsequently develop complications. Our approach is based on the following factors: (1) 30 to 40 percent of patients observed over a long period of time will develop complications related to the hypercalcemic state with no criteria to predict which ones [173, 179]; (2) parathyroid surgery in the elderly performed by an experienced surgeon has a low morbidity and mortality similar to that found in younger patients and is also curative in a very high proportion of cases [63, 180–183]; and (3) there is a high prevalence of metabolic bone disease (osteoporosis) as well as a risk that PTH will accelerate the rate of loss of appendicular bone in elderly women [184–186]. Therefore, we generally recommend surgery for all of our elderly patients with an established diagnosis of primary hyperparathyroidism unless other serious diseases (unrelated malignancy, advanced cardiovascular disease) associated with a limited life expectancy exist [187]. Patients who refuse or are judged unsuitable candidates for surgery should be followed closely. A significant number of these patients will have a relatively benign long-term course [188]. For those who have or develop symptoms or complications of the disease, medical therapy, at best inadequate and potentially dangerous, can be offered [189, 190].

In the elderly hyperparathyroid woman, conjugated estrogens (0.625 to 2.6 mg per day) can be used. These drugs lower the serum calcium by acting directly on bone resorption through receptors located on the osteoblasts and on the parathyroid glands, reducing their response to a hypocalcemic stimulus [191]. Serum concentrations of calcitonin and free $1,25(OH)_2D_3$ are not affected by this treatment [192, 193]. Patients with an intact uterus should, in addition to the estrogen, receive medroxyprogesterone acetate, 10 mg per day for 7 to 10 days every 2 to 3 months, and should undergo regular gynecologic follow-up [194]. Instead of the combination therapy referred to above, good results can be obtained by using norethindrone, 5 mg per day [193, 195]. This drug may be preferable in the elderly because it has the added advantage of not producing undesirable effects on the uterus or blood clotting. Since both estradiol and progesterone can stimulate PTH release, such therapy has the potential to worsen the bone disease over the long term [196].

For males and females who are inoperable and fail to respond to either the estrogen and intermittent progesterone combination or norethindrone, the equivalent of 1,500 mg of elemental phosphorus given in four divided doses should be tried [197]. The serum calcium, fasting Ca excretion, and urinary hydroxyproline may decrease with this therapy, whereas PTH either increases or remains unchanged. Since approximately 65 percent of the administered phosphorus is reabsorbed, this form of therapy is probably not safe in patients with pre-existing renal insufficiency or in those with a serum calcium above 11.5 mg per dl.

Oral diphosphonates represent another alternative to controlling hypercalcemia in hyperparathyroidism. Further studies are required to confirm their long-term benefits [198]. Gallium nitrate has been found to lower serum calcium in patients with refractory hypercalcemia of parathyroid carcinoma [199]. This drug acts by antagonizing the effect of PTH on bone resorptive activity. WR-2721 is an experimental drug that is being used to protect normal tissues against the toxic effects of radiation and chemotherapy. One of the side effects of the drug is hypocalcemia, which appears to be secondary to the inhibition of parathyroid hormone secretion [200]. This agent may ultimately become useful in the management of parathyroid disease.

OTHER. Drug-induced hypercalcemia is best managed by discontinuing the offending agent. Short-term corticosteroid therapy may hasten recovery in patients with vitamin D intoxication. In hypercalcemia-associated tuberculosis and fungal infections or endocrinopathies, adequate therapy of the underlying disease is usually curative. Prednisone (40–60 mg with subsequent tapering) is used in patients with sarcoidosis. The hypercalcemia of benign familial hypercalcemia can be managed conservatively because complications related to the elevated calcium per se are rare.

HYPOCALCEMIA

INCIDENCE AND PREVALENCE
In 485 consecutive patients admitted to a geriatric unit for long-term care, Sorva and Tilvis [47] found hypocalcemia (serum calcium less than 8.5 mg per dl) in 10 (2 percent), which is similar to the 2.8 percent rate seen in the elderly at our own institution.

ETIOLOGY
Patients with chronic renal insufficiency or hypoalbuminemia comprise more than 60 percent of the cases of hypocalcemia seen in our elderly hospital population. Other causes, in decreasing order of frequency, include hypomagnesemia, acute pancreatitis, hypoparathyroidism, malabsorption syndrome, acute renal failure, alkalosis, and osteoblastic metastatic malignancy.

CLINICAL MANIFESTATIONS AND PATHOGENESIS
In most patients, the clinical manifestations are usually those of the underlying disease rather than of hypocalcemia per se. Nevertheless,

hypocalcemia may be associated with a variety of neurologic or neuro-muscular disturbances including apprehension, depression, irritability, anxiety, paresthesias of the hands and feet, increased muscle irritability, carpopedal and laryngeal spasm, and tetany. In addition, patients may have nonspecific gastrointestinal complaints or abdominal pain.

Hypocalcemia of Chronic Renal Insufficiency
See Chap. 11 on chronic renal insufficiency.

Hypocalcemia of Hypoalbuminemia
Since the calcium measured in most hospital and commercial laborato-ries is the total calcium, including that portion bound to albumin, hypocalcemia is often seen with hypoalbuminemia. In general, the lower the serum albumin, the lower the serum calcium. Ionized calcium, the physiologically important fraction, is usually normal in such pa-tients, and the hypocalcemia is usually asymptomatic. In some patients, however, the ionized fraction is also low. Such patients usually are acutely ill with sepsis and various other complications [201]. The hypo-calcemia in this setting is multifactorial and results from parathyroid in-sufficiency, renal 1-alpha-hydroxylase or vitamin D deficiency [202]. Mortality is quite high in this group.

Hypocalcemia of Hypomagnesemia
Hypocalcemia develops when the serum magnesium decreases below 0.3 mmol/liter (0.7 mg per dl). The hypocalcemia reflects an inappropri-ate response of the parathyroid gland to the low calcium level [203] as well as a direct effect of hypomagnesemia on bone metabolism, resulting in a relative reduction of calcium release [204]. In addition, hypomag-nesemia can interfere with the metabolism of vitamin D, since magne-sium is required for its hepatic 25-hydroxylation [205]. Serum phosphate is usually normal. Symptoms and signs of hypocalcemia occur in 30 to 40 percent of these patients.

Hypocalcemia of Acute Pancreatitis
During acute pancreatitis, large amounts of calcium may be deposited in areas of fat necrosis. Those patients in whom hypocalcemia develops have been found to have an inadequate parathyroid hormone response to the hypocalcemia [206]. The serum Mg and albumin should also be measured, particularly in patients with alcohol-induced pancreatitis. Clinical manifestations are those of acute pancreatitis, with a small num-ber of patients showing evidence of increased muscle irritability [207].

Hypocalcemia of Hypoparathyroidism
In 64 percent of elderly patients with hypoparathyroidism, the condition is secondary to surgical removal of the glands during thyroid surgery. In

the remaining 37 percent, no specific reason for the gland's inability to produce enough PTH to maintain normal extracellular calcium is found [208, 209]. Often the patient presents with symptoms related to hypocalcemia, and Trousseau's and Chvostek's signs are elicited on physical examination. In these patients the hypocalcemia is frequently associated with hyperphosphatemia; the 25(OH)D$_3$ level is usually normal, and 1,25(OH)$_2$D$_3$ is low [209].

Hypocalcemia of Malabsorption

In the elderly with malabsorption and related hypocalcemia, the clinical manifestations are those of the underlying gastrointestinal disease. The hypocalcemia is due to a decrease in both calcium and vitamin D absorption. The unabsorbed free fatty acids form insoluble calcium soaps in the intestinal lumen, making less calcium ions available for absorption. Vitamin D, being fat soluble, cannot be absorbed adequately owing to the unavailability of bile salts. Plasma levels of phosphorus and 25(OH)$_2$D$_3$ are decreased. PTH and alkaline phosphatase are increased, and 1,25(OH)$_2$D$_3$ is usually normal. Clinical or radiologic evidence of osteomalacia may be seen in a small number of patients.

Hypocalcemia of Acute Renal Failure

The hypocalcemia of acute renal failure is rarely clinically significant. Its pathogenesis is the same as that of chronic renal insufficiency (see Chap. 11). Hypocalcemia tends to be more severe in acute renal failure accompanying rhabdomyolysis owing to metastatic calcification in the involved muscle and a decrease in the serum concentration of 1,25(OH)$_2$D$_3$ [210].

Hypocalcemia of Alkalosis

Hypocalcemia due to a decrease in the ionized serum calcium fraction, severe enough to cause symptoms, can occur occasionally in the elderly person who is subjected to a rapid rise in blood pH.

Hypocalcemia in Patients with Osteoblastic Metastatic Malignancy

Patients with osteoblastic metastatic tumors from the prostate or breast can occasionally present with hypocalcemia. In addition to bone pain due to extensive metastases, patients may rarely present with manifestations of hypocalcemia [211]. They differ from those with oncogenic osteomalacia (see later section on hypophosphatemia) in that their serum phosphorus level is either normal or elevated. Hypomagnesemia may occasionally be present. An elevated alkaline phosphatase is universally found. This syndrome may represent an inability of PTH (usually elevated) to maintain an adequate serum calcium concentration in response to excessive bone calcium accretion. The role of the various forms of vitamin D or a humoral substance produced by the tumor is unclear and deserves further study [212].

TREATMENT AND PROGNOSIS

Emergency Therapy

The symptomatic patient should receive parenteral therapy in the form of calcium gluconate. It can be used either intermittently or continuously with the dose adjusted according to the clinical response and serum calcium level.

Specific Therapy

Except in patients with hypoparathyroidism, hypocalcemia is the consequence of another disease process. Therefore, the prognosis and treatment are those of the underlying disease. In the hypoparathyroid elderly patient with mild hypocalcemia (Ca 7.5–8.5 mEq per dl), chlorthalidone (50 mg daily), a thiazide diuretic, together with a low-sodium (50–100 mEq per day) diet will raise the total and ionized calcium concentrations [213]. This effect results from a direct action of the drug on calcium release by the bone [137] and a decrease in urinary calcium excretion [135]. In patients with more severe hypocalcemia, oral calcium and vitamin D supplementation will be needed. There are several preparations available, but the authors prefer calcium carbonate because of its high concentration of elemental calcium (40 percent) per tablet. We usually start with 250 mg 3 times a day with meals in order to lower the serum phosphorus as well (which is usually elevated) by binding ingested phosphate and making it unavailable for absorption. Twenty-four-hour urine calcium excretion should be monitored so that hypercalciuria may be detected and corrected to prevent the formation of stones or nephrocalcinosis. The maintenance dose in the elderly is between 500 and 1,000 mg per day. Vitamin D supplementation can be provided either as 1-alpha(OH)D_3 (hytacherol), 0.5–1.0 μg per day, or as 1-alpha 25(OH)$_2$D$_3$ (calcitriol), 0.25–1.0 μg per day. Both act by increasing calcium absorption from the gut, although a direct effect on bone is quite probable. These drugs are, in general, well tolerated and relatively safe. The serum calcium should be monitored regularly during therapy because hypercalcemia is not uncommon with the combination [208, 214].

PHOSPHORUS METABOLISM

NORMAL PHYSIOLOGY

Ninety percent of the total body phosphorus serves as a structural component of bones and teeth. The remaining 10 percent is found intracellularly in soft tissues and in body fluids in the form of organic phosphate compounds that contribute to the formation of phospholipids, nucleic acids, and phosphoprotein macromolecules. The phosphate ion is essential for carbohydrate, lipid, and protein metabolism, serves as a cofactor in a variety of enzyme systems, and plays an important role in acid-base metabolism, both intracellularly and in the blood.

The serum phosphorus concentration is maintained in the range of 2.8 to 4.5 mg per dl, with 90 percent in the free form, complexed with mono- and divalent anions. The remaining 10 percent is protein bound. That serum pool is in dynamic equilibrium with phosphorus entry and exit from the gastrointestinal tract, bone, kidneys, and soft tissue. Two-thirds of the 1,000 to 1,500 mg of daily phosphorus ingested is absorbed in the duodenum and jejunum, a process that is active, sodium dependent, and stimulated by vitamin D. The remaining third is excreted in the stools [215].

Since 90 percent of the serum phosphorus exists in its free form, the kidneys play an important role in phosphorus homeostasis through filtration and reabsorption. Eighty to ninety percent of the filtered load is reabsorbed in the proximal tubule, with the distal convoluted tubule accounting for another 5 to 10 percent. The participation of the cortical collecting tubule and the medullary collecting ducts in phosphorus reabsorption in humans is not clear. Several factors, both intrinsic and extrinsic to the tubules, may modulate the rate of phosphorus reabsorption [216]. The renal tubule has an intrinsic ability to respond to phosphate availability independent of any extrarenal influences. The exact mechanism by which this adaptive phenomenon takes place is not known. Small changes in intracellular phosphate availability may play a role, however [217].

PTH is the most important of the extrinsic factors known to regulate tubular phosphorus transport. It acts by blocking the reabsorption of phosphorus in the proximal tubule as well as in the distal portions of the nephron [218, 219]. It also modulates the phosphaturia seen with volume expansion. If PTH is absent during volume expansion most of the phosphorus that escapes reabsorption in the proximal tubule is reabsorbed in the distal tubule, and only a small amount appears in the urine. On the other hand, in the presence of PTH distal phosphorus reabsorption is decreased, and significant phosphaturia ensues [220]. Other hormones (glucocorticoids, growth hormone, thyrocalcitonin), vitamin D, acid-base balance, and the serum concentration of divalent ions (calcium and magnesium) have also been implicated in the regulation of phosphate balance by the kidneys [216].

Serum phosphorus changes with aging, decreasing in the male and increasing in the female [221]. The decrease in serum phosphorus in the male is associated with a 14 percent drop in total body phosphorus from the third to the sixth decade and a 10 percent drop from the sixth to the seventh decade [222]. In normal individuals the kidney maintains the serum phosphorus concentration at a value close to the tubular phosphorus threshold (called the TmP/GFR*) [224], and therefore the latter also decreases in the male, suggesting a progressive tubular defect in phosphorus reabsorption with age. This defect may be secondary to the increase in PTH that occurs with age or to a decrease in the number or turnover rate of the phospate carriers located in the proximal tubule [225]. Age-related biochemical and biophysical alterations in the luminal brush border membrane have also been reported [226]. The mean TmP/GFR seen in 10 elderly men at our institution was 2.9 ± 0.7 mg per dl (range 2.2–4.0 mg per dl) compared with 3.7 ± 0.6 mg per dl (range 2.5–4.2 mg per dl) in 10 men under 50 years.

In females there is an 18 percent drop in total body phosphate from the third to the fifth decade; however, in contrast to men, serum phosphorus increases by 3 percent from the fifth to the sixth decade and by 9 percent from the sixth to the seventh decade. There is an 8 percent increase from the seventh to the eighth decade [222]. The mechanisms for the decrease in total body phosphorus is not clear, but a positive association has been found with the serum $1,25(OH)_2D_3$ level [227]. As might be expected, the TmP/GFR tends to be higher in the postmenopausal woman (range 2.8–4.5 mg per dl) compared with their younger counterparts (range 2.5–4.2 mg per dl). Plasma phosphorus as well as TmP/GFR may be lowered to the normal male level after administration of estrogen [228]. Therefore, the hypoestrogenemia that accompanies menopause most likely contributes to phosphorus retention [229].

HYPERPHOSPHATEMIA

INCIDENCE AND PREVALENCE
Hyperphosphatemia is found in 3 to 4 percent of elderly patients admitted to our hospital. The incidence in a given general hospital population encompassing all age groups is 2.8 percent [230].

ETIOLOGY
Renal insufficiency, both acute and chronic, is responsible for most (50 percent) cases of hyperphosphatemia in the elderly. Other less common

---

*TmP/GFR expresses phosphorus reabsorption as a function of both serum phosphorus concentration and glomerular filtration. It is the best index of renal tubular phosphorus reabsorption as long as GFR is above 40 ml per minute. A nomogram is available that allows calculation of the TmP/GFR from the simultaneous determination of creatinine and phosphorus concentrations in both serum and urine [223].

causes, in decreasing frequency, include pseudohyperphosphatemia, hypoparathyroidism, neoplastic diseases, and phosphate-containing enemas.

CLINICAL MANIFESTATIONS AND PATHOGENESIS
The clinical manifestations associated with hyperphosphatemia are generally those of the underlying disease processes.

Acute and Chronic Renal Failure
See Chapters 10 and 11.

Pseudohyperphosphatemia
This diagnosis should be suspected in any elderly patient who is otherwise well but presents with hyperphosphatemia (range 10–20 mg per dl) and normal serum calcium and kidney function (creatinine ≤ 1.5 mg per dl). Two processes may be responsible for the hyperphosphatemia. The first is hemolysis, in which intracellular phosphate is released from destroyed red cells and is measured as inorganic phosphorus. A concomitantly elevated serum K may help in making this diagnosis. The second is the presence of a paraprotein in the serum that spuriously raises the phosphorus level if the colorimetric assay technique is used prior to removal of serum proteins [231]. Since hyperglobulinemia is not invariably associated with hyperphosphatemia, it is quite possible that unique physicochemical characteristics of the specific abnormal globulin may also account for the spurious hyperphosphatemia [232]. A low anion gap, which is often found in these patients, should alert the clinician to the probability of a paraproteinemia. The diagnosis can be confirmed by serum protein electrophoresis, immunoelectrophoresis, or a repetition of the phosphorus measurement after the serum specimen has been deproteinated [233].

Hypoparathyroidism
The clinical manifestations associated with hypoparathyroidism are those of hypocalcemia (see previous section on hypocalcemia). The hyperphosphatemia is usually mild to moderate (6.0–9.0 mg per dl) and is secondary to a decrease in the renal tubular reabsorption of phosphorus.

Neoplastic Diseases
Tumor lysis syndrome is characterized by the development of severe hyperphosphatemia (10–20 mg per dl) with or without symptomatic hypocalcemia, hyperuricemia, hyperkalemia, and acute renal failure following chemotherapy for highly responsive tumors. This syndrome, although more prevalent in younger patients, does occur in the elderly and is due to a rapid release of intracellular phosphate into the extra-

cellular fluid [234, 235] and decreased phosphate excretion if volume contraction or acute renal failure is present.

Phosphate Enemas

Hyperphosphatemia can develop in elderly patients who abuse sodium phosphate–containing enemas for control of constipation. Pre-existing renal insufficiency is usually present. Symptomatic hypocalcemia (tetany, carpopedal spasm) associated with hypokalemia and a non–anion gap metabolic acidosis (due to K and HCO_3 losses through the gastrointestinal tract) suggest this diagnosis [236]. The hyperphosphatemia represents increased absorption of phosphate from the gastrointestinal tract (108 ml of enema contains 19 g of sodium biphosphate and 7 g of sodium phosphate) together with decreased excretion due to the presence of renal insufficiency. In addition, by suppressing intracellular phosphorylation, the accompanying acidosis may be responsible for a transcellular shift of the ion from the intra- to the extracellular space [237, 238].

TREATMENT AND PROGNOSIS

The treatment and prognosis of hyperphosphatemia are those of the underlying disease. Phosphate binders should be used in patients with renal failure (see Chap. 10) as well as in those with hypoparathyroidism. Hyperphosphatemia secondary to tumor lysis can be prevented by judicious volume expansion and control of the serum uric acid level with allopurinol to prevent development of acute renal failure. Volume expansion, correction of the acidosis, and calcium infusion for control of symptoms (care should be used not to raise the serum calcium level too high to avoid inducing metastatic calcification) are used in overabusers of phosphate enemas in addition to discontinuing the enemas. Dialysis may be indicated in the presence of superimposed acute renal failure.

HYPOPHOSPHATEMIA

INCIDENCE AND PREVALENCE

Hypophosphatemia occurs in 4 percent of elderly hospitalized patients, similar to the 3.2 to 4.7 percent rate reported by different groups for the general population [239, 240]. Mild hypophosphatemia (1.6–2.4 mg per dl) is most common, present in 67 percent of patients, followed by moderate hypophosphatemia (1.1–1.5 mg per dl) in 20 percent. The remaining 13 percent have a phosphorus level of less than 1.0 mg per dl [241, 242].

ETIOLOGY

The different causes of hypophosphatemia in our elderly population, in decreasing frequency, include dextrose infusion and refeeding after starvation, alcohol withdrawal, treatment for diabetic ketoacidosis, phosphate binders, respiratory alkalosis, and oncogenic osteomalacia. It should be noted, however, that in most patients with severe hypophosphatemia more than one of these factors is usually present.

CLINICAL MANIFESTATIONS AND PATHOGENESIS
Patients with mild to moderate hypophosphatemia are usually asymptomatic. In patients with a serum phosphorus of less than 1 mg per dl, CNS dysfunction ranging from irritability to coma and death, muscle weakness, rhabdomyolysis, elevated creatine phosphokinase [CPK], hemolysis, and white blood cell and platelet dysfunction may be seen [243].

Apart from an increase in CPK found in 10 to 15 percent of elderly patients with a serum phosphorus of less than 1 mg per dl, the other manifestations have been rather rare, an observation also made by others [244].

Dextrose Infusion and Refeeding After Starvation
In these patients, who are usually admitted to the hospital with multiple organ failure and starvation, a decision is subsequently made to initiate either enteral or parenteral feeding. Hypophosphatemia ensues as phosphorus is used for tissue repair in a previously phosphorus-depleted patient. Quite often phosphate supplementation in the enteral or parenteral preparation has been insufficient.

Alcohol Withdrawal
The clinical picture here is primarily that of alcohol withdrawal. Hypophosphatemia in the alcoholic depends on several factors including poor intake, use of antacids (for those with accompanying gastritis), alcoholic ketoacidosis, respiratory alkalosis, and a low TmP/GFR suggestive of a renal leak that is apparently related to hypomagnesemia [245]. This group of patients is prone to develop rhabdomyolysis. CPK should be monitored, and if found to be elevated, good hydration should be maintained and the urine alkalinized to prevent development of acute renal failure.

Therapy for Diabetic Ketoacidosis
Patients with diabetic ketoacidosis often are found to have a normal phosphorus level on admission despite a decrease in total body phosphorus. As insulin therapy is initiated and the acidosis corrected, the extracellular phosphate ion moves with glucose and potassium intracellularly, unmasking the hypophosphatemia [246]. Urinary losses that occur during the osmotic diuresis that accompanies glycosuria also play a role.

Phosphate Binders
Phosphate binders are most commonly encountered in patients using either aluminum- or calcium-containing antacids. Hypophosphatemia results from phosphate binding in the gut by those cations.

Respiratory Alkalosis
Respiratory alkalosis develops during prolonged and intense hyperventilation, and hypophosphatemia is due partly to a shift of phosphorus from the blood to skeletal muscle cells. Such a shift results from an increase in muscle glycolytic activity [247]. Factors that increase muscle glycolysis such as dextrose administration may also increase the severity of the hypophosphatemia.

Oncogenic Osteomalacia
This syndrome, although more common in younger patients, has been described in the elderly [248]. These patients present with bone and muscle pain and weakness involving mainly the proximal musculature. Besides mild to moderate hypophosphatemia and a low TmP/GFR suggestive of renal phosphate wasting, $1,25(OH)_2D_3$ is also decreased, and serum calcium is normal or mildly decreased. PTH and $25(OH)D_3$ are normal. Looser zones, which consist of bands crossing the bones and representing microfractures or pseudofractures, can be found on x-ray. Bone biopsy after tetracycline labeling reveals changes compatible with osteomalacia. Vascular (hemangiopericytoma), prostatic, and lung tumors have been associated with the syndrome [249–251]. It is postulated that a factor produced by the tumor blocks either the activity or the synthesis of 25-hydroxy-l-hydroxylase, thus accounting for the low $1,25(OH)_2D_3$. A decrease in the tubular transport of phosphate by such a factor or factors could also account for the phosphate leak [252]. The nephron site where this transport inhibition takes place is not yet known. It should be noted that in patients with prostatic cancer on estrogen therapy, the latter drug rather than oncogenic osteomalacia may be responsible for the hypophosphatemia [253]. A normal $1,25(OH)_2D_3$ should help to differentiate between these two possibilities.

TREATMENT AND PROGNOSIS
Once the diagnosis of hypophosphatemia has been made, a specific etiology should be sought and adequate corrective measures taken. In patients with oncogenic osteomalacia, pharmacologic amounts of vitamin D result only in partial improvement of the bone disease. Removal of the tumor may be followed by a lasting remission. Phosphate supplementation should be reserved for patients with severe hypophosphatemia (serum phosphorus ≤ 1.0 mg per dl) or for those with hypophosphatemia of varying degrees of severity and respiratory fail-

ure. In such cases the hypophosphatemia might be contributing to respiratory muscle weakness, rendering weaning from mechanical ventilation difficult [240]. In our elderly patients we use the approach suggested by Vannatta et al [254], in which 4 ml of intravenous phosphate (in the form of potassium phosphate with 2 mmol of phosphorus and 3 mmol of K per ml) is infused every 12 hours; serum phosphorus is monitored before each dose. This treatment has worked well in all of our patients within 72 hours. An oral preparation (K-Phos), which provides 125.6 mg of phosphorus, 44.5 mg of potassium, and 67 mg of sodium per tablet, is also available for chronic use.

MAGNESIUM

NORMAL PHYSIOLOGY

Magnesium (Mg) is mainly an intracellular cation. Sixty-five percent of magnesium is found in the skeleton, 34 percent is intracellular in other tissues, and only 1 percent is found in the extracellular fluid [255]. The skeletal Mg pool has a very low turnover rate, and the small extracellular pool has a rapid turnover. The intracellular pool has a turnover rate about half that of the extracellular pool.

The average diet contains 20 to 30 mEq of Mg per day (240–360 mg), of which 25 to 65 percent is normally absorbed [256], mainly in the small intestine. In certain circumstances, such as in disorders of the small intestine and during enema administration, the colon can also absorb Mg [257]. The exact mechanism of transcellular intestinal transport is controversial; however, there is some indirect evidence suggesting that the intestine can absorb Mg against an electrochemical gradient [258]. The proportion of Mg absorbed by the gut varies directly with its content in the diet. Mg absorption decreases in subjects with renal insufficiency, most likely as a result of the deficiency in $1,25(OH)_2D_3$ and an increase in intra- and extracellular Mg [259]. During Mg-depleted states, Mg absorption varies inversely with the calcium content of the diet.

Normally, serum Mg level is 1.5 to 3.0 mg per dl. Seventy-five to eighty percent of Mg exists in the ionic and complexed form and therefore is freely filtered at the glomerulus. The remaining 20 to 25 percent is protein bound. Only 3 to 5 percent of the filtered Mg appears in the urine [260]. During magnesium deprivation or hypomagnesemia, urinary Mg excretion decreases to less than 1 mEq per 24 hours (12 mg). In contrast, during parenteral Mg infusion or with a high Mg intake, urinary excretion of Mg is elevated. In normal subjects the Tm Mg has been found to be 1.4 mg per dl GFR per 1.73 m^2 for the ionized portion, or 2.0 mg per dl GFR per 1.73 m^2 for total serum Mg [261]. The average daily

Mg excretion is 100 mg per day in men and 90 mg per day in women (range 50–225 mg).

The proximal tubule reabsorbs 20 to 30 percent of the filtered Mg. The exact mechanism is not known, but the reabsorption depends on Na and water transport and intraluminal Mg concentration. Fifty to sixty percent of Mg is reabsorbed in the loop of Henle by a voltage-dependent mechanism that is secondary to active chloride transport. This portion also constitutes the major nephron segment where various hormones such as PTH, calcitonin, glucagon, and ADH modulate Mg reabsorption. Only a small portion of the remaining filtered Mg (approximately 20 percent) is reabsorbed by the distal tubule. Extracellular fluid volume expansion, osmotic diuresis, diuretic therapy, hypercalcemia, and alcohol ingestion are known to decrease tubular reabsorption of Mg [262].

CHANGES IN Mg METABOLISM IN THE ELDERLY

The plasma Mg level tends to decrease with age, as shown by Hollifield [263]. This concurs with our own observations in a small number of elderly of both sexes. In the 60- to 69-year-old age group the serum Mg was 1.6 to 2.2 mg per dl, in the 70- to 79-year age group it was 1.5 to 2.1 mg per dl, and in the 80- to 89-year age group it was 1.5 to 1.9 mg per dl. A decreased dietary intake has been implicated as a cause of the decrease with age [264]. These findings have not been universal because some authors have not found an age-related decrease [265], whereas others have found a significant increase in serum Mg in postmenopausal women associated with an increase in urinary excretion, which is reversible by estrogen administration [266]. The exact mechanism by which estrogen exerts its effect is unclear. Further studies dealing with Mg absorption, total body Mg, and Tm Mg/GFR in a large number of elderly subjects (both male and female) are needed before any definite conclusions can be reached about what happens to this cation with aging.

HYPERMAGNESEMIA

The incidence of hypermagnesemia in the elderly is not known. Since clinical manifestations associated with an elevated Mg level are not unique and do not constitute a syndrome that is readily recognizable, the serum Mg is not usually measured. In a survey of 621 patients of different ages, hypermagnesemia was found in 9.3 percent [267]. A somewhat lower incidence of 5.6 percent was found in another study [268]. Increased intake in the presence of renal insufficiency accounts for practically all the instances of hypermagnesemia seen in the elderly at our hospital. Mg-containing antacids have been responsible for most of the cases, although on occasion we have seen hypermagnesemia in cathartic abusers [269]. Mild hypermagnesemia has also been reported in patients with hypocalciuric familial hypercalcemia (see earlier section in this chapter on hypercalcemia). Patients with hypermagnesemia are usually asymptomatic except when the condition is severe (Mg > 10 mg per dl), at which point hypotension, bradycardia, changes in mentation, respiratory failure, and hypocalcemia have been described [270, 271]. Treatment in such cases should include calcium chloride infusion and other supportive measures, including dialysis.

HYPOMAGNESEMIA

INCIDENCE AND PREVALENCE
Since serum Mg is not routinely measured, the true incidence of hypomagnesemia (as is true for hypermagnesemia) is not really known in the elderly. In the same study noted earlier [267] in which the Mg concentration was determined in 621 randomly selected subjects, hypomagnesemia was found to be present in 11 percent. The incidence in Whang's study [268] was 6.9 percent. Nineteen percent of elderly patients evaluated by Martin and Milligan [272] had a serum Mg of 1.6 mg per dl or less. In our own study, in which serum magnesium was measured in 40 elderly patients, hypomagnesemia (< 1.5 mg per dl) was found in 4 (10 percent). These findings most likely underestimate the problem because significant Mg depletion can be present despite a normal serum Mg level.

ETIOLOGY
Hypomagnesemia in the elderly is generally due to (1) increased urinary losses due to diuretics or other drugs; (2) increased gastrointestinal losses associated with malabsorption or laxative abuse; (3) a combination of factors (see earlier discussion) such as the hypomagnesemia of alcoholism; and (4) endocrine disturbances including hyperthyroidism, hyperaldosteronism, and diabetes mellitus.

CLINICAL MANIFESTATIONS AND PATHOGENESIS
Magnesium is the second most prevalent intracellular cation and is therefore involved in the activation of various enzyme systems that play key roles in intermediary metabolism and phosphorylation. Therefore, it is not surprising that symptoms of hypomagnesemia may involve several organ systems. Clinical manifestations that may be seen when the serum Mg is less than 1 mg per dl include difficulty with concentration, confusion, disorientation, hallucinations, neuromuscular irritability, tingling, numbness, tremor, twitching, anorexia, diarrhea, abdominal

pain, constipation, cardiac arrhythmias (mainly ventricular), hypotension, and sudden cardiac death.

Obviously, most of those symptoms may be very easily attributed to the accompanying disease state rather than to hypomagnesemia per se. Therefore, it is advisable to measure Mg in patients at risk (see earlier section on etiology) as well as in those with acute respiratory failure, hypokalemia, hypophosphatemia, hyponatremia, and hypocalcemia, since such abnormalities have been found to be associated with a significantly high incidence of hypomagnesemia [273, 274]. Since the correlation between extracellular fluid Mg and intracellular Mg stores is poor, we suggest that urinary Mg be measured in patients who are at risk of developing hypomagnesemia but who have a normal serum Mg level. A value of less than 12 mg per 24 hours should be taken as evidence of Mg depletion.

Drug-Induced Hypomagnesemia

DIURETICS. Thirty to forty-eight percent of elderly patients on diuretics develop hypomagnesemia [263, 275]. Diuretic-induced renal losses are responsible for 75 percent of cases of hypomagnesemia seen in the elderly [263, 272]. Both the thiazide and "loop" diuretics interfere with distal nephron Mg reabsorption. As might be expected, the losses are more significant with the loop diuretics. Hypokalemia, which may be correctable only after magnesium repletion, is also common in these patients. It is postulated that Mg deficiency alters cell membrane permeability to K either directly or through a decrease in activation of Na-K-ATPase [276]. Mg-depleted patients are also at risk of developing cardiac arrhythmias (extrasystole, torsade de pointes), particularly if they are receiving digitalis concomitantly [277]. The exact mechanisms for this complication are not known, but it is possible that Mg deficiency leads to an alteration in the response of myocardial cells to digitalis [278]. Also, K depletion very likely potentiates the arrhythmogenic effect of Mg depletion.

OTHER DRUGS. Hypomagnesemia may be seen in elderly patients taking cisplatin (usually women who are being treated for ovarian cancer) owing to a decrease in renal tubular Mg reabsorption [279]. A large percentage of these patients are brought to medical attention because of the development of symptoms and signs of increased muscle irritability due in part to hypocalcemia (see earlier section on hypocalcemia of hypomagnesemia). The development of hypomagnesemia depends on the cumulative dose of cisplatin used [280].

Twenty-five percent of patients taking aminoglycoside antibiotics develop hypomagnesemia, which occurs early during therapy (average,

2.8 ± 0.5 days) and is due to decreased tubular reabsorption of Mg, since urinary Mg excretion is elevated [281]. Hypocalcemia may also be present. The concomitant presence of hypophosphatemia, hypokalemia, and hypouricemia in some patients suggests that the defect is located in the proximal tubule, most likely as a direct result of the toxicity of the aminoglycoside [282]. An indirect effect, through hyperaldosteronism, has also been postulated [283]. Hypomagnesemia due to renal losses has also been reported with amphotericin B [284].

Malabsorption
Severe hypomagnesemia can occur in patients with a malabsorption syndrome as well as in those abusing laxatives. The hypomagnesemia is secondary to the formation of Mg soaps and their subsequent loss in the stool. Urinary magnesium is low in such patients.

Alcoholism
Hypomagnesemia in alcoholics is multifactorial and results from decreased intake, decreased intestinal absorption (diarrhea, pancreatic insufficiency), starvation ketosis, and increased urinary losses either secondary to a direct suppressive effect of ethanol on the renal tubule or through binding of luminal Mg with lactate [285], making it unavailable for reabsorption.

Endocrine Disorders
Hypomagnesemia can occur in patients with thyrotoxicosis, although the mechanism is not known [286]. In those with hyperaldosteronism the hypomagnesemia is due to an increase in Mg excretion. It is not clear whether this represents a direct effect of aldosterone on Mg reabsorption or is a reflection of some degree of volume expansion with a resulting increase in delivery of Na and Mg to the distal tubule, where mineralocorticoids may enhance sodium reabsorption without affecting Mg transport [287]. The hypomagnesemia of hyperaldosteronism is reversed by spironolactone (Aldactone) administration. In uncontrolled diabetes mellitus urinary Mg losses occur because of the osmotic diuresis associated with glycosuria. In these patients serum Mg may be normal despite severe deficiency; however, during insulin therapy the extracellular Mg enters the cell, causing a subsequent drop in serum Mg.

TREATMENT AND PROGNOSIS
Since part of the decrease in serum Mg with age reflects poor dietary intake, any elderly person who is at increased risk of developing hypomagnesemia should be encouraged to consume foods rich in Mg such as vegetables, cereals, seafood, and so on. In symptomatic patients and in

those with severe hypomagnesemia, therapy can be started with a loading dose of 4 g (32.4 mEq) of 10 percent magnesium sulfate ($MgSO_4$) administered intravenously over a 10- to 20-minute period [288]. Deep tendon reflexes should be followed during treatment, and the infusion should be stopped if they decrease in intensity. Repeated doses of 1 g can be given hourly for a maximum of 8 g. Despite cellular depletion, only approximately 50 percent of each administered dose of $MgSO_4$ is retained, so that oral therapy in the form of magnesium oxide 300 mg (24.7 mEq) every 6 hours should be continued, generally for 4 to 5 days, or longer if the reason for the hypomagnesemia persists [289]; for example, cisplatin-induced hypomagnesemia might persist long after the drug has been discontinued. Diarrhea, which constitutes the most common side effect, may be controlled by lowering the dose. The recently available magnesium chloride (Slow-Mag) tablets, which provide 64 mg of elemental magnesium per tablet, are an even better alternative. For those patients who require continuous diuretic treatment, consideration should be given to adding either amiloride, 5 mg per day, or triamterene, 50 to 100 mg per day, because Mg sparing has been reported for both these agents [290, 291]. The hypomagnesemia that occurs during therapy for diabetic ketoacidosis is usually mild and of short duration and rarely requires therapy.

REFERENCES

1. Moore EW: Ionized calcium in normal serum, ultrafiltrates and whole blood determined by ion-exchange electrodes. *J Clin Invest* 49:318–334, 1970.
2. Sherwood LM, et al: Regulation of parathyroid hormone secretion: proportional control by calcium, lack of effect of phosphate. *Endocrinology* 83:1043–1051, 1968.
3. Yamamoto M, et al: Hypocalcemia increases and hypercalcemia decreases the steady-state level of parathyroid hormone messenger RNA in the rat. *J Clin Invest* 83:1053–1056, 1989.
4. Fuleihan GEH, et al: Calcium dependent release of N-terminal fragments and intact immunoreactive parathyroid hormone by human pathological parathyroid tissue in vitro. *J Clin Endocrinol Metab* 69:860–867, 1989.
5. Naveh-Many T, et al: Calcium regulates PTH messenger ribonucleic acid (mRNA) but not calcitonin mRNA in vivo in the rat. Dominant role of 1,25-dihydroxyvitamin D. *Endocrinology* 125:275–280, 1979.
6. Brown EM: Regulation of synthesis, metabolism and actions of parathyroid hormone. In *Contemporary Issues in Nephrology*, Vol. II. New York: Churchill-Livingstone, 1983. Pp 151–188.
7. Habener JF, Rosenblatt M, and Potts JT Jr: Parathyroid hormone: biochemical aspects of biosynthesis, secretion, action and metabolism. *Physiol Rev* 64:985–1053, 1984.

8. Morel F: Sites of hormone action in the mammalian nephron. *Am J Physiol* 240:F159–F164, 1981.

9. Martin KJ, et al: Selective uptake of the synthetic aminoterminal fragment of bovine parathyroid hormone by isolated perfused bone. *J Clin Invest* 62:256–261, 1978.

10. Peacock M, Robertson WG, and Nordin BEC: Relation between serum and urinary calcium with particular reference to parathyroid activity. *Lancet* 1:384–388, 1969.

11. Hollander D, Muralidhara KS, and Zimmerman A: Vitamin D_3 intestinal absorption in vivo: influence of fatty acids, bile salts and perfusate pH on absorption. *Gut* 19:267–272, 1978.

12. Holick MF, et al: Photosynthesis of previtamin D_3 in human skin and the physiologic consequences. *Science* 210:203–205, 1980.

13. Bell NH, Shaw S, and Turner RT: Evidence that 1,25-dihydroxyvitamin D_3 inhibits the hepatic production of 25-hydroxyvitamin D in man. *J Clin Invest* 74:1540–1544, 1984.

14. Baran DT and Milne ML: 1,25-dihydroxyvitamin D increases hepatocyte cytosolic calcium levels. A potential regulator of vitamin D-25 hydroxylase. *J Clin Invest* 77:1622–1626, 1986.

15. Norman DA, et al: Jejunal and ileal adaptation to alterations in dietary calcium. Changes in calcium and magnesium absorption and pathogenetic role of parathyroid hormone and 1,25-dihydroxyvitamin D. *J Clin Invest* 67:1599–1603, 1981.

16. Audran M and Kumar R: The physiology and pathophysiology of vitamin D. *Mayo Clin Proc* 60:851–866, 1985.

17. Tanaka Y and DeLuca HF: Bone mineral mobilization activity of 1,25-dihydroxycholecalciferol, a metabolite of vitamin D. *Arch Biochem Biophys* 146:574–578, 1971.

18. Hughes MR and Haussler MR: 1,25 dihydroxycholecalciferol receptors in parathyroid glands. *J Biol Chem* 253:1065–1069, 1978.

19. Silver J, et al: Regulation by vitamin D metabolites of messenger ribonucleic acid for preproparathyroid hormone in isolated bovine parathyroid cells. *Proc Natl Acad Sci USA* 82:4270–4273, 1985.

20. Heath H IV and Sizemore GW: Plasma calcitonin in normal man. Differences between men and women. *J Clin Invest* 60:1135–1140, 1977.

21. Torring O, Bucht E, and Sjöberg HE: Plasma calcitonin response to a calcium clamp. Influence of sex and age. *Horm Metab Res* 17:536–539, 1985.

22. Chapuy MC, Durr F, and Chapuy P: Age-related changes in parathyroid hormone and 25-hydroxycholecalciferol levels. *J Gerontol* 38:19–22, 1983.

23. Marcus R, Madirg P, and Young G: Age-related changes in parathyroid hormone and parathyroid hormone action in normal humans. *J Clin Endocrinol Metab* 58:223–230, 1984.

24. Greenblatt DJ: Reduced serum albumin concentration in the elderly: A report from the Boston Collaborative Drug Surveillance Program. *J Am Geriatr Soc* 27:20–22, 1979.

25. Wiske PS, et al: Increase in immunoreactive parathyroid hormone with age. *N Engl J Med* 300:1419–1421, 1979.

26. Orwoll ES and Meier D: Alterations in calcium, vitamin D and parathyroid hormone physiology in normal man with aging: Relationship to the development of senile osteopenia. *J Clin Endocrinol Metab* 63:1262–1269, 1986.

27. Endras DB, et al: Age-related changes in serum immunoreactive parathyroid hormone and its biological action in healthy men and women. *J Clin Endocrinol Metab* 65:724–736, 1979.

28. Gallagher JC, et al: Intestinal calcium absorption and serum vitamin D metabolites in normal subjects and osteoporotic patients. *J Clin Invest* 64: 729–736, 1979.
29. Francis RM, et al: Calcium malabsorption in the elderly: The effect of treatment with oral 25-hydroxyvitamin D_3. *Eur J Clin Invest* 13:391–396, 1983.
30. Malm OJ: Calcium requirement and adaptation in adult men. *Scand J Clin Lab Invest* 10 (Suppl 36):1–289, 1958.
31. Ireland P and Fordtran JS: Effect of dietary calcium and age on jejunal calcium absorption in humans studied by intestinal perfusion. *J Clin Invest* 52:2672–2681, 1973.
32. Gallagher JC and Riggs LB: Current concepts in nutrition. Nutrition and bone disease. *N Engl J Med* 298:193–195, 1978.
33. Paillard M, Patron P, and Gardin JP: Determinants of circulating levels of 1,25-dihydroxyvitamin D_3 in primary hyperparathyroidism (PHPT). *Min Electrol Metab* 11:334, A79, 1985.
34. Bouillon RA, et al: Vitamin D status in the elderly: seasonal substrate deficiency causes 1,25 dihydroxycholecalciferol deficiency. *Am J Clin Nutr* 45:755–763, 1987.
35. Mori S, et al: Bone fracture in elderly female with primary hyperparathyroidism: relationship among renal function, vitamin D status and fracture risk. *Horm Metabol Res* 19:183–185, 1897.
36. Armbrecht HJ, Forte LR, and Halloran BP: Effect of aging and dietary calcium on renal 25-hydroxyvitamin D metabolism, serum 1,25(OH)$_2$D and PTH. *Am J Physiol* 246:E266–E270, 1984.
37. Armbrecht HJ, Forte LR, and Wongsurawat N: Forskolin increases 1,25-dihydroxyvitamin D_3 production by rat renal slices in vitro. *Endocrinology* 114:644–649, 1984.
38. Ishida M, et al: Hydroxylation of 25-hydroxyvitamin D_3 by renal mitochondria from rats of different ages. *Endocrinology* 121:443–448, 1987.
39. Silverberg SJ, et al: Abnormalities in parathyroid hormone secretion and 1,25-dihydroxyvitamin D_3 formation in women with osteoporosis. *N Engl J Med* 320:277–289, 1989.
40. Editorial: Vitamin D supplementation in the elderly. *Lancet* 1:306–307, 1987.
41. Toss G and Sörbo B: Serum concentrations of 25-hydroxyvitamin D and vitamin D-binding protein in elderly people. *Acta Med Scand* 220:273–277, 1986.
42. Goldray D, et al: Vitamin D deficiency in elderly patients in a general hospital. *J Am Geriatr Soc* 37:589–592, 1989.
43. Sommerville PJ, Lien JWK, and Kaye M: The calcium and vitamin D status in an elderly female population and their response to administered supplemental vitamin D_3. *J Gerontol* 32:659–663, 1977.
44. Maclaughlin J and Holick MF: Aging decreases the capacity of human skin to produce vitamin D_3. *J Clin Invest* 76:1536–1538, 1985.
45. Christensson T, et al: Prevalence of hypercalcemia in a health screening in Stockholm. *Acta Med Scand* 200:131–137, 1976.
46. Grero PS and Hodkinson HM: Hypercalcemia in elderly hospital inpatients: Values of discriminant analysis in differential diagnosis. *Age Aging* 6:14–20, 1977.
47. Sorva A and Tilvis R: Survival and calcemic status of geriatric inpatients. *Lancet* 1:799, 1987.
48. Mallete LE: Review: Primary hyperparathyroidism, an update: Incidence, etiology, diagnosis and treatment. *Am J Med Sci* 293:239–249, 1987.

49. Marx SJ: New insights into primary hyperparathyroidism. *Hosp Pract* 19:55–63, 1984.
50. Taffet GE, et al: Elevated parathyroid hormone in elderly males. *J Am Geriat Soc* 34:906A, 1986.
51. Tibblin S, Pälsson N, and Rydberg J: Hyperparathyroidism in the elderly. *Ann Surg* 197:135–138, 1983.
52. Carnevale N, Samson R, and Bennett BP: Multiple parathyroid adenomas. *JAMA* 246:1332–1333, 1981.
53. Black BK: Carcinoma of the parathyroid. *Ann Surg* 139:355–363, 1954.
54. Holmes EC, Morton DL, and Ketcham AS: Parathyroid carcinoma: A collective review. *Ann Surg* 169:631–640, 1969.
55. Shane E and Bilezikian JP: Parathyroid carcinoma: A review of 62 patients. *Endocrine Rev* 3:218–226, 1982.
56. Murray TM, et al: Non-autonomy of hormone secretion in primary hyperparathyroidism. *Clin Endocrinol* 1:235–239, 1972.
57. Brown EM, et al: Dispersed cells from human parathyroid glands: Distinct calcium sensitivity of adenomas vs primary hyperplasia. *J Clin Endocrinol Metab* 46:267–275, 1978.
58. Dietel M, et al: Abnormal calcium distribution in human parathyroid adenomas as possible cause of primary hyperparathyroidism. *Horm Metab Res* 19:177–181, 1987.
59. Bellorin-Font E, et al: Altered adenylate cyclase kinetics in hyperfunctioning human parathyroid glands. *J Clin Endocrinol Metab* 52:499–507, 1981.
60. Juhlin C, et al: Monoclonal antiparathyroid antibodies revealing defect expression of a calcium receptor mechanism in hyperparathyroidism. *World J Surg* 12:552–558, 1988.
61. Parfitt AM: Equilibrium and disequilibrium hypercalcemia. New light on an old concept. *Metab Bone Dis* 1:279–283, 1979.
62. Stewart AF: Is there a role for parathyroid hormone in humoral hypercalcemia of malignancy? *Min Electrol Metab* 8:215–226, 1982.
63. Heath DA, et al: Surgical treatment of hyperparathyroidism in the elderly. *Br Med J* 280:1406–1408, 1980.
64. Brothers TA and Thompson NW: Surgical treatment of primary hyperparathyroidism in elderly patients. *Acta Clin Scand* 153:175–178, 1987.
65. Joborn C, et al: Primary hyperparathyroidism in patients with organic brain syndrome. *Acta Med Scand* 219:91–98, 1986.
66. Joborn C, et al: Psychiatric morbidity in primary hyperparathyroidism. *World J Surg* 12:476–481, 1988.
67. Patten BM, et al: Neuromuscular disease in primary hyperparathyroidism. *Ann Intern Med* 80:182–193, 1974.
68. Broadus AE, et al: The importance of circulating 1,25-dihydroxyvitamin D in the pathogenesis of hypercalciuria and renal stone formation in primary hyperparathyroidism. *N Engl J Med* 302:421–426, 1980.
69. Pak CYC, et al: A lack of unique pathophysiologic background for nephrolithiasis of primary hyperparathyroidism. *J Clin Endocrinol Metab* 53:536–542, 1981.
70. Lafferty FW: Primary hyperparathyroidism. Changing clinical spectrum, prevalance of hypertension and discriminant analysis of laboratory tests. *Arch Intern Med* 141:1761–1766, 1981.
71. Diamond TW, et al: Parathyroid hypertension. A reversible disorder. *Arch Intern Med* 146:1709–1712, 1986.
72. Salahudeen AK, et al: Hypertension and renal dysfunction in primary hyperparathyroidism: Effect of parathyroidectomy. *Clin Sci* 76:289–296, 1989.

73. Ganguly A, et al: The renin-angiotensin system and hypertension in primary hyperparathyroidism. *Metabolism* 31:595–600, 1982.
74. Richards AM, et al: Hormone, calcium and blood pressure relationship in primary hyperparathyroidism. *J Hypert* 6:747–752, 1980.
75. Vlachakis ND, et al: Sympathetic system function and vascular reactivity in hypercalciuric patients. *Hypertension* 4:452–458, 1982.
76. Daniels J and Goodman DA: Hypertension and hyperparathyroidism. Inverse relation of serum phosphate level and blood pressure. *Am J Med* 75:17–23, 1983.
77. Payne RL Jr and Fitchett CW: Hyperparathyroid crisis. A survey of the literature and a report of two additional cases. *Ann Surg* 161:737–747, 1965.
78. Mundy GR, Cove DH, and Fisken R: Primary hyperparathyroidism: Changes in the pattern of clinical presentation. *Lancet* 1:1317–1320, 1980.
79. Fitzpatrick LA and Bilezikan JP: Acute primary hyperparathyroidism. *Am J Med* 82:275–282, 1987.
80. Raisz LG, et al: Comparison of commercially available parathyroid immunoassays in the differential diagnosis of hypercalcemia due to primary hyperparathyroidism or malignancy. *Ann Intern Med* 91:739–740, 1979.
81. Boyd JC and Ladenson JH: Value of laboratory tests in the differential diagnosis of hypercalcemia. *Am J Med* 77:863–872, 1984.
82. Lufkin EG, Kao PC, and Heath H III: Parathyroid hormone radioimmunoassays in the differential diagnosis of hypercalcemia due to primary hyperparathyroidism or malignancy. *Ann Intern Med* 106:559–560, 1987.
83. Martin KJ, et al: Clinical utility of radioimmunoassay for parathyroid hormone. *Min Electrol Metab* 3:283–290, 1980.
84. Mallette LE, et al: Radioimmunoassay for the middle region of human parathyroid hormone using an homologous antiserum with a caroxyterminal fragment of bovine PTH as radioligand. *J Clin Endocrinol Metab* 54:1017–1024, 1982.
85. Broadus AE and Rasmussen H: Clinical evaluation of parathyroid function. *Am J Med* 70:475–478, 1981.
86. Rude RK, et al: Urinary and nephrogenous adenosine 3'5'-monophosphate in the hypercalcemia of malignancy. *J Clin Endocrinol Metab* 52:765–771, 1981.
87. Torring O, et al: Urinary cyclic AMP corrected for glomerular filtration rate in the differential diagnosis of hypercalcemia. *Acta Med Scand* 211:401–405, 1982.
88. Sample WF, Mitchell SP, and Bledsoe RC: Parathyroid ultrasonography. *Radiology* 127:485–490, 1978.
89. Gatekunst R, et al: Parathyroid localization. *J Clin Endocrinol Metab* 63:1390–1393, 1986.
90. Krudy AG, et al: The detection of mediastinal parathyroid glands by computed tomography, selective arteriography and various sampling. *Radiology* 140:739–744, 1981.
91. Kovarik J, et al: The value of computed tomography as a noninvasive method for preoperative localization of parathyroid adenomas of the neck in primary hyperparathyroidism. *Min Electrol Metab* 5:228–232, 1981.
92. Cates JD, et al: CT evaluation of parathyroid adenomas. Diagnostic criteria and pitfalls. *J Comput Assist Tomogr* 12:626–629, 1988.
93. Clark OH, et al: Localization studies in patients with persistent or recurrent hyperparathyroidism. *Surgery* 98:1083–1094, 1985.
94. Young AE, et al: Location of parathyroid adenomas by thallium-201 and technetium-99m subtraction scanning. *Br Med J* 286:1384–1386, 1983.

95. Skibber JM, et al: Computerized technetium/thallium scans and para-thyroid reoperation. *Surgery* 98:1077–1082, 1985.
96. Levin KE, et al: Localizing studies in patients with persistent or recurrent hyperparathyroidism. *Surgery* 102:917–925, 1987.
97. Aufferman W, et al: Diagnosis of recurrent hyperparathyroidism: Comparison of MR imaging and other imaging techniques. *AJR* 150:1027–1033, 1988.
98. Farr HW: Hyperparathyroidism and cancer. *CA* 26:66–74, 1976.
99. Wajngot A, et al: Occurrence of pituitary adenomas and other neoplastic diseases in primary hyperparathyroidism. *Surg Gynecol Obstet* 151:401–403, 1980.
100. Ljunghall S, et al: Dynamic tests of parathyroid function for diagnosis of primary hyperparathyroidism in malignancy. *Clin Endocrinol* 27:163–170, 1987.
101. Ljunghall S, et al: Improved differential diagnosis of hypercalcemia by hypocalcemic stimulation of parathyroid hormone. *World J Surg* 12:496–502, 1988.
102. Bensen L, et al: A stimulation test with calcitonin for differential diagnosis of hypercalcemia. *Acta Endocrinol* 107:237–244, 1984.
103. Rasbach DA and Hammond JM: Pancreatic islet cell carcinoma with hypercalcemia. Primary hyperparathyroidism or humoral hypercalcemia of malignancy. *Am J Med* 78:337–342, 1985.
104. Gardin JP and Paillard M: Normocalcemic primary hyperparathyroidism: Resistance to PTH effect on tubular reabsorption of calcium. *Min Electrol Metab* 10:301–308, 1984.
105. Myers WPL: Hypercalcemia in neoplastic disease. *Arch Surg* 80:308–310, 1960.
106. Burt ME and Brennan MF: Incidence of hypercalcemia and malignant neoplasm. *Arch Surg* 115:704–707, 1980.
107. Mundy GR and Martin TJ: The hypercalcemia of malignancy: Pathogenesis and management. *Metabolism* 31:1247–1277, 1982.
108. Ray AK and Rao DB: Hypercalcemia and malignant disease in the elderly: Magnesium sulfate therapy. *J Am Geriatr Soc* 22:413–415, 1974.
109. Levine MM and Kleeman CR: Hypercalcemia: Pathophysiology and treatment. *Hosp Pract* 22:93–110, 1987.
110. Ralston S, et al: Hypercalcemia and metastatic bone disease: Is there a causal link? *Lancet* 2:903–905, 1982.
111. Eilon G and Mundy GR: Effects of inhibition of microtubule assembly on bone mineral release and enzyme release by human breast cancer cells. *J Clin Invest* 67:69–76, 1981.
112. Mundy GR, Ibbotson KJ, and D'Souza SM: Tumor products and the hypercalcemia of malignancy. *J Clin Invest* 76:391–394, 1985.
113. Goldfarb S and Agus ZS: Mechanism of the polyuria of hypercalcemia. *Am J Nephrol* 4:69–76, 1984.
114. Lins LE: Renal function in hypercalcemia. A clinical and experimental study. *Acta Med Scand* Suppl 632:1–46, 1979.
115. Stewart AF, et al: Biochemical evaluation of patients with cancer-associated hypercalcemia. Evidence for humoral and nonhumoral groups. *N Engl J Med* 303:1377–1383, 1980.
116. Skrabanek P, McPartlin J, and Powell D: Tumor hypercalcemia and "ectopic hyperparathyroidism." *Medicine* 59:262–289, 1980.
117. Harris RC, et al: Evidence for glomerular actions of epidermal growth factor in the rat. *J Clin Invest* 82:1028–1038, 1988.
118. Insogna KL, et al: Native and a synthetic analogue of the malignancy-

associated parathyroid hormone-like protein have in vitro transforming growth factor-like properties. *J Clin Invest* 83:1057–1060, 1989.

119. Ralston SH, et al: Hypercalcemia of malignancy. Evidence for non-parathyroid humoral agent with an effect on renal tubular handling of calcium. *Clin Sci* 66:187–197, 1984.

120. Tuttle KR, Mundy GR, and Kunau RT: Renal tubular calcium (Ca) reabsorption is uniformly increased in hypercalcemia of malignancy (HCM). *Clin Res* 37:463A, 1989.

121. Ralston SH: The pathogenesis of humoral hypercalcemia of malignancy. *Lancet* 2:1443–1446, 1987.

122. Mundy GR: The hypercalcemia of malignancy. *Kidney Int* 31:142–155, 1987.

123. Mundy GR, et al: The hypercalcemia of cancer. Clinical implications and pathogenic mechanisms. *N Engl J Med* 310:1718–1727, 1984.

124. Suva LJ, et al: A parathyroid hormone related protein implicated in malignant hypercalcemia: Cloning and expression. *Science* 237:893–896, 1987.

125. Broadus A, et al: Humoral hypercalcemia of cancer. Identification of a novel parathyroid hormone-like peptide. *N Engl J Med* 319:556–563, 1988.

126. Budayr AA, et al: Increased serum levels of parathyroid hormone-like protein in malignancy-associated hypercalcemia. *Ann Intern Med* 111:807–812, 1989.

127. Kukreja SC, et al: Antibodies to parathyroid hormone-related protein lower serum calcium in athymic mouse models of malignancy-associated hypercalcemia due to human tumors. *J Clin Invest* 82:1798–1802, 1988.

128. Mundy GR: Hypercalcemia of malignancy revisited. *J Clin Invest* 82:1–6, 1988.

129. Ross Garrett I, et al: Production of lymphotoxin, a bone-resorbing cytokine by cultured human myeloma cells. *N Engl J Med* 317:526–532, 1987.

130. Gowan M, et al: An interleukin-1 like factor stimulates bone resorption in vitro. *Nature* 306:378–380, 1983.

131. Breslay NA, et al: Hypercalcemia associated with increased serum calcitriol levels in three patients with lymphoma. *Ann Intern Med* 100:1–7, 1984.

132. Zaloga GP, Eil C, and Medberry CA: Humoral hypercalcemia in Hodgkin's disease. *Arch Intern Med* 145:155–157, 1985.

133. Mundy GR and Bertolini DR: Bone destruction and hypercalcemia in plasma cell myeloma. *Semin Oncol* 13:291–299, 1986.

134. State RM, et al: Hydrochlorothiazide effects on serum calcium and immunoreactive parathyroid hormone concentrations. Studies in normal subjects. *Ann Intern Med* 77:587–591, 1972.

135. Costanzo LS and Windhagen EE: Calcium and sodium transport by the distal convoluted tubule of the rat. *Am J Physiol* 235:F492–F506, 1978.

136. Koppel JH, et al: Thiazide-induced rise in serum calcium and magnesium in patients on maintenance hemodialysis. *Ann Intern Med* 72:895–901, 1970.

137. Malluche HH, et al: Evidence for a direct effect of thiazide on bone. *Min Electrol Metab* 4:89–96, 1980.

138. Christensson T, Hellström K, and Wengle B: Hypercalcemia and primary hyperparathyroidism. Prevalence in patients receiving thiazides as detected in a health screen. *Arch Intern Med* 137:1138–1142, 1977.

139. Frame B, et al: Hypercalcemia and skeletal effects in chronic hypervitaminosis A. *Ann Intern Med* 80:44–48, 1974.

140. Editorial. Osteoporosis. *Lancet* 2:833–835, 1987.

141. Schwartzman MS and Franck WA: Vitamin D toxicity complicating the treatment of senile postmenopausal and glucocorticoid induced osteoporosis. *Am J Med* 82:224–230, 1987.

142. Mawber EB, et al: Vitamin D metabolism in patients intoxicated with ergo-calciferol. *Clin Sci* 68:135–141, 1985.

143. Reichel H, et al: Regulation of 1,25-dihydroxyvitamin D_3 production by cultured alveolar macrophages from normal human donors and from patients with pulmonary sarcoidosis. *J Clin Endocrinol Metab* 65:1201–1209, 1987.

144. Strewler GJ and Nissenson RA: Nonparathyroid hypercalcemia. *Adv Intern Med* 32:235–258, 1987.

145. Marx SJ, et al: The hypocalciuric or benign variant of familial hypercalcemia: Clinical and biochemical features in fifteen kindreds. *Medicine* 60:397–412, 1981.

146. Marx SJ, et al: Divalent cation metabolism. Familial hypocalciuric hypercalcemia versus typical primary hyperparathyroidism. *Am J Med* 65:235–242, 1978.

147. Law WM Jr, et al: High-resolution parathyroid ultrasonography in familial benign hypercalcemia (Familial hypocalciuric hypercalcemia). *Mayo Clin Proc* 59:153–155, 1984.

148. Marx SJ, et al: Circulating parathyroid hormone activity. Familial hypocalciuric hypercalcemia versus typical primary hyperparathyroidism. *J Clin Endocrinol Metab* 47:1190–1197, 1978.

149. Bouillon R, Muls E, and DeMoor P: Influence of thyroid function on the serum concentration of 1,25-dihydroxyvitamin D_3. *J Clin Endocrinol Metab* 51:793–797, 1980.

150. Mosekilde L and Christensen MS: Decreased parathyroid function in hyperthyroidism: Interrelationships between serum parathyroid hormone, calcium-phosphorous metabolism and thyroid function. *Acta Endocrinol* 84:566–575, 1977.

151. Suki WN, et al: Acute treatment of hypercalcemia with furosemide. *N Engl J Med* 283:836–840, 1970.

152. Edwards BR, et al: Micropuncture study of diuretic effects on sodium and calcium reabsorption in the dog nephron. *J Clin Invest* 52:2418–2427, 1978.

153. Ralston SH, et al: Comparison of amino hydroxypropylidene, diphosphonate, mithramycin and corticosteroid calcitonin in treatment of cancer-associated hypercalcemia. *Lancet* 2:907–910, 1985.

154. Malatino LS, et al: Acute effects of salmon calcitonin in man include stimulation of the renin-angiotensin-aldosterone system. *Min Electrol Metab* 13:316–322, 1987.

155. Wener JA, Gorton SJ, and Raisz LG: Escape from inhibition of resorption in cultures of fetal bone treated with calcitonin and parathyroid hormone. *Endocrinology* 90:752–759, 1972.

156. Binstock ML and Mundy GR: Effect of calcitonin and glucocorticoids in combination in malignant hypercalcemia. *Ann Intern Med* 93:269–272, 1980.

157. Suda T, Testa NG, and Allen TD: Effects of hydrocortisone on osteoclasts generated in cat bone marrow cultures. *Calcif Tissue Int* 35:82–86, 1983.

158. Kanis JA, et al: Effects of intravenous etidronate disodium on skeletal and calcium metabolism. *Am J Med* 82 (Suppl 2A):55–70, 1987.

159. Hasling C, Charles P, and Mosekilde L: Etidronate disodium in the management of malignancy-related hypercalcemia. *Am J Med* 82 (Suppl 2A):51–54, 1987.

160. Evans RA: Hypercalcemia, what does it signify? *Drugs* 31:64–74, 1986.

161. Singer FR and Fernandez M: Therapy of hypercalcemia of malignancy. *Am J Med* 82 (Suppl 2A):34–41, 1987.

162. Rinenberg QS and Ritch PS: Efficacy of oral administration of etidronate

disodium in maintaining normal serum calcium levels in previously hypercalcemic cancer patients. *Clin Ther* 9:1–8, 1987.

163. Van-Holten-Verzantvoort AT, et al: Reduced morbidity from skeletal metastases in breast cancer patients during long term biphosphonate (APD)
treatment. *Lancet* 2:983–985, 1987.

164. Bruining HA, et al: Causes of failure in operations for hyperparathyroidism. *Surgery* 101:562–565, 1987.

165. Spiegel AM, et al: Intraoperative measurements of urinary cyclic AMP to
guide surgery for primary hyperparathyroidism. *N Engl J Med* 303:1457–
1460, 1980.

166. Gonzalez-Villapando C, et al: Vitamin D metabolism during recovery from
severe osteitis fibrosa cystica of primary hyperparathyroidism. *J Clin Endocrinol Metab* 51:1180–1183, 1980.

167. Niederle B, et al: Successful parathyroidectomy in primary hyperparathyroidism: A clinical follow-up study of 212 consecutive patients. *Surgery*
102:903–909, 1987.

168. Deaconson TF, Wilson SD, and Lemann J Jr: The effect of parathyroidectomy on the recurrence of nephrolithiasis. *Surgery* 102:910–913, 1987.

169. Schatz A and Castleman B: Parathyroid carcinoma: A study of 70 cases.
Cancer 31:600–605, 1973.

170. McCance DR, et al: Parathyroid carcinoma: A review. *J R Soc Med*
80:505–514, 1987.

171. Heath H III, Hodgson SF, and Kennedy MA: Primary hyperparathyroidism: incidence, morbidity and potential economic impact in a community.
N Engl J Med 302:189–193, 1980.

172. Coe FL and Favus MJ: Does mild, asymptomatic hyperparathyroidism require surgery? *N Engl J Med* 302:224–225, 1980.

173. Scholz DA and Purnell DC: Asymptomatic primary hyperparathyroidism.
Ten year prospective study. *Mayo Clin Proc* 56:473–478, 1981.

174. Hodgson SF and Heath H III: Asymptomatic primary hyperparathyroidism: Treat or follow? *Mayo Clin Proc* 56:521–522, 1981.

175. Lueg MC: Asymptomatic primary hyperparathyroidism. *Hosp Pract*
17:29–39, 1982.

176. Amorosa LF and Amorosa JK: Hyperparathyroidism with asymptomatic
hypercalcemia. *Hosp Pract* 18:223–246, 1983.

177. Pearson MW: Asymptomatic primary hyperparathyroidism in the elderly.
Age Aging 13:1–5, 1984.

178. Van't Hoff W, Ballardi FW, and Bicknell EJ: Primary hyperparathyroidism:
The case for medical management. *Br Med J* 287:1605–1608, 1983.

179. Corlew DS, et al: Observations on the course of untreated primary hyperparathyroidism. *Surgery* 98:1064–1070, 1985.

180. Alveryd AS, et al: Indication for surgery in the elderly patient with primary
hyperparathyroidism. *Acta Chir Scand* 142:491–494, 1976.

181. Lifschitz BM and Barzel US: Parathyroid surgery in the aged. *J Gerontol*
36:573–575, 1981.

182. Peskin GW, Greenberg GA, and Salk RP: Expanding indications for early
parathyroidectomy in the elderly female. *Am J Surg* 136:45–48, 1978.

183. Brothers TE and Thompson NW: Surgical treatment of primary hyperparathyroidism in elderly patients. *Acta Chir Scand* 153:175–178, 1987.

184. Kochersberger G, et al: What is the clinical significance of bone loss in primary hyperparathyroidism? *Arch Intern Med* 147:1951–1953, 1987.

185. Wilson RJ, et al: Mild asymptomatic primary hyperparathyroidism is not a
risk factor for vertebral fractures. *Ann Intern Med* 109:959–962, 1988.

186. Block MA, Daily GE III, and Muchmore DE: Bone demineralization, a factor of increasing significance in the management of primary hyperparathyroidism. *Surgery* 106:1063–1069, 1989.
187. Block MA, Xavier A, and Brush BE: Management of primary hyperparathyroidism in the elderly. *J Am Geriatr Soc* 23:385–389, 1975.
188. Sampson MJ, Van't Hoff W, and Bicknell EJ: The conservative management of primary hyperparathyroidism. *Q J Med* 65:1009–1014, 1987.
189. Bilezikian JP: The medical management of primary hyperparathyroidism. *Ann Intern Med* 96:198–202, 1982.
190. Editorial: Medical management of primary hyperparathyroidism. *Lancet* 2:727–728, 1984.
191. Eriksen EF, et al: Evidence of estrogen receptors in normal human osteoblast-like cells. *Science* 241:84–86, 1988.
192. Marcus R, et al: Conjugated estrogens in the treatment of postmenopausal women with hyperparathyroidism. *Ann Intern Med* 100:633–640, 1984.
193. Selby PL and Peacock M: Ethinyl estradiol and norethindrone in the treatment of primary hyperparathyroidism in postmenopausal women. *N Engl J Med* 314:1481–1485, 1986.
194. Judd HL, et al: Estrogen replacement therapy. *Obstet Gynecol* 58:267–275, 1981.
195. Horowitz M, et al: Treatment of postmenopausal hyperparathyroidism with norethindrone. Effects on biochemistry and forearm mineral density. *Arch Intern Med* 147:681–685, 1987.
196. Duarte B, Hargis GK, and KuKreja SC: Effects of estradiol and progesterone on parathyroid tissue. *J Clin Endocrinol Metab* 66:584–587, 1988.
197. Broadus AE, et al: A detailed evaluation of oral phosphate therapy in selected patients with primary hyperparathyroidism. *J Clin Endocrinol Metab* 56:953–961, 1983.
198. Shane E, Baquiran DC, and Bilezikian JP: Effects of dichloromethylene diphosphonate on serum and urinary calcium in primary hyperparathyroidism. *Ann Intern Med* 95:23–27, 1981.
199. Warrell RP Jr, et al: Gallium nitrate for treatment of refractory hypercalcemia from parathyroid carcinoma. *Ann Intern Med* 107:683–686, 1987.
200. Glover D, et al: Hypocalcemia and inhibition of parathyroid hormone secretion after administration of WR-2721 (a radioprotective and chemoprotective agent). *N Engl J Med* 309:1137–1141, 1983.
201. Desai TK, Carlson RW, and Gehab MA: Prevalence and clinical implications of hypocalcemia in acutely ill patients in a medical intensive setting. *Am J Med* 84:209–214, 1988.
202. Zaloga GP and Chernow B: The multifactorial basis for hypocalcemia during sepsis. Studies of the parathyroid hormone-vitamin D axis. *Ann Intern Med* 107:36–41, 1987.
203. Chase LR and Slatopolsky E: Secretion and metabolic efficacy of parathyroid hormone in patients with severe hypomagnesemia. *J Clin Endocrinol Metab* 38:363–371, 1974.
204. Rude RK, Oldham SB, and Singer FR: Functional hyperparathyroidism and parathyroid hormone end-organ resistance in human magnesium deficiency. *Clin Endocrinol* 5:209–224, 1976.
205. Rosler A and Rabinowitz D: Magnesium-induced reversal of vitamin D resistance in hyperparathyroidism. *Lancet* 1:803, 1973.
206. Robertson GM Jr, et al: Inadequate parathyroid response in acute pancreatitis. *N Engl J Med* 294:512–516, 1976.

207. Haldeman B, et al: Renal function and blood levels of divalent ions in acute pancreatitis. *Min Electrol Metab* 3:190–199, 1980.
208. Breslau NA and Pak CYC: Hypoparathyroidism. *Metabolism* 28:1261–1276, 1979.
209. Fourman P, et al: Parathyroid insufficiency after thyroidectomy. Review of 46 cases with the study of the effects of hypocalcemia on the electroencephalogram. *Br J Surg* 50:608–619, 1963.
210. Llach F, Felsenfeld AJ, and Haussler MR: The pathophysiology of altered calcium metabolism in rhabdomyolysis-induced acute renal failure. *N Engl J Med* 305:117–123, 1981.
211. Riancho JA, et al: The clinical spectrum of hypocalcemia associated with bone metastases. *J Intern Med* 226:449–452, 1989.
212. Smallbridge RC, Wray HL, and Schaef M: Hypocalcemia with osteoblastic metastases in a patient with prostate carcinoma. A cause of secondary hyperparathyroidism. *Am J Med* 71:184–188, 1981.
213. Porter RH, et al: Treatment of hypoparathyroid patients with chlorthalidone. *N Engl J Med* 298:577–581, 1978.
214. Davies M, et al: 1,25-dihydroxycholecalciferol in hyperparathyroidism. *Lancet* 1:55–59, 1977.
215. Wasserman RH: Intestinal absorption of calcium and phosphorus. *Fed Proc* 40:68–72, 1981.
216. Mizgala CL and Quamme GA: Renal handling of phosphate. *Physiol Rev* 65:431–466, 1985.
217. Mühlbauer RC, Bonjour JP, and Fleisch H: Tubular localization of adaptation to dietary phosphate in rats. *Am J Physiol* 233:F342–F348, 1977.
218. Dennis VW, Bello-Reuss E, and Robinson R: Response of phosphate transport to parathyroid hormone in segments of rabbit nephron. *Am J Physiol* 233:F28–F38, 1977.
219. Pastoriza-Muñoz E, et al: Effect of parathyroid hormone on phosphate reabsorption in rat distal convolution. *Am J Physiol* 235:321–330, 1978.
220. Beck LH and Goldberg M: Mechanism of the blunted phosphaturia in saline-loaded thyroparathyroidectomized dogs. *Kidney Int* 6:18–23, 1974.
221. Garry PJ, et al: Clinical chemistry reference intervals for healthy elderly subjects. *Am J Clin Nutr* 50:1219–1230, 1989.
222. Cohen SH, et al: Changes in body chemical composition with age measured by total-body neutron activation. *Metabolism* 25:85–95, 1976.
223. Walton RJ and Bijvoet OLM: Normogram for derivation of renal threshold phosphate concentration. *Lancet* 2:309–310, 1975.
224. Bijvoet OLM: Relation of plasma phosphate concentration to renal tubular reabsorption of phosphate. *Clin Sci* 37:23–36, 1969.
225. Kiebzak GM and Saktor B: Effect of age on renal conservation of phosphate in the rat. *Am J Physiol* 251:F399–F407, 1986.
226. Levi M, Jameson DM, and Van Der Meer WB: Role of brush border membrane lipid composition and fluidity in impaired renal Pi transport in aged rats. *Am J Physiol* 256:F85–F94, 1989.
227. Aloia JF, et al: Total body phosphorus in postmenopausal women. *Min Electrol Metab* 10:73–76, 1984.
228. Young MM and Nordin BEC: Some effects of ethinyl oestradiol on calcium and phosphorus metabolism in osteoporosis. *Clin Sci* 34:411–417, 1968.
229. Tschöpe W, et al: Decreased plasma phosphate under hormonal contraceptives. *Min Electrol Metab* 10:88–91, 1984.
230. Betro MG and Pain RW: Hypophosphatemia and hyperphosphatemia in a hospital population. *Br Med J* 1:273–276, 1972.

231. Busse JC, et al: Pseudohyperphosphatemia and dysproteinemia. *Arch Intern Med* 147:2045–2046, 1987.
232. Adler SG, et al: Hyperglobulinemia may seriously elevate measured serum inorganic phosphate levels. *Am J Kidney Dis* II:260–263, 1988.
233. Weinberg J and Adler AJ: Spurious hyperphosphatemia in patients with dysglobulinemia. *Min Electrol Metab* 15:185–186, 1989.
234. Muggia FM, Chia GA, and Mickley DA: Hyperphosphatemia and hypocalcemia in neoplastic disorders. *N Engl J Med* 290:857–858, 1974.
235. Tsokos GC, et al: Renal and metabolic complications of undifferentiated and lymphoblastic lymphomas. *Medicine* 60:218–229, 1981.
236. Goldfinger P: Hypokalemic metabolic acidosis and hypocalcemic tetany in a patient taking laxatives. *J Mt Sinai Hosp* 36:113–116, 1969.
237. Pitts RF, et al: The renal regulation of acid-base balance in man. I: The nature of the mechanism of acidifying the urine. *J Clin Invest* 27:48–61, 1948.
238. Barsotti G, et al: The role of metabolic acidosis in causing uremic hyperphosphatemia. *Min Electrol Metab* 12:103–106, 1986.
239. Larsson L and Sörbo B: Hypophosphatemia: A neglected electrolyte disturbance. *Min Electrol Metab* 6:249A, 1981.
240. Gravelyn TR, et al: Hypophosphatemia-associated respiratory muscle weakness in a general inpatient population. *Am J Med* 84:870–876, 1988.
241. Juan D and Elrazak MA: Hypophosphatemia in hospitalized patients. *JAMA* 242:163–164, 1979.
242. Larsson L, Rebel K, and Sorbo B: Severe hypophosphatemia. A hospital survey. *Acta Med Scand* 214:221–223, 1983.
243. Knochel JP: Hypophosphatemia. *Clin Nephrol* 7:131–137, 1977.
244. King AL, et al: Severe hypophosphatemia in a general hospital population. *South Med J* 80:831–835, 1987.
245. Adler AJ, Gudis S, and Berlyne GM: Reduced renal phosphate threshold concentration in alcoholic cirrhosis. *Min Electrol Metab* 10:63–66, 1984.
246. Kebler R, McDonald FB, and Cadnapaphornchai P: Dynamic changes in serum phosphorus levels in diabetic ketoacidosis. *Am J Med* 79:571–576, 1985.
247. Brautbar N, Leibovici H, and Massry SG: On the mechanism of hypophosphatemia during hyperventilation: Evidence for increased muscle glycolysis. *Min Electrol Metab* 9:45–50, 1983.
248. Ryan EA and Reiss E: Oncogenous osteomalacia. Review of the world literature of 42 cases and report of 2 new cases. *Am J Med* 77:501–512, 1984.
249. Lyles KW, et al: Hypophosphatemic osteomalacia: Association with prostatic carcinoma. *Ann Intern Med* 93:275–278, 1980.
250. Taylor HC, Fallon MD, and Velasco ME: Oncogenic osteomalacia and inappropriate antidiuretic hormone secretion due to oat-cell carcinoma. *Ann Intern Med* 101:786–788, 1984.
251. McClure J and Smith PS: Oncogenic osteomalacia. *J Clin Pathol* 40:446–453, 1987.
252. Mirjauchi A, et al: Hemangiopericytoma-induced osteomalacia: Tumor transplantation in nude mice causes hypophosphatemia, and tumor extracts inhibit renal 25(OH)D 1-alpha-hydroxylase activity. *J Clin Endocrinol Metab* 67:46–53, 1988.
253. Citrin DL, et al: Decreased serum phosphate levels after high dose estrogens in metastatic prostate cancer. Possible implications. *Am J Med* 76:787–793, 1984.
254. Vannatta JB, Whang R, and Papper S: Efficacy of intravenous phosphorus

therapy in the severely hypophosphatemic patient. *Arch Intern Med* 141: 885–887, 1981.

255. Levine BS and Cobern JW: Magnesium, the mimic/antagonist of calcium. *N Engl J Med* 310:1253–1254, 1984.

256. Wacker WEC and Parisi AF: Magnesium metabolism. *N Engl J Med* 278:658–663, 712–717, 772–776, 1968.

257. Seelig MS: Perspectives in nutrition. The requirement of magnesium by the normal adult. *Am J Clin Nutr* 14:342–390, 1964.

258. Brannan PG, et al: Magnesium absorption in the human small intestine. Results in normal subjects, patients with chronic renal disease and patients with absorptive hypercalciuria. *J Clin Invest* 57:1412–1418, 1976.

259. Spencer H, et al: Magnesium absorption and metabolism in patients with chronic renal failure and in patients with normal renal function. *Gastroenterology* 79:26–34, 1980.

260. Massry SG: Pharmacology of magnesium. *Ann Rev Pharmacol Toxicol* 17:67–82, 1977.

261. Rude RK, Bethume JF, and Singer FR: Renal tubular maximum for magnesium in normal, hyperparathyroid and hypoparathyroid man. *J Clin Endocrinol Metab* 51:1425–1431, 1980.

262. Quamme GA and Dirks JH: The physiology of renal magnesium handling. *Renal Physiol* 9:257–259, 1966.

263. Hollifield JW: Magnesium depletion, diuretics and arrhythmias. *Am J Med* 82 (Suppl 3A):30–37, 1987.

264. Lindsay R, Hart DM, and Forrest C: Effect of a natural and artificial menopause on serum, urinary and erythrocyte magnesium. *Clin Sci* 58:255–257, 1980.

265. Keating RF Jr, et al: The relation of age and sex to distribution of values in healthy adults of serum calcium, inorganic phosphorus, magnesium, alkaline phosphatase, total proteins, albumin and blood urea. *J Lab Clin Med* 73:825–834, 1969.

266. McNair P. Christiansen C, and Transbol IB: Effect of menopause and estrogen substitutional therapy on magnesium metabolism. *Min Electrol Metab* 10:84–87, 1984.

267. Wong ET, et al: A high prevalence of hypomagnesemia and hypermagnesemia in hospitalized patients. *Am J Clin Pathol* 79:348–352, 1983.

268. Whang R: Magnesium deficiency: Pathogenesis, prevalence and clinical implications. *Am J Med* 82 (Suppl 3A):24–29, 1987.

269. Smilkstein MJ, et al: Severe hypermagnesemia due to multiple-dose cathartic therapy. *West Med* 148:208–210, 1988.

270. Mordes JP, Swartz R, and Arky RA: Extreme hypermagnesemia as a cause of refractory hypotension. *Ann Intern Med* 83:657–658, 1975.

271. Fassler CA, et al: Mg toxicity as a cause of hypotension and hypoventilation. Occurrence in patients with normal renal function. *Arch Intern Med* 145:1604–1606, 1985.

272. Martin BJ and Milligan K: Diuretic-associated hypomagnesemia in the elderly. *Arch Intern Med* 147:1768–1771, 1987.

273. Fiaccadori E, et al: Muscle and serum magnesium in pulmonary intensive care unit patients. *Crit Care Med* 16:751–760, 1988.

274. Whang R, et al: Predictors of clinical hypomagnesemia. Hypokalemia, hypophosphatemia, hyponatremia and hypocalcemia. *Arch Intern Med* 145:1086–1089, 1985.

275. Petri M, Cumber P, and Grimes L: The metabolic effects of thiazide therapy in the elderly: A population study. *Age Aging* 15:151–155, 1986.

276. Whang R, et al: Magnesium depletion as a cause of refractory potassium repletion. *Arch Intern Med* 145:1086–1089, 1985.
277. Dyckner T and Wester P: Relation between potassium and magnesium in cardiac arrhythmias. *Acta Med Scand* (Suppl) 647:163–169, 1981.
278. Roden DM and Iansmith DHS: Effects of low potassium or magnesium concentrations on isolated cardiac tissue. *Am J Med* 82 (Suppl 3A):18–23, 1987.
279. Schlisky RL and Anderson T: Hypomagnesemia and renal magnesium patients receiving cis-platin. *Ann Intern Med* 90:929–931, 1979.
280. Buckley JE, et al: Hypomagnesemia after cisplatin combination chemotherapy. *Arch Intern Med* 144:2347–2348, 1984.
281. Chernow B, et al: Aminoglycoside induced hypomagnesemia: A prospective study. *Clin Res* 30:863A, 1982.
282. Keating MJ, et al: Hypocalcemia with hypoparathyroidism and renal tubular dysfunction associated with aminoglycoside therapy. *Cancer* 39:1410–1414, 1977.
283. Patel R and Savage A: Symptomatic hypomagnesemia associated with gentamicin therapy. *Nephron* 23:50–52, 1979.
284. Barton CH, et al: Renal magnesium wasting associated with amphotericin B therapy. *Am J Med* 77:471–474, 1984.
285. Sullivan JF, Lankford HG, and Robertson P: Renal excretion of lactate and magnesium in alcoholism. *Am J Clin Nutr* 18:231–237, 1966.
286. Doe RP, Flink EB, and Prased AS: Magnesium metabolism in hyperthyroidism. *J Lab Clin Med* 54:805–810, 1959.
287. Horton R and Biglieri EG: Effect of aldosterone on the metabolism of magnesium. *J Clin Endocrinol Metab* 22:1187–1192, 1962.
288. Oster JR and Epstein M: Management of magnesium depletion. *Am J Nephrol* 8:349–354, 1988.
289. Elin RJ: Magnesium metabolism in health and disease. *DM* 34:166–218, 1988.
290. Ryan MP: Diuretics and potassium/magnesium depletion. Directions for treatment. *Am J Med* 82 (Suppl 3A):38–47, 1987.
291. Dyckner T, Wester PO, and Widman L: Amiloride prevents thiazide-induced intracellular potassium and magnesium losses. *Acta Med Scand* 224:25–30, 1988.

6 PRIMARY GLOMERULAR DISEASE

THE KIDNEY BIOPSY

Because the kidney biopsy is the primary method of diagnosing glomerulonephritis and other parenchymal disease of the kidney, and because there is a general reluctance to perform biopsies in older patients due to a perceived increased risk of complications, we have reviewed our experience in 90 consecutive biopsies performed in patients over the age of 60 between 1968 and 1987. We found a complication rate of 7 percent (of which 80 percent was bleeding), which is similar to the experience of the Mayo Clinic [1]. There were no deaths, but two patients required a nephrectomy because of persistent bleeding.

In an analysis of 1,000 consecutive kidney biopsies at the Mayo Clinic, the incidence of complications was 7.9 percent in the 164 patients 60 years and older, 8.1 percent for the remaining 836 patients, and 8.1 percent for the group as a whole [1]. Bleeding (hematuria, both micro- and macroscopic, or perirenal hematoma) was the most frequently encountered complication (88 percent). Associated conditions such as hypertension and renal insufficiency increased the risk of complications.

INCIDENCE

Primary glomerular diseases are not uncommon in the elderly. Of 379 patients aged 14 to 89 years diagnosed as having a primary glomerular disease in our hospital during the past 20 years, 67 (18 percent) were over 60 years old (Fig. 6-1); this rate is similar to the 19 percent reported by Cameron [2]. Figure 6-2 shows the sex distribution according to age; there were 35 males (52 percent) and 32 females (48 percent). Our indications for kidney biopsy are identical to those reported by others and include significant proteinuria (usually more than 1 g per 24 hours) with or without renal insufficiency in a nondiabetic, unexplained renal failure, and hematuria with renal insufficiency or significant proteinuria. The histopathologic diagnosis in elderly patients with primary glomerular disease derived from our own experience and the literature is shown in Table 6-1.

Proteinuria with or without the nephrotic syndrome, edema, hyper-

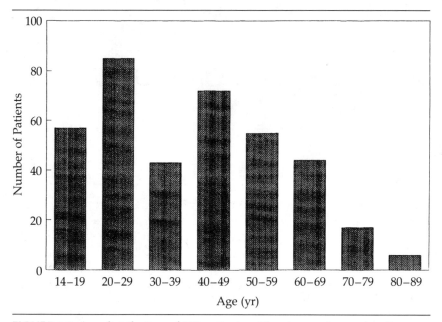

FIGURE 6-1. Age distribution of 379 patients with primary glomerular disease seen at the Brookdale Hospital Medical Center (1968–1987).

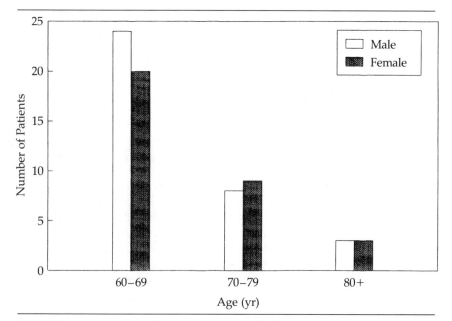

FIGURE 6-2. Age and sex distribution of 67 elderly patients with primary glomerular disease.

TABLE 6-1. The histopathologic diagnosis
in 284 elderly patients with primary glomerular disease

Glomerular disease	No. patients	Percentage (%)
Membranous nephropathy[a]	73	(26)
Extracapillary glomerulonephritis	50	(12)
Minimal change disease	37	(13)
Other proliferative glomerulonephritis[b]	34	(12)
Mesangiocapillary glomerulonephritis	29	(10)
Chronic glomerulonephritis	24	(8)
Focal segmental glomerulosclerosis	24	(8)
Acute endoproliferative glomerulonephritis	13	(5)
	284	(100)

[a] Only patients with idiopathic membranous nephropathy are included.
[b] Including IgA glomerulonephritis and other mesangial proliferative disease as well as focal proliferative glomerulonephritis.

tension, hematuria (gross or microscopic), and renal insufficiency constitute the clinical hallmarks of primary glomerular disease.

PROTEINURIA
In normal adults, protein excretion is usually less than 150 mg per 24 hours. Friedman et al [3] measured 24-hour urine protein excretion in 21 patients over 60 years old and found the same normal range. We studied protein excretion in 40 elderly patients (aged 60 to 90 years) using a single-voided urine sample. A normal protein-creatinine ratio of less than 0.2 as reported by Ginsberg and colleagues [4] was found in all these patients. All of these patients had a serum creatinine of less than 1.5 mg per dl and no evidence of infection, decompensated congestive heart failure, or hypertension.

In experimental studies the following factors have been shown to play a role in the glomerular filtration of protein:

Size
Smaller proteins filter more easily than larger ones. It has been estimated that the normal glomerular capillary wall acts as a membrane that has uniform pores with a radius of approximately 50 Å. Macromolecules that have a molecular radius of less than 24 Å have a clearance identical to that of the glomerular filtration rate, whereas molecules greater than 60 Å are completely excluded from the glomerular filtrate.

Charge
The backbone of the glomerular basement membrane is composed mainly of type IV collagen to which are attached negatively charged

glycoproteins and proteoglycans. Electrostatic interactions at the glomerular capillary wall tend to retard the filtration of polyanions such
as albumin while enhancing the filtration of polycations, as shown by
Rennke et al [5].

Hemodynamic Factors

Conditions associated with a decrease in glomerular plasma flow such as
congestive heart failure are associated with an increase in protein excretion [6]. Molecular configuration may also play a role.

With this background, the specific mechanism or mechanisms responsible for the increased permeability of the glomerular capillary to plasma
protein in different forms of glomerulopathy may be examined. Blau and
Haas [7], using cytochemical techniques, have shown severe depletion
of the fixed negatively charged components of the glomerular capillary
wall in virtually all proteinuric disorders of man. More recently, Myers
and associates [8] have postulated that in patients with selective proteinuria (mostly excreting albumin) there is a loss of the fixed negative
charge in the glomerular wall. In patients with nonselective proteinuria,
the glomerular capillary wall becomes a heteroporous membrane with a
bimodal pore-size distribution; a large-pore ultra-filter develops that is
responsible for the increased filtration of large molecules (such as IgG)
with varying charges [9].

EDEMA

The edema of nephrotic syndrome is due to salt retention with both extrarenal and renal factors implicated in its pathogenesis.

Extrarenal Factors

PLASMA VOLUME. According to the traditional view, hypoalbuminemia,
by lowering the plasma oncotic pressure, favors the movement of water
from the intravascular to the interstitial space, resulting in a decrease in
plasma volume, which then leads to renal salt and water retention. The
plasma volume is usually low in patients with severe hypoalbuminemia
(serum albumin less than 1.0 g per dl); however, in the majority of patients with nephrotic syndrome, the plasma volume is either normal or
increased [10–12]. Furthermore, plasma volume expansion with hyper-
oncotic albumin does not necessarily induce natriuresis [13]. Finally, in
patients with nephrotic syndrome who undergo water immersion, the
urinary excretion of sodium peaks toward the end (third or fourth hour)
of immersion, when volume expansion has presumably been present for
some time [14, 15]. It appears that intravascular hypovolemia per se is
not solely responsible for the salt retention of nephrotic syndrome.

SALT-REGULATING HORMONES. The renin-angiotensin-aldosterone system is frequently activated in patients with nephrotic syndrome; however, it may be normal in a substantial number of patients [16]. Moreover, patients with nephrotic syndrome who are placed on a high-salt diet may continue to retain salt despite a lowering of plasma renin and aldosterone levels [17]. Also, captopril, 50 mg 3 times a day, orally, given to nephrotic patients with elevated plasma aldosterone does not induce natriuresis despite lowering the aldosterone level [18]. Identical results were also reported with infusion of saralasin (an angiotensin II competitive inhibitor that lowers plasma aldosterone) [19].

Many animal studies have confirmed the role of catecholamines in increasing renal sodium reabsorption [20]. Oliver et al [21] found an increase in catecholamine excretion in patients with the nephrotic syndrome. This, however, was not confirmed by Geers and associates [22]. They measured plasma noradrenalin in normal subjects and in patients with nephrotic syndrome and found it identical in both groups.

Since the kidneys play an important role in the catabolism of atrial natriuretic peptides (ANP) [23], the plasma concentration of these peptides tends to vary in direct proportion to the glomerular filtration rate (GFR). In patients with glomerular disease but normal kidney function, plasma ANP is similar to that in normal controls, whereas in those with renal insufficiency the ANP level is increased [24, 25]. During the phase of active renal salt retention in nephrotics, a blunted natriuretic response of the inner medullary collecting duct to ANP has been found [26]. During the maintenance phase of edema or in the nonedematous patient with glomerular disease, the response reverts back to normal [27].

Renal production of prostaglandin E_2, a natriuretic substance, is suppressed in nephrotic patients [28]. The significance of the observation in relation to the salt retention characteristic of nephrotic syndrome is not clear, however.

Renal Factors

The GFR is frequently decreased in patients with the nephrotic syndrome [29], but a significant number of patients with minimal change disease have a normal GFR despite the presence of massive edema. Also, during water immersion, natriuresis may be dissociated from any change in GFR. Using a model of unilateral puromycin aminonucleoside–induced albuminuria in the rat, Ichikawa et al [30] demonstrated that only the proteinuric kidney retained salt, but the specific mechanism responsible for the salt retention was not defined. Using a variety of methods, most investigators have placed the site of increased salt reabsorption in the distal nephron [31]; however, evidence of increased proximal reabsorption has also been provided by Koomans and associates [13].

In summary, the edema and salt retention characteristic of the nephrotic syndrome is the consequence of multiple factors, one or several of which may be present at any time in a given patient. These factors include a decreased plasma volume, the renin-angiotensin-aldosterone system, other vasoactive hormones, a decrease in GFR, and other, still undefined renal mechanisms [30].

HYPERTENSION

Hypertension is frequently present in patients with a glomerular disease. In the majority of these patients renal insufficiency (defined as a serum creatinine greater than 1.5 mg per dl) is present. It has been suggested that the hypertension represents a trade-off necessary for the restoration of sodium balance [32]. Although hypertension is secondary to renal disease in most of these patients, some may have essential hypertension. Also, given the prevalence of atheromatous renovascular disease in the elderly, one should always keep in mind the possibility that the hypertension is secondary to renal artery stenosis, and clues to this diagnosis such as evidence of peripheral vascular disease, an abdominal bruit, or a discrepancy in kidney size should be looked for carefully.

HEMATURIA

Hematuria, either microscopic (more than 5 RBC per high-power field) or macroscopic, is frequently present in patients with glomerular disease. In the elderly, in whom even intermittent hematuria may be due to other serious conditions of the genitourinary tract [33], the decision has to be made whether the red blood cells originate from the glomeruli or from more distal portions of the urinary tract. The presence of red blood casts usually means that the blood comes from the glomeruli. In the absence of casts, red blood cell morphology may help to determine the origin of the cells. More than 90 percent of patients with glomerular disease have distorted, dysmorphic red blood cells in their urine, unlike the more uniform red blood cell morphology found in patients with hematuria due to other causes [34–36]. To evaluate red cell morphology the simple "Sedicolor" staining procedure of the urinary sediment can be used [37]. Briefly, 10 ml of fresh clean-voided urine is centrifuged at 1,500 revolutions per minute for 5 minutes. Two drops of the stain are added to the sediment. Examination is done by light microscopy under oil immersion. It should be noted, however, that a close correlation (as reported above) between red cell morphology and diagnosis has not been found by all observers [38]. Nevertheless, as a rule less than 15 percent of dysmorphic red cells in a sediment specimen makes a renal cause of hematuria unlikely [39]. When in doubt, lesions of the urinary tract should be adequately ruled out using imaging techniques and cystoscopic examination.

SPECIFIC GLOMERULOPATHIES

MEMBRANOUS NEPHROPATHY

Membranous nephropathy is the most common form of primary glomerular disease in the elderly [2, 40–44] (Table 6-1). Of 80 patients with membranous nephropathy seen in our hospital during the past 15 years, 14, or 17.5 percent, were over the age of 60. This proportion is similar to that reported by Noel et al [45], who noted that 21 of 116 patients (18 percent) with membranous nephropathy were over the age of 60. There was a slight preponderance of males over females (57 to 43 percent). In our series, an attempt was made to include only patients with the idiopathic variety; however, it should be emphasized that in certain patients, particularly when the disease is associated with carcinoma, the nephropathy may develop before the underlying disease becomes apparent.

Pathology

LIGHT MICROSCOPY. The characteristic finding is thickening of the glomerular capillary walls. In the early stages of the disease the walls may appear normal, however. By means of special stains (silver, trichrome), the thickening of the basement membrane can be seen to be due to the presence of subepithelial deposits. The mesangium is usually not affected, although in a small percentage of patients mild to moderate cellular proliferation has been described.

ELECTRON MICROSCOPY. The capillary changes have been divided into four stages by Ehrenreich and Churg [46]:

Stage I. This stage is characterized by the presence of small scattered subepithelial electron-dense deposits.
Stage II. The deposits are more numerous and are separated by projections arising from and having the appearance of the lamina densa.
Stage III. The spikes fuse over the deposits incorporating them into the basement membrane.
Stage IV. Most of the deposits disappear, leaving an irregularly thickened lamina densa.

It is possible to see more than one stage in the same biopsy specimen.

FLUORESCENCE MICROSCOPY. Fluorescence microscopy reveals the presence of evenly distributed granular deposits of IgG and C3 along the glomerular capillary wall.

Pathogenesis
The nature and source of the deposits found in patients diagnosed as having idiopathic membranous nephropathy are not clear and are still a matter of controversy. Two major hypotheses have been proposed: circulating immune complexes and in situ immune complexes. In the former the complexes are formed by antibodies of low avidity with an overall cationic charge that become entrapped in the subepithelium [47]. This may account for the infrequent finding of circulating immune complexes by conventional methods in patients with membranous nephropathy. According to the hypothesis of in situ immune complexes, antibody binds to either a fixed glomerular antigen or a planted antigen. Even though there is considerable experimental evidence in favor of this mechanism [48], which is also compatible with the general absence of circulatory immune complexes, the nature of the antigens and antibodies responsible for the human disease remains to be determined.

Clinical Manifestations
Nephrotic syndrome (i.e., proteinuria of more than 3.0 to 3.5 g per 24 hours and hypoalbuminemia) constituted the initial presentation in 91 percent of our elderly patients with membranous nephropathy. The remaining 9 percent had non-nephrotic proteinuria (less than 3.0 g per 24 hours). Renal insufficiency, defined as a serum creatinine of more than 1.5 mg per dl or a creatinine clearance of less than 50 ml per minute, was present in 37 percent of the patients. Examination of the urinary sediment revealed hematuria in 78 percent. Hypertension (blood pressure over 160/90) was detected in 49 percent. There is not enough information in the literature to suggest a specific association between the presence of renal insufficiency and a specific histologic appearance; however, among our 14 patients, all those with a serum creatinine of over 1.5 mg per dl had either stage II or stage III disease. Hypertension was found more frequently in patients with renal failure.

Natural History and Treatment
Because of the varying natural history in patients with idiopathic membranous nephropathy, it has been very difficult to assess the results of therapeutic interventions in this disease. Moreover, there have been no studies specifically addressing the disease in the elderly. In general, membranous nephropathy in adults has the following natural history.

In approximately 25 percent the disease undergoes a spontaneous remission, and in the same percentage persistent proteinuria (usually non-nephrotic range) without progressive renal failure occurs. In the remaining 50 percent of patients renal insufficiency develops, usually progressing slowly (reaching end-stage kidney disease in 20 or more years) but in others progressing relatively rapidly and reaching end-stage renal disease in 5 to 7 years [45].

Patients with less than 2 g of proteinuria per 24 hours tend to do better than those with nephrotic-range proteinuria, and those with more advanced stages of the disease generally do worse. There are many exceptions, however, so that it is not easy to prognosticate. Although there have been suggestions that early glomerular sclerosis, increases in mesangial cellularity, or chronic tubulointerstitial changes may portend a worse prognosis [49], these associations have not been definitely proved. In most reported series in adults, except the one by Davison and co-workers [50] in which older patients fared less well, age per se has not been found to have important prognostic implications, so our approach to the disease in the elderly is similar to that in other adults.

PATIENTS WITH NON-NEPHROTIC PROTEINURIA. Because these patients usually have a benign course, therapy is recommended only for those in whom the disease subsequently progresses to nephrotic proteinuria or who develop renal failure (approximately 20 percent) [51].

PATIENTS WITH NEPHROTIC SYNDROME AND NORMAL GFR. Since the results of the U.S. collaborative study have shown better results in steroid-treated patients [52], we administer a two-month course of alternate-day prednisone (125 mg orally) with tapering on a weekly or biweekly basis for two additional months. If there is a relapse or an exacerbation, we re-treat. We have not encountered any significant side effects in the elderly using this regimen during the past several years.

Ponticelli and colleagues [53] have also shown benefits from therapy in a controlled, prospective study. Their regimen consists of a 3-day course of 1 g of methylprednisolone administered intravenously followed by oral methylprednisolone, 0.4 mg per kg per day, for 27 days (cycle A), alternating with chlorambucil, 0.2 mg per kg per day, for 1 month (cycle B). These cycles are repeated 3 times for a total treatment period of 6 months. The incidence of remission in terms of proteinuria in patients with a serum creatinine of less than 1.7 mg per dl was significantly higher in the treated group. Two of their treated patients were over the age of 60. One was still nephrotic after 1 year of follow-up, and the other had a relapse after 5 years of sustained remission. No significant side effects were noted. A follow-up study of these patients, some of whom have had repeated kidney biopsies, has been reported recently

[54, 55]. It appears that this treatment schedule increases the likelihood of remission, complete or partial.

PATIENTS WITH RENAL INSUFFICIENCY. There are no published results of a prospective study in this patient group. A striking finding in our retrospective analysis was that none of the untreated patients had a remission of proteinuria, and in 92 percent the renal failure was progressive [51]. In the treated group, by contrast, 53 percent had complete or partial remission or improved renal function, whereas renal function became progressively worse in 37 percent. Based on these findings, we recommended an initial course of prednisone, as described earlier. If well tolerated, the prednisone may be continued for a longer period of time, with tapering of the dose depending on the response. Whether the addition of a cytotoxic drug to the prednisone in the unresponsive patient will be beneficial is not yet known.

It should be cautioned that the therapeutic regimen outlined above represents the authors' views, and many authorities still do not consider steroid therapy with or without the addition of cytotoxic agents beneficial in patients with membranous nephropathy [56–58]. Based on current available data [51], we do not recommend the use of cytotoxic agents alone in the therapy of the disease; however, in a recently published prospective study, cyclophosphamide (mean 1.5 mg per kg per day for a 23-month period) was found to be of benefit [59]. Six of the nine treated patients did receive glucocorticoid (five received it concomitantly with the cyclophosphamide), however.

So far we have discussed patients with the idiopathic form of the disease. It should be noted that in 15 percent of patients with membranous nephropathy a variety of infections, multisystemic diseases, neoplasms, or drugs may be associated with the disease, and these will be dealt with in another section of this chapter.

EXTRACAPILLARY GLOMERULONEPHRITIS

Incidence
Extracapillary or crescentic glomerulonephritis was found in 18 percent of reported elderly patients with primary glomerular disease who underwent biopsy (see Table 6-1). A significant percentage of patients with crescentic disease originally classified as idiopathic may at a later time develop clinical evidence of a systemic vasculitis [60, 61]. (See Chap. 7.)

Pathology
The light microscopic findings are identical in all the patients and are characterized by epithelial cell proliferation and mononuclear and polymorphonuclear cell infiltration during the active phase of the disease.

These cells eventually disappear as the crescents become fibrous. Tubular degeneration may be present. On electron microscopy fibrin is seen in Bowman's space or the capillary lumen. The capillary walls may show "breaks" in the areas of crescents or elsewhere. On occasion translucent deposits may occupy the lamina rara interna. Frequently no deposits are seen. On the basis of fluorescent microscopy, idiopathic crescentic glomerulonephritis can usually be subdivided into two groups. In one group there is linear capillary wall staining with IgG and C3. In the other there is granular capillary wall or mesangial staining with a variety of immunoglobulins and C3. Actually, there is a third group in whom no staining is seen with immunoglobulins or C3. Whether these latter patients comprise a distinct group is still a matter of controversy [62–64], as is the frequency and the significance of this finding. In all patients fibrin is seen in Bowman's space, the crescents, and the capillary tufts.

In the elderly, either no deposits or granular deposits are seen approximately 3 times more often than linear deposits of immunoglobulins, which are most commonly found in Goodpasture's syndrome and represent deposits of antiglomerular basement membrane (anti-GBM) antibodies [65, 66].

Pathogenesis
The mechanism responsible for the development of anti-GBM antibody in patients with linear deposits is not clear. The proposed hypotheses have been summarized by Lewis and Schwartz [67] and include release into the systemic circulation of cross-reacting endogenous nonrenal antigen (alveolar basement membrane) or exogenous antigen (microorganisms), which elicits an immune response at the glomerular level, or an abnormality (congenital or acquired) in the antigenic structure of the glomerular basement membrane that leads to antibody formation.

Whatever the pathogenic mechanism, there is experimental evidence that complement and leukocytes participate in the clinical manifestations of the disease [68]. Leukocyte depletion with irradiation can prevent the decrease in the ultrafiltration coefficient (LpA or Kf) and single-nephron GFR in a rat model of antiglomerular basement membrane antibody nephritis [69]. Locally produced lytic factors have also been found to participate in the damage to the glomerular basement membrane [70].

For those patients with granular or no deposits, the pathogenesis of the disease is even less clear; however, there is experimental evidence that suggests that soluble immune complexes that do not deposit in glomeruli may be primary mediators of damage to the glomeruli [71]. Also, as noted by Cohen et al [64], the absence of deposits at the time of biopsy does not necessarily rule out a pathologic process involving humoral immunity. Indeed, Olsen and associates [72] reported a patient in whom the initial biopsy was free of deposits, but 12 days later a nephrectomy specimen disclosed granular deposits of immunoglobulins and complement.

Clinical Manifestations

As noted earlier, the presence of linear deposits on biopsy is less common in the elderly. Of 17 such patients reported in the literature, nine were males and eight were females. Acute renal failure was the initial presentation in all patients, with pulmonary hemorrhage a less frequent occurrence. All patients had hematuria (microscopic or macroscopic) with red blood cell casts. Protein excretion generally ranged between 500 to 1,000 mg per 24 hours. One patient had a history of hydrocarbon exposure [62, 64, 73–76].

In 50 elderly patients gleaned from the literature who had granular or no deposits, there were 30 males and 20 females. The most common presentation was acute renal failure (78 percent), and the patients usually complained of malaise and gross hematuria. All the patients had macroscopic or microscopic hematuria with or without RBC casts. Twenty-two percent had chronic renal failure, and 10 percent had hypertension. Protein excretion ranged between 200 and 3,000 mg per 24 hours [62–64, 73, 74, 77–81].

Natural History and Treatment

It is very difficult to decide whether or not treatment is beneficial in the elderly with crescentic disease because there is still no reported double-blind prospective study comparing any given therapeutic regimen with no therapy. In general, older patients do worse than younger ones [65, 82]. In most series therapy has not been uniform. Although the great majority of patients reported received some form of treatment, in those with granular or no deposits 74 percent either died or were placed on dialysis in a relatively short period of time (weeks to months). The remaining 26 percent either recovered renal function or had stable chronic renal insufficiency. The outcome appears to be just as severe in patients with linear deposits, although the number of such elderly patients reported is quite small. The presence of oliguria, a high percentage of crescents on initial renal biopsy, and high entry serum creatinine levels are usually associated with a poor outcome.

Even though there is no proof that therapy alters the course of the disease, most authors suggest early institution of intensive plasma exchange and immunosuppression for patients with antiglomerular basement membrane antibody disease (linear deposits). Johnson et al [83] used 4 liters exchange with type-specific frozen plasma together with saline or a saline-albumin solution every 3 days. Plasma exchange was continued until the anti-GBM antibody titer was less than 5 percent binding or the patient required maintenance hemodialysis for longer than 30 days. Alternate-day or daily exchange regimens have also been used. Immunosuppressive treatment usually consists of predisone, 2 mg per kg daily for 1 week, followed by 1 mg per kg daily for the next 3 weeks, and then tapered to alternate-day dosage for the next 3 months. In addition, cyclophosphamide, 2 mg per kg per day, is frequently recommended.

Episodes of pulmonary hemorrhage are best managed with high-dose intravenous prednisone (30 mg per kg to a maximum single dose of 3 g) infused over 20 minutes on alternate days for three treatments (1 g can also be used on a daily basis for 3 days). Attention should be paid to avoiding volume overload and treating superimposed infection because these factors have been shown to precipitate hemorrhage [75].

In the majority of elderly patients with granular or no deposits on biopsy, high-dose intravenous methylprednisolone followed by maintenance oral therapy (see regimen described earlier) is the preferred treatment [65, 78–80].

More recently, Niva and colleagues [84], in a preliminary report, have noted a beneficial effect of prostaglandin E_1 infusion in patients with crescentic glomerulonephritis.

MINIMAL CHANGE GLOMERULOPATHY (LIPOID NEPHROSIS)

Incidence
Minimal change disease is found in 13 percent of elderly patients with primary glomerular disease (Table 6-1).

Pathology
On light microscopy the glomeruli appear normal, although the mesangium may be slightly widened with increased matrix and a mild increase in mesangial cells. Completely sclerosed glomeruli are frequently present and at times may be quite significant (see Chap. 1). The tubules exhibit the usual findings of nephrotic syndrome—i.e., hyaline casts, hyaline droplets in the cytoplasm, and small areas of calcification. On electron microscopy the main finding is the loss or effacement (fusion) of the foot processes of the epithelial cells. This is a nonspecific finding seen in all forms of glomerular disease.

Immunofluorescence microscopy is usually completely negative. On occasion, a small amount of immunoglobulin such as IgM may be found in the mesangium. The significance of such deposits is a matter of controversy. It is not clear whether these patients should be classified as having mesangial nephritis (see following section, "Diffuse Mesangial or Focal Proliferative Glomerulonephritis") or considered a special category of minimal change disease with a different and worse prognosis. There are arguments on both sides [85, 86].

Pathogenesis
Increased suppressor cell function has been found in patients in relapse with minimal change disease [87]. The activity of one of the products of the activated suppressor T cell, the lymphokine-soluble immune response suppressor (SIRS), has been found to be increased in the urine of patients with minimal change disease that disappears after steroid treatment [88]. Whether these lymphokines are responsible for the generalized loss of the membrane negative charge reported in patients with minimal change disease [89] is not clear, but there is experimental evidence that lymphocytes may mediate depletion of glomerular polyanion [90]. Some type of allergic manifestation is found in 40 to 70 percent of patients with minimal change disease [91]. Indeed, serum IgE is frequently increased in these patients. Such patients, after exposure to a contact allergen, demonstrate lymphocyte (T or B cell?) stimulation, with subsequent production of a lymphokine. The latter has been named the vascular permeability factor; its exact role in modifying the sialoproteins of glomerular capillary walls is not known.

Clinical Manifestations
In an experimental model of minimal change disease (puromycin-induced proteinuria) GFR was decreased, apparently secondary to a decrease in the surface areas available for filtration (Kf or LpA) [92]. In patients with minimal change disease a strong inverse correlation between GFR and the degree of foot process fusion was found by Bohman et al [93], lending support to the possibility that in the human disease the decreased GFR may also be due to a decrease in Kf. A similar conclusion has been reached by Bridges and colleagues [94]. Since the effective pore size was not changed, these authors concluded that the decreased Kf most likely represents a reduction in the number of pores. Patients with minimal change disease have a reduction in the concentration of fixed negative charges in the glomerular membrane. Therefore, the proteinuria appears to be mainly a consequence of defective electrostatic function of the glomerular barrier to protein filtration [95].

In 44 elderly patients reported from the literature with minimal change disease, 26 (59 percent) were males, and all had proteinuria in the nephrotic range [40, 41, 43, 96–99]. Microscopic hematuria was seen in 8 (18 percent), hypertension in 31 (71 percent), and renal insufficiency in 18 (41 percent).

Natural History and Treatment
The prognosis of minimal change disease in the elderly is rather good in terms of progression to end-stage kidney disease. In our experience and that of others the response to immunosuppressive therapy tends to be slower compared to that in younger patients [100, 101]. The survival of elderly patients was only 50 percent at 10 years in the series of Nolasco

and colleagues [100]; however, only 5 of 15 deaths were related to complications of the nephrotic syndrome per se. From an analysis of the reported cases there is a 9 percent rate of spontaneous remission. The high incidence of ischemic changes found on biopsy by Cameron et al [98] in their patients 60 years and older did not seem to have any prognostic significance. Moreover, this histologic picture has not been universally observed [40, 41].

Eighty-seven percent of patients treated with steroids or cytotoxic agents (cyclophosphamide, azathioprine, chlorambucil) undergo complete remission; however, among these, 35 percent have one or more relapses at varying intervals (sometimes several years later). A subsequent course of therapy usually again induces a remission. Generally, long-lasting therapy is well tolerated by the elderly. Based on these data, we recommend an 8-week course of prednisone (60 mg daily) followed by tapering over a 4-week period. In those patients who fail to respond to this regimen, we usually continue therapy for at least 4 months. If the patient does not have a remission or manifests severe steroid side effects such as proximal muscle weakness, cyclophosphamide (3 mg per kg per day for 8 weeks) can be used, usually with rather good results [100]. There is not enough experience with azathioprine or chlorambucil in the elderly with minimal change disease to recommend their routine use.

DIFFUSE MESANGIAL OR FOCAL PROLIFERATIVE GLOMERULONEPHRITIS

Incidence

Diffuse mesangial or focal proliferative glomerulonephritis was found in 12 percent of patients (see Table 6-1). The majority of these patients were reported by Kingswood et al [41], who classified 17 patients as having diffuse mesangial proliferative and 10 with focal segmental glomerulonephritis. Only two of the patients in the series of Zech and colleagues [43] and seven in Moorthy and Zimmerman's series [40] had mesangial proliferative glomerulonephritis. We have rarely found this form of glomerulonephritis in elderly patients. There are several possible reasons for this disparity. Most of these patients probably have IgA nephropathy, and this disease is known to have an irregular geographic distribution, with a higher incidence in Asia and Europe [102]. In fact, Kingswood's patients [41] were from the United Kingdom, where IgA nephropathy is relatively common [103]. Because hematuria is one of the most common clinical manifestations of mesangial nephritis, which is more common in males, it is quite possible that some elderly male patients with the disease may be labeled as prostatic bleeders. Thus, the true incidence of diffuse mesangial or focal proliferative glomerulonephritis in the elderly is not known.

Mesangial nephritis consists of a heterogeneous group of diseases in which IgA, IgM, or C3 may be seen in the mesangium with a varying degree of electron-dense deposits [104, 105]. Since IgA nephropathy is the most common form of the disease and the best studied, the following discussion will deal mainly with this form of mesangial proliferative nephritis. Among 244 adult patients with mesangial IgA nephropathy reported by Nicholls et al [106], nine (3.7 percent) were over the age of 60. In Clarkson et al's series of 50 patients [107], four (8 percent) were over the age of 60, a figure similar to the incidence reported by Neela-Kantappa et al [108]. Boyce and colleagues [109] found that 14 percent of patients were over the age of 60. Eighty-three percent of elderly patients with IgA nephropathy are males [106–109].

Pathology

According to Sinniah (110), the pathology of mesangial nephritis can be classified as follows:

Class I. Minimal lesions appearing "normal" on light microscopy.

Class II. Minor changes with widening of the mesangium and increased cellularity in groups of up to three cells per area in the periphery of the glomerulus.

Class III. Focal and segmental glomerulonephritis with less than 50 percent of the glomeruli showing localized or segmental sclerosis and mesangial cell proliferation; the remaining glomeruli show minor changes only.

Class IV. Diffuse mesangial cell proliferation. Segmental crescents may be found.

Class V. Diffuse sclerosing glomerulonephritis in which more than 80 percent of the glomeruli are involved.

Focal interstitial edema with lymphocytic cell infiltrates may also be present, as well as fibrosis, which varies with the severity of the glomerular lesions. In patients with IgA nephropathy, C3, IgM, or IgG may also be present along the glomerular capillary wall, a finding associated with a rather poor prognosis [111, 112].

A modified classification with only three stages of disease has been published more recently [109]:

Class I. Mesangial matrix expansion alone.

Class II. Diffuse or focal segmental mesangial cell proliferation.

Class III. Diffuse or focal segmental mesangial proliferation with or without segmental necrosis, synechiae, sclerosis, or crescent formation.

Pathogenesis

As with other glomerular diseases, the pathogenesis of IgA nephropathy is still not clear; however, increased levels of IgA have been found in the plasma in more than 20 percent of the patients [113]. This finding suggests that in these immunologically susceptible patients a specific clone (or clones) of lymphocytes produces an increased amount of IgA when challenged with an exogenous antigen (e.g., virus or bacteria); the resulting antigen-antibody complexes are deposited in the mesangium [113]. The nature of the genetic defect and the reason for the mesangial location of the immune complexes are not clear, although factors such as the multimeric nature of IgA, the formation of IgA complexes, and the anionic charge of IgA have been suggested as possibilities [114]. Also, there remains the possibility that the whole reaction may be secondary to the formation of in situ immune complexes in response to planted or "trapped" antigens.

Clinical Manifestations
Indications for kidney biopsy in 36 elderly patients reported in the different series described above were nephrotic syndome (15 patients), proteinuria or hematuria (13 patients), acute renal failure (5 patients), and chronic renal failure (5 patients). It is not clear whether the episodes of acute renal failure were reversible or whether the renal failure was associated with bouts of macroscopic hematuria, as recently reported [15].

Natural History and Treatment
The natural history of mesangial nephritis in the elderly has not been adequately studied. According to Kobayashi and associates [111], patients with renal failure at the time of biopsy are usually older. Also, factors such as hypertension, severe histologic grade, and the presence of nephrotic syndrome, which are known to alter the course of the disease unfavorably, have been found with higher frequency in older patients [106–108, 115–119]. Thus, it appears that the disease has a worse prognosis when it is discovered in the elderly.

Because of the probable role of IgA in the pathogenesis of the disease and the known effect of phenytoin in reducing serum IgA levels, this drug has been tried but has shown no apparent therapeutic success [120, 121]. This may be explained by the absence of any effect of this drug on IgA-containing circulating immune complexes [122].

Mustonen et al [123], Kobayashi et al [124], and Lai et al [118] reported remissions in patients with proteinuria and IgA nephropathy treated with corticosteroids. Brown et al [125] noted a similar beneficial response to steroids, reporting complete remission in 10 of 12 patients with mesangial proliferative glomerulonephritis.

Given the fact that most elderly patients with mesangial nephritis present with nephrotic syndrome and that a short course of steroids (8–12 weeks of 120 mg given on alternate days) is usually well tolerated in this age group, we suggest that such a course be tried unless class V disease is found on biopsy, keeping in mind that evidence of long-term benefit is lacking. Plasma exchange and large-dose steroids have also been tried in patients with crescentic disease [126, 127], as has dipyridamole (300 mg per day), danazole (200 mg per day), and cyclosporine [128, 129]. Only a small number of patients have been treated, so no definite comment can be made about the therapeutic benefit of these agents. The acute renal failure that occurs during episodes of macroscopic hematuria tends to be reversible and should be managed with supportive therapy, dialysis when indicated, and antibiotics when bacterial infection is present.

MESANGIOCAPILLARY (MEMBRANOPROLIFERATIVE) GLOMERULONEPHRITIS

Incidence
As shown in Table 6-1, mesangiocapillary glomerulonephritis was present in 10 percent of elderly patients with primary glomerular disease. Although this form of primary glomerulonephritis is seen predominantly in the second and third decades of life [130], our experience has been somewhat different. Of the 22 adults with idiopathic mesangiocapillary glomerulonephritis in our series of primary glomerular disease, 11 (50 percent) were over the age of 60. The reason for this discrepancy is not clear; however, a high incidence (27 percent) of mesangiocapillary glomerulonephritis was also reported by Nuñez et al [131] in their series of 74 patients over the age of 50 with a primary glomerulopathy.

Pathology
Mesangiocapillary glomerulonephritis has been divided into three different types.

TYPE I. Light microscopy reveals the presence of increased mesangial cells and matrix. Polymorphonuclear leukocytes may be present, often in large numbers. One characteristic feature of the disease is the thickening of the capillary wall, which on special stains such as periodic acid-Schiff (PAS) has a "double contour," i.e., two dark lines separated by a pale zone. Crescents are also commonly present. On electron microscopy one sees increased cells, matrix, and electron-dense deposits in the expanded mesangium. Deposits may also be seen in the subendothelial space. On immunofluorescence IgG and C3 may be found.

TYPE II. This disease is also called "dense deposit disease" because of the presence of electron-dense deposits in the lamina densa of the capillary basement membrane. Deposits may also be seen in the mesangium. On immunofluorescence microscopy the most constant finding is the extensive deposition of C3 in the mesangium. The light microscopic changes are similar to those seen in type I.

TYPE III. This is a variant of type I mesangiocapillary glomerulonephritis and is characterized by the presence of extensive subepithelial deposits with intervening projections of basement membrane–like material in conjunction with the lesions described for type I disease [132]. On immunofluoresence microscopy, C3 is almost invariably present in a granular pattern along the capillary wall. Other components of the complement cascade (C1q, C4, C2) may also be present along with immunoglobulins of the IgG, IgM, or IgA types.

There are not enough data in the literature concerning the incidence of type II mesangiocapillary glomerulonephritis in the elderly, although some of the patients described by Cameron and associates [130] were over the age of 55. In any case, type II disease is rare in the elderly, and most (if not all) elderly patients with mesangiocapillary glomerulonephritis have type I disease.

Pathogenesis

The pathogenesis of mesangiocapillary glomerulonephritis is not known. Since circulating immune complexes have been found in some patients with the disease [133, 134], an immune mechanism seems likely. The specific antigen responsible for the activation of the process has not yet been identified. Whatever the precise mechanism might be, the complement system is probably involved, with activation of both the classic and alternate pathways [135, 136].

Clinical Manifestations

Nephrotic syndrome was the initial clinical manifestation in 9 of our 11 patients (six females, five males), and acute nephritis was the first sign in the remaining two. Hematuria with red blood cell casts was present in every patient. Seven were hypertensive. Renal insufficiency of varying severity was found in eight patients. Complement levels (C3 and C4) were measured in nine patients; all had a normal C3, and C4 was normal in seven and decreased in two.

Natural History and Therapy

Mesangiocapillary glomerulonephritis usually progresses to end-stage renal failure; however, the clinical course is extremely variable. Therefore, the efficacy of a therapeutic regimen becomes difficult to assess unless one is dealing with a well-controlled prospective study involving a large number of patients followed for a long period of time.

All of our 11 patients were treated with corticosteriods (60 mg per day) for long periods of time (6 months to 1 year), with follow-up varying from 1 to 10 years. Two patients have moderate renal insufficiency after 10 years of follow-up. Five patients reached end-stage renal disease in 6 months to 3 years. Four were lost to follow-up after approximately 1 year and were still nephrotic with renal insufficiency at the time of last follow-up.

Two prospective studies dealing with therapy of mesangiocapillary glomerulonephritis have appeared recently. Zimmerman et al [137] reported a trial of warfarin (at a dose adjusted to keep the prothrombin time 1.5 to 2 times the control value) and dipyridamole (100 mg 4 times a day). Thirteen patients served as their own control, having had both a control and a treatment year. The age of the patients was 28.5 ± 4.5. The treatment appeared to slow the rate of decline in GFR and decreased the proteinuria. Bleeding complications were rather high, with one death from an intracerebral hemorrhage and two serious bleeding episodes. Given the propensity for the elderly to develop subdural hematomas and other bleeding complications, such therapy should probably be avoided in patients over the age of 60.

In the second study, reported from the Mayo Clinic, dipyridamole, 75 mg, and aspirin, 325 mg, were administered one-half hour before meals 3 times daily for 1 year [138]. GFR (estimated by iothalamate clearance) was better maintained in the treated group, although no difference could be found between groups in the level of proteinuria, degree of hematuria, urinary sediment, or serum complement levels. The treated patients varied in age from 6 to 72 years. Treatment was well tolerated by most patients without any major bleeding complications.

Because the latter regimen was so well tolerated, we think it is worth trying in the elderly patient with mesangiocapillary glomerulonephritis. One should keep in mind that longer follow-up is needed before a definite conclusion can be reached about the efficacy of these drugs in altering the long-term natural history of type I mesangiocapillary glomerulonephritis. It should be emphasized that because this therapy was used in patients with rather well-preserved kidney function, it is not clear whether those who already have renal insufficiency at the time of diagnosis will be equally benefitted.

FOCAL SEGMENTAL GLOMERULOSCLEROSIS

Incidence

Focal segmental glomerulosclerosis was present in 8 percent of elderly patients with primary glomerular disease who underwent biopsy (Table 6–1). This glomerulopathy is much more common in younger patients; for example, of 40 patients from the Mayo Clinic with focal glomerulosclerosis only 2 were over the age of 60 [139].

Pathology

Light microscopy of these lesions is characterized by focal mesangial expansion and collapse of the capillaries. The sclerotic lesions involve only a portion of the glomerular tuft (segmental), most often in the juxtamedullary glomeruli. The areas of sclerosis contain hyaline material, and the sclerotic segment is frequently adherent to Bowman's capsule. The percentage of involved glomeruli varies according to the severity of the disease. Tubular atrophy, interstitial fibrosis, and inflammatory cells are commonly present. On electron microscopy, there is foot process fusion, capillary collapse, and areas of epithelial detachment with formation of subepithelial zones containing fibrillar material. Electron-dense deposits may be found in the mesangium or in the subendothelial or intraluminal space. On immunofluorescence microscopy, most often no immune deposits are found; when present, they are seen in the sclerotic areas and in the mesangium of the affected glomeruli, with IgM and C3 the most common constituents.

Pathogenesis

Focal glomerulosclerosis is the most common isolated glomerular disease in drug addicts and patients with human immunodeficiency virus (HIV) infections [140]. It also is the histologic picture seen in patients with nephrotic syndrome associated with reflux nephropathy [141]. The remaining patients are usually classified as having the "idiopathic" form of the disease, which is the predominant form of focal glomerulosclerosis seen in the elderly. The pathogenesis of this disease is unknown; however, the fact that it can recur early after renal transplantation suggests that a humoral factor is responsible, at least in some patients [142]. Abnormalities of cell-mediated immunity such as increased concanavalin A–induced suppressor cell activity have been described [143]. Whether these activated cells secrete a lymphokine capable of injuring the glomerulus is not clear. Genetic factors or overloading of phagocytic mechanisms in the mesangium, with sclerotic glomerular lesions a consequence of increased glomerular permeability, may also play a role [142]. There is controversy over whether focal glomerulosclerosis represents a specific disease entity or a variant of minimal change disease [105].

Clinical Manifestations

In the 29 elderly patients with focal glomerulosclerosis culled from the literature and combined with our own experience, 19 (66 percent) were males [41, 43, 139, 144]. Twenty-two (76 percent) had hypertension, and 22 (76 percent) had renal insufficiency (serum creatinine greater than 1.5 mg per dl). The decrease in GFR in patients with focal glomerulosclerosis has been attributed to a reduction in the filtering surface area.

The proteinuria, which consists mainly of albumin, is thought to be secondary to a defect in the electrostatic barrier due to a depletion of glomerular polyanion [145].

Natural History and Treatment

Age per se has been found in one study [146] but not in others [147–149] to affect the prognosis negatively. The presence of renal insufficiency, large amounts of proteinuria, and severe tubulointerstitial changes at the time of diagnosis are usually associated with progressive renal failure [147–150]. Since 76 percent of the elderly patients with focal glomerulosclerosis referred to earlier presented with both nephrotic-range proteinuria and renal insufficiency, the prognosis appears to be poor in this age group. In the series of Beaufils et al [151], which included younger patients, the incidence of nephrotic-range proteinuria was 56 percent, compared with non-nephrotic proteinuria of 56 to 44 percent. These authors noted a 10-year renal survival rate of only 45 percent in the group with nephrotic syndrome compared to 91 percent in those with non-nephrotic proteinuria. Such data are unfortunately not available in the elderly.

Some adult patients with focal segmental glomerulosclerosis and nephrotic proteinuria respond to corticosteroids. Those who respond usually have a significantly more favorable prognosis than nonresponders and patients who are not treated [148, 149]. Since at present there are no clinical or histologic grounds on which to predict who will respond, our approach is to administer a short course of prednisone, 120 mg on alternate days for 8 weeks followed by gradual tapering, to every elderly patient with focal glomerulosclerosis and nephrotic proteinuria unless it is absolutely contraindicated. This regimen, as previously noted, is relatively well tolerated. Thirty percent of our patients responded with a decrease in proteinuria below 1 g. Various other drugs, namely chlorambucil, cyclophosphamide, azathioprine, and cyclosporine have been tried in patients with focal glomerulosclerosis resistant to corticosteroids [152]. Their use in the elderly is rather limited and therefore cannot be recommended.

More recently, meclofenamate, a nonsteroidal anti-inflammatory agent, has been tried in 16 patients with focal glomerulosclerosis who have shown persistent nephrotic syndrome after having received daily prednisone (1 mg per kg body weight) for at least 6 weeks [153]. The starting dose is 50 mg orally twice a day, gradually increasing to 50 mg every 6 hours. Eight patients were classified as responders (a 40 percent or greater decrease in protein excretion) and six as nonresponders. Drug side effects, requiring discontinuance of the therapy, developed in the remaining two patients. The rationale for using meclofenamate in preference to other nonsteroidal anti-inflammatory drugs has been reviewed

[154]. The drug not only inhibits the synthesis of prostaglandins but also may block the prostaglandin receptors of the effector cells. Furthermore, meclofenamate can block the increase in capillary permeability that usually follows administration of the so-called vascular permeability factor, which has been isolated from patients with minimal change disease (see section on minimal change disease).

These results are encouraging, and a prospective double-blind study with a large number of patients appears worthwhile. One should remember, however, that the elderly are more susceptible to serious side effects from nonsteroidal anti-inflammatory agents than younger patients and will require close follow-up if such therapy is undertaken.

CHRONIC GLOMERULONEPHRITIS
Twenty-four patients (8 percent of reported elderly with glomerular disease) were diagnosed as having nonclassifiable chronic glomerulonephritis (Table 6-1). This does not represent the true incidence of this entity in the elderly because patients with the same clinical picture who have small kidneys at the time of diagnosis usually do not undergo biopsy. Histologically, the diagnosis of chronic glomerulonephritis is made when there is so much scarring that the original disease is no longer discernible. The glomeruli are sclerosed with extensive tubular atrophy associated with interstitial fibrosis and lymphocytic infiltration. On electron microscopy, basement membrane wrinkling is usually seen. There is no constant pattern as far as the presence of immunoglobulins and complement are concerned.

Clinical Manifestations
Renal insufficiency of varying severity and proteinuria (more than 2 g per 24 hours) were present in all our patients at time of diagnosis. Seventy-five percent of them were also hypertensive. Hematuria was found in 20 percent.

Natural History and Treatment
The disease is usually progressive, and management is identical to that for any patient with chronic renal insufficiency (see Chap. 11).

ACUTE ENDOPROLIFERATIVE GLOMERULONEPHRITIS

Incidence
Acute endoproliferative glomerulonephritis accounts for the remaining 5 percent of elderly patients with primary glomerular disease (Table 6-1).

Pathology
On light microscopy all glomeruli exhibit diffuse endothelial cell proliferation. There is also increased cellularity, with both mononuclear

cells and polymorphonuclear leukocytes. Crescent formation and adhesions between the loops and Bowman's capsule may be present. On immunofluorescence microscopy, granular deposits of complement and frequently immunoglobulins (IgG) are found. Electron microscopy is characterized by the presence of subepithelial electron-dense, humplike deposits.

Pathogenesis
The current evidence strongly suggests that acute endoproliferative glomerulonephritis is an immune complex disease. Serum complement level is depressed in the majority of the patients, with a pattern suggesting activation of the alternate pathway; C4 is normal in all patients and C3 is depressed in over 85 percent [155, 156]. Circulating immune complexes, as measured by C1q-binding activity, have been found in the serum of two-thirds of the patients in the first week of the disease [157, 158]. The antigen responsible for the disease (which is supposedly of bacterial origin) could induce disease by stimulating antibody production, with the resulting antigen-antibody complex deposited in the glomerulus, or the antigen could be planted in the glomerulus, triggering an in situ immune reaction [159]. Factors such as electrical charge could influence the location of the antigen [160].

A role for antiglobulin antibodies has been postulated, but the exact mechanism whereby immunoglobulins become autoantigenic is not clear. Circulating anti-immunoglobulins have been detected in the serum in a large percentage of patients with acute poststreptococcal glomerulonephritis [161].

Clinical Manifestations
The clinical manifestations of the disease in the elderly do not differ from those seen in other age groups [162]. A history of antecedent streptococcal infection can be elicited from most of the patients (83 percent), with pharyngeal involvement in 50 percent and skin involvement in 33 percent. In 17 percent a nonstreptococcal infection precedes the onset (usually pulmonary). Heart failure constitutes the initial presentation in 40 percent of the elderly. Renal insufficiency of varying severity is present in more than 90 percent, and hypertension is present in 83 percent. Hematuria, either microscopic or macroscopic, is a universal finding, as is proteinuria. The latter varies in degree from non-nephrotic (74 percent) to nephrotic levels (26 percent). ASO titer is elevated in only 56 percent of patients [155, 163–167]. The relatively low incidence of an elevated ASO titer may be related to the fact that when the streptococcal infection originates in the skin the antibody response may be blunted, and the ASO titer may not rise because of binding of antigen by lipids present in the skin [168]. According to Montoliu et al [169], the immune

response to deoxyribonuclease B is more constant and diagnostically helpful. As noted earlier, serum C4 is usually normal, whereas C3 is depressed in more than 85 percent of patients.

Clinical Course

Severe azotemia may occur in the elderly with acute endocapillary glomerulonephritis, with a significant number of the patients requiring dialytic intervention, most frequently for control of fluid overload [163–167, 170]. The course can be protracted, lasting weeks or months; however, the prognosis is usually good, with clinical recovery being the rule, and only a minority of patients are left with mild to moderate impairment of kidney function, particularly those who present initially with the nephrotic syndrome [171]. Therefore, an aggressive approach should be adopted and dialysis used as necessary to sustain these patients through the acute phase of their illness.

If a patient is seen early in the course of the disease or if streptococci are recovered from the throat or skin, penicillin or one of its derivatives should be administered. Antibiotics are not necessary for patients seen late or for those who have negative cultures. Fluid and sodium restriction and bed rest are usual until signs of circulatory overload disappear. Blood pressure and serum potassium must be monitored regularly (particularly when the patient is oliguric), and hypertension and hyperkalemia must be treated. Corticosteroid therapy is not recommended in the management of patients with acute endoproliferative glomerulonephritis.

SPECIAL PROBLEMS ASSOCIATED WITH PRIMARY GLOMERULAR DISEASE IN THE ELDERLY

HYPOALBUMINEMIA AND EDEMA

In our experience, most elderly patients tolerate moderate hypoalbuminemia as well as younger patients, so our approach to management is no different from that suggested for nephrotics in general [172]. On occasion, some patients may develop severe edema associated with discomfort or abdominal pain when the serum albumin is very low (< 1.5 g per dl). We usually admit these patients to the hospital and treat them with a salt-poor albumin infusion followed by furosemide, with the dose tailored to the level of kidney function. In patients in whom diuresis fails to occur with this regimen, the addition of furosemide directly to the albumin has been found to enhance the response greatly [173]. This approach is continued until the patient is euvolemic. To date we have not noted any adverse side effect from this regimen.

The majority of patients do well on salt restriction (2–3 g per day) with or without an oral diuretic. When needed, our preference is to use furosemide, administered on an alternate-day basis. Attention should be paid to potassium balance, particularly in those patients receiving concomitant digitalis. We also recommend a diet with moderate protein restriction of high biologic value, approximately 0.90 to 1.0 g per kg plus urinary losses for proteinuria of more than 5 g per 24 hours, in patients with normal kidney function. (For patients with renal insufficiency see Chap. 11.)

Despite these measures, a small number of elderly (10 percent in our experience) will continue to be incapacitated by edema and hypoalbuminemia. In such cases, a cyclo-oxygenase inhibitor (e.g., indomethacin, meclofenanate) can be tried, keeping in mind that these drugs may precipitate acute renal failure, especially in this age group. These drugs reduce proteinuria by decreasing the GFR as well as by restoring the barrier size selectivity of the glomerular basement membrane [174]. We do not routinely recommend these drugs for reducing proteinuria in the elderly, but if a decision is made to use them, the guidelines issued by Velosa and Torres [175] should be followed: (1) Restrict their use to patients with a GFR greater than 50 ml per minute; (2) continue long-term treatment only when the patient shows either a doubling of serum albumin or a reduction in proteinuria greater than 40 percent of baseline; (3) start treatment with a low dose, gradually reaching the desired dose over a 1- to 2-week period; (4) maintain the patient on a low-sodium diet (< 90 mEq per day); and (5) follow serum creatinine weekly during the first month and every 1 to 2 months thereafter. Another, and perhaps safer, alternative for such patients is the use of a converting enzyme inhibitor. We recommend that guidelines similar to those outlined above be applied to the use of these agents as well [176–178].

HYPERLIPIDEMIA

The incidence of hyperlipidemia in the elderly patient with nephrotic syndrome has not been addressed specifically; however, if one extrapolates from published studies in adult nephrotics in general, it occurs in 50 to 70 percent of patients [179, 180]. Primarily, the plasma cholesterol is elevated with lesser changes in triglyceride levels. Lipoprotein profiles reveal that most of the subjects fall into three groups, type II (IIa, IIb), type III, and type V [181]. Lipoprotein fractionation shows that the cholesterol is mainly in the low-density lipoprotein (LDL) fraction, with a smaller proportion in very low density (VLDL) and high-density lipoprotein (HDL). Whereas plasma LDL and VLDL were elevated in most of the patients reported by Appel and colleagues [180], HDL was either normal or low. The presence of a normal total HDL, however, does not rule out an abnormality in the metabolism of this lipoprotein.

As shown by Short and associates [182], the HDL_3 subfraction of HDL may be elevated in nephrotic patients, whereas the HDL_2 subfraction is reduced. The latter is probably the one most closely associated with decreasing risk of ischemic heart disease. Hyperlipidemia is probably the result of both altered catabolism and enhanced synthesis of lipoproteins [183]. The stimulus for increased synthesis is mainly the low plasma albumin concentration and oncotic pressure. It is also quite possible that renal losses of macromolecules such as lipoprotein lipase contribute to the altered rate of removal and processing of VLDL [184]. The relatively low concentration of HDL_2 may reflect, in part, its loss in the urine through its major protein moiety, apolipoprotein AI [185, 186].

The role of hyperlipidemia in the incidence of atherosclerotic heart disease in nephrotic patients is still a matter of controversy [187, 188]. Based on the data available, suggesting a positive correlation between elevated LDL cholesterol and the risk of myocardial infarction, and the fact that HDL (which appears to be protective) is decreased in the majority of patients with nephrotic syndrome [189–191], we suggest the following approach: (1) both fasting plasma cholesterol and triglycerides should be measured in elderly patients with the nephrotic syndrome; (2) for those with elevated values, the lipoproteins should be fractionated; (3) if the LDL/HDL cholesterol ratio is above 3 (or if HDL is < 35 mg per dl), dietary manipulation is advised [192].

If hyperlipidemia is not controlled by diet and if there are associated risk factors such as cigarette smoking, diabetes mellitus, hypertension, or obesity, a more aggressive approach with pharmacologic intervention should be undertaken [193]. Colestipol (15 to 25 mg per day in divided doses), probucol (500 mg twice a day administered with food), and gemfibrozil (600 mg twice daily) have recently been found to be efficient and well tolerated in nephrotic patients with abnormal lipid values [194]. We have found lovastatin, an HMG-CoA reductase inhibitor, to be effective in our elderly patients. The usual starting dose is 20 mg per day. Most patients require 20 to 40 mg twice a day [195–198].

CALCIUM AND VITAMIN D

The elderly nephrotic is more prone than younger patients to alterations in calcium and vitamin D metabolism. Besides the increased losses of both $25(OH)D_3$ and $1,25(OH)_2D_3$ in the urine attributable to the nephrotic state per se, calcium absorption as well as plasma levels of $1,25(OH)_2D_3$ are decreased as a function of aging [199–201] (see Chap. 5 on Ca metabolism). Thus, it is not surprising that both osteomalacia and hyperparathyroid bone disease have been found on bone biopsies in these patients, more so in those with superimposed renal insufficiency [202, 203]. Finally, glucocorticoids, which are commonly used in treating elderly patients with glomerular diseases, decrease intestinal calcium and phosphorus absorption by a mechanism not yet fully elucidated, and also increase the rate of bone resorption, exceeding that of bone formation [204]. As a consequence, this therapy facilitates either the new development or the exacerbation of pre-existing osteoporosis [205]. Therefore, it has been our policy to administer vitamin D supplementation to our elderly nephrotic patients in the form of either vitamin D_3 (400 IU per day) or calcitriol (1.0 to 2.5 μg per day) [206]. Elemental calcium supplementation, 500 to 1,000 mg daily, can be added if calcium intake is judged inadequate [207]. The 24-hour urine calcium excretion should be monitored, together with plasma Ca and 25(OH)D_3 levels.

RENAL VEIN THROMBOSIS

The incidence of renal vein thrombosis in the elderly with nephrotic syndrome is not known. This complication, which is most common in patients with membranous nephropathy, seems to be less common in elderly than in younger patients. We have seen only two cases of renal vein thrombosis in our series of elderly patients—1 in 14 with membranous glomerulopathy and 1 in 11 with mesangiocapillary glomerulonephritis. In 27 patients with membranous glomerulopathy reported by Wagoner et al [208], 20 were younger than 60 years; of those 20, 11 had renal vein thrombosis compared with 2 of 7 older patients. Four of the 31 (13 percent) elderly patients with membranous nephropathy reported by Zech et al [43] had renal vein thrombosis. Finally, in most of the reported series of patients with renal vein thrombosis, the majority were less than 60 years of age [209–211].

In addition to an abrupt decline in renal function, other clinical manifestations of renal vein thrombosis include development of pulmonary embolism and new onset of hematuria. Other thrombotic complications such as deep vein thrombosis and arterial thrombosis have also been reported [212].

The hypercoagulable state of nephrotic syndrome is caused by several abnormalities of the coagulation cascade and of platelet function. The predisposition to thrombosis in a given patient varies depending on the balance of procoagulant and anticoagulant factors. Plasma concentration of the natural anticoagulant protein C (an inhibitor of both factor V and factor VIII) and its cofactor protein S have been found to be either normal or elevated in proteinuric patients [213, 214]. The reason for such variability may be related to the type of glomerular disease studied or the technique used (bound or unbound fraction measured) [215]. In recent studies involving mainly the unbound fraction of this protein, both qualitative (decreased specific activity) and quantitative (decreased plasma level) defects have been found that may contribute to the increased incidence of thrombosis in nephrotics [216]. Du et al [217] have postulated that an increased level of alpha-antiplasmin may be a factor in determining susceptibility to renal vein thrombosis in nephrotic patients. An increase in platelet aggregability is also present in patients with nephrotic syndrome [218], related to the hypoalbuminemia, hypercholesterolemia, and high plasma fibrinogen accompanying the nephrotic state [219].

The diagnosis of renal vein thrombosis depends on the demonstration of clots in the renal veins by venography. Noninvasive techniques, such as gray-scale ultrasonography, have been tried with variable success [220, 221]. Avasthi and associates [222] have suggested the potential usefulness of the Doppler flowmetric method for the diagnosis and follow-up of patients with renal vein thrombosis.

There remains the question of whether to perform renal venography routinely in nephrotic patients. As we discussed, the incidence of renal vein thrombosis in elderly patients with primary glomerular disease (even those with membranous nephropathy) is sufficiently low that renal venography can be reserved for those in whom the clinical suspicion of thrombosis is increased by any of the symptoms or signs described above [223].

Once the diagnosis of renal vein thrombosis has been made, anticoagulant therapy should be started. A 7- to 10-day course of heparin followed by warfarin constitutes the therapy of choice. This regimen has been found to result in significant improvement in creatinine clearance in patients presenting with rapid worsening in GFR [210]. There is not enough information about how long anticoagulation should be continued in such patients. We have used 3 months as a guideline, keeping in mind the higher susceptibility of the elderly to bleeding. Longer term therapy should be considered in patients with recurrent pulmonary embolism. Success with fibrinolytic therapy (streptokinase) has been reported [224]; however, further experience with a large number of patients is needed before its routine use can be recommended.

ACUTE RENAL FAILURE

Acute renal failure (ARF) as an initial presentation or a subsequent complication of nephrotic syndrome has been reported in more than 62 adult patients. Although the true incidence is not clear, it is probably not a common phenomenon. Esparza et al [225] found four patients with nephrotic syndrome out of 102 patients in whom a renal biopsy was performed for ARF. Whatever its true incidence, the condition seems to be more prevalent in the elderly. Of the 62 patients reported in the literature, 34 (55 percent) were older than 60 years [100, 225–235].

In addition to edema and other stigmata of nephrotic syndrome, patients with ARF were usually oliguric, and the fractional excretion of sodium (FENa) was less than 1 percent in the patients reported by Lowenstein et al [229]. Some patients require dialysis because of uremic complications. Kidney biopsy reveals minimal change nephropathy in over 87 percent, with focal glomerulosclerosis and membranous glomerulopathy in the remaining 13 percent. Since the histologic findings were not severe enough to explain the change in renal function, several hypotheses have been proposed to explain the renal failure. In some cases, a temporal association has been found between the use of analgesics or nonsteroidal anti-inflammatory drugs [234]. Small vessel thrombosis in the nephrotic kidney made ischemic by hypotension [225], and nephrosarca with subsequent increased intratubular pressure [229] are among the mechanisms proposed. Contrary to previous suggestions, hypovolemia per se does not appear to play a role in the ARF associated with the nephrotic syndrome unless the patient has been aggressively diuresed without the support of a volume expander such as albumin.

Every patient with ARF and the nephrotic syndrome should receive albumin infusion with or without a diuretic to induce diuresis, which has been associated with prompt remission in some patients. In others, the course may be quite protracted. Since minimal change disease is by far the most commonly found histologic diagnosis in these patients, steroid therapy should also be initiated. (See previous section, "Minimal Change Glomerulopathy [Lipoid Nephrosis].") Seventy-nine percent of the patients reported recovered kidney function eventually. The remaining patients either expired (mainly those in whom acute renal failure was the presenting manifestation of the nephrotic syndrome) or did not improve and had to be maintained on dialysis.

SUPERIMPOSED CRESCENTIC GLOMERULONEPHRITIS

In some patients with a known primary glomerular disease, a rapid decline in renal function may supervene due to the development of crescentic glomerulonephritis. The incidence of this complication is not known, but it has been reported in patients with membranous glomerulopathy, mesangiocapillary glomerulonephritis, mesangial nephritis, and focal glomerulosclerosis [236–240]. Antiglomerular basement membrane antibodies have been found in some patients. It is postulated that pre-existing immune complexes along the glomerular basement membrane may render the glomerulus more susceptible to additional injury. A repeat kidney biopsy is necessary to confirm the diagnosis. The prognosis, as expected, is usually poor. We suggest plasmapheresis for those with anti-GBM antibody and pulse steroid therapy for those without [240]. There are, however, no data to support such an approach in the elderly.

MALIGNANCY

A final consideration in patients with nephrotic syndrome is that of associated malignancy. Lee et al [241] reported 11 cases of an underlying malignancy among 101 patients older than 40 years of age with de novo onset of nephrotic syndrome. In a review of 48 patients with malignancy and nephrotic syndrome, 33 had membranous glomerulopathy, four had membranoproliferative glomerulonephritis, three had minimal change disease, two had amyloid, and six had various other glomerulopathies [242].

In five reports, which included 103 elderly patients with membranous glomerulopathy, 12 patients (12 percent) had a malignancy [40, 41, 43, 243, 244]. More than 50 percent of patients with lymphomas and nephrotic syndrome have been found to have minimal change disease on biopsy. Crescentic glomerulonephritis has been more commonly associated with solid tumors [245, 246]. Although tumor-associated antigen-antibody complex deposition (for patients with solid tumors) and production of a humoral substance (lymphokines in patients with lymphomas) have been suggested as pathogenetic factors in the development of the glomerular injury associated with neoplasia, direct proof has been lacking in the great majority of cases.

The nephrotic syndrome can develop concurrently or may preceed the diagnosis of malignancy by several months. If the neoplasm is diagnosed concurrently with the nephrotic syndrome, treatment of the former could result in remission of the latter. We do not think that an extensive search for malignancy should be undertaken in the elderly patient with either membranous nephropathy or minimal change disease. We believe in performing a detailed history and physical examination in such patients to alert us to the possibility of a malignancy. Since lung and bowel cancer are the most common tumors associated with membranous nephropathy, a chest x-ray and serial examination of stools for occult blood are recommended. In a long-term follow-up of a large number of patients in the U.S. Collaborative Study of Nephrotic Syndrome (C. Coggins, personal communication) as well as in the study of Lund et al [247], the development of malignancy has not been found to be a significant problem.

REFERENCES

1. Diaz-Buxo JA and Donadio JV Jr: Complications of percutaneous renal biopsy: An analysis of 1,000 consecutive biopsies. *Clin Nephrol* 4:223–227, 1975.
2. Cameron JS: The nephrotic syndrome and its complications. *Am J Kidney Dis* 10:157–171, 1987.
3. Friedman SA, et al: Functional defects in the aging kidney. *Ann Intern Med* 76:41–45, 1972.
4. Ginsberg JM, et al: Use of single voided urine samples to estimate quantitative proteinuria. *N Engl J Med* 309:1543–1546, 1983.
5. Rennke HG, Patel Y, and Venkatachalam MA: Effect of molecular charge on

glomerular permeability to proteins in the rat: Clearance studies using neutral, anionic and cationic horseradish peroxidase. *Kidney Int* 13:278, 1983.

6. Bohrer MP, et al: Mechanism of angiotensin II-induced proteinuria in the rat. *Am J Physiol* 223:F13–F21, 1977.

7. Blau EB and Haas JE: Glomerular sialic acid and proteinuria in human renal disease. *Lab Invest* 28:477–481, 1973.

8. Myers BD, et al: Mechanisms of proteinuria in human glomerulonephritis. *J Clin Invest* 70:732–746, 1982.

9. Dean WM, et al: Heteroporous model of glomerular size selectivity: Application to normal and nephrotic humans. *Am J Physiol* 249:F374–F389, 1989.

10. Dorhout Mees EJ, et al: Observations on edema formation in the nephrotic syndrome in adults with minimal lesions. *Am J Med* 67:378–384, 1979.

11. Krishna GG and Danovitch GM: Effects of water immersion on renal function in the nephrotic syndrome. *Kidney Int* 21:395–401, 1982.

12. Dorhout Mees EJ, et al: Changes in plasma volume and renin activity during correction of edema in the nephrotic syndrome. *Kidney Int* 25:163A, 1984.

13. Koomans HA, et al: Effects of plasma volume expansion on renal salt handling in patients with the nephrotic syndrome. *Am J Nephrol* 4:227–234, 1984.

14. Berlyne GM, et al: Renal salt and water handling in water immersion in the nephrotic syndrome. *Clin Sci* 61:605–610, 1981.

15. Berlyne GM, et al: Water immersion in nephrotic syndrome. *Arch Intern Med* 141:1275–1278, 1981.

16. Meltzer JI, et al: Nephrotic syndrome: Vasoconstriction and hypovolemic types indicated by renin-sodium profiling. *Ann Intern Med* 91:688–696, 1979.

17. Chonko AM, et al: The role of renin and aldosterone in the salt retention of edema. *Am J Med* 63:881–889, 1977.

18. Brown EA, et al: Evidence that some mechanism other than the renin system causes sodium retention in nephrotic syndrome. *Lancet* 2:1237–1239, 1982.

19. Dusing R, Vetter H, and Kramer HJ: The renin-angiotensin-aldosterone system in patients with nephrotic syndrome. Effects of 1 sar-8-ala-angiotensin II. *Nephron* 25:187–192, 1980.

20. Kopp UC and DiBona GF: Neural Control of Volume Homeostasis. In Brenner BM and Stein JH (eds): *Body Fluid Homeostasis*, Vol 16. *Contributions in Nephrology*. New York, Churchill-Livingstone, 1987.

21. Oliver WJ, Kelch RC, and Chandler JP: Demonstration of increased catecholamine excretion in the nephrotic syndrome. *Proc Soc Exp Biol Med* 125:1176–1180, 1967.

22. Geers AB, et al: Postural changes in the nephrotic syndrome (NS). *Kidney Int* 25:165A, 1984.

23. Hollister AS, et al: Clearance of atrial natriuretic factor by lung, liver and kidney in human subjects and the dog. *J Clin Invest* 83:623–628, 1989.

24. Yamamoto Y, et al: Plasma concentration of human atrial natriuretic polypeptide in patients with impaired renal function. *Clin Nephrol* 27:84–86, 1987.

25. Daniels H and Pederson EB: Atrial natriuretic peptide, angiotensin II and aldosterone in plasma in chronic glomerulonephritis during basal conditions and during exercise. *Acta Med Scand* 224:61–67, 1988.

26. Zietse R and Schalekamp NA: Effect of synthetic human atrial natriuretic peptide (102–106) in nephrotic syndrome. *Kidney Int* 34:717–724, 1988.

27. Peterson C, et al: Atrial natriuretic peptide and the renal response to hypervolemia in nephrotic humans. *Kidney Int* 34:828–831, 1988.

28. Pedersen EB, et al: Urinary prostaglandin E_2 and F_{2a} excretion in nephrotic syndrome during basal conditions, after water loading, and after remission of the syndrome. *Acta Med Scand* 224:69–77, 1988.

29. Shapiro MD, et al: Role of glomerular filtration rate in the impaired sodium and water excretion in patients with the nephrotic syndrome. *Am J Kidney Dis* 8:81–87, 1986.

30. Ichikawa I, et al: Role for intrarenal mechanisms in the impaired salt excretion of experimental nephrotic syndrome. *J Clin Invest* 71:91–103, 1983.

31. Gransz H, Lieberman R, and Earley LE: Effect of plasma albumin on sodium reabsorption in patients with nephrotic syndrome. *Kidney Int* 1:47–54, 1972.

32. Koomans HA, et al: Sodium balance in renal failure. A comparison of patients with normal subjects under extreme sodium intake. *Hypertension* 71:714–722, 1985.

33. Messing EM, et al: The significance of asymptomatic microhematuria in men 50 or more years old. Findings of a home screening study using urinary dipsticks. *J Urol* 137:919–922, 1987.

34. Rizzoni G, Braggion F, and Zacchello G: Evaluation of glomerular and nonglomerular hematuria by phase-contrast microscopy. *J Pediatr* 103:370–374, 1983.

35. Birch DF, et al: Urinary erythrocyte morphology in the diagnosis of glomerular hematuria. *Clin Nephrol* 20:78–84, 1983.

36. Fassett RG, et al: Scanning electron microscopy of glomerular and nonglomerular red blood cells. *Clin Nephrol* 20:11–16, 1983.

37. Haughstaine D, Bollens W, and Michielsen R: Detection of glomerular bleeding using a simple staining method for light microscopy. *Lancet* 2:761, 1982.

38. Raman GV, et al: A blind controlled trial of phase-contrast microscopy by two observers for evaluating the source of hematuria. *Nephron* 44:304–308, 1986.

39. Pollack C, et al: Dysmorphism of urinary red blood cells. Value in diagnosis. *Kidney Int* 36:1045–1049, 1989.

40. Moorthy AV and Zimmerman SW: Renal disease in the elderly: Clinicopathologic analysis of renal disease in 115 elderly patients. *Clin Nephrol* 14:223–229, 1980.

41. Kingswood JC, et al: Renal biopsy in the elderly: Clinicopathological correlations in 143 patients. *Clin Nephrol* 22:183–187, 1984.

42. Fawcett TW, et al: Nephrotic syndrome in the elderly. *Br Med J* 2:387–388, 1971.

43. Zech P, et al: The nephrotic syndrome in adults aged over 60: Etiology, evolution and treatment of the cases. *Clin Nephrol* 5:232–236, 1982.

44. Boner G, et al: Nephrotic syndrome in patients over 60 years of age. Abstract Seventh International Congress of Nephrology, June 18–26, 1978.

45. Noel LH, et al: Long-term prognosis of idiopathic membranous glomerulonephritis. Study of 116 untreated patients. *Am J Med* 66:82–90, 1979.

46. Ehrenreich T and Churg J: Pathology of membranous nephropathy. *Pathol Ann* 3:145–186, 1968.

47. Gallo GR, Caulin-Glaser T, and Lamm ME: Charge of circulating immune complexes as a factor in glomerular basement membrane localization in mice. *J Clin Invest* 67:1305–1313, 1981.

48. Couser WG and Salant DJ: Immunopathogenesis of Glomerular Capillary Wall Injury in Nephrotic States. In Brenner BM and Stein JH (eds): *Contemporary Issues in Nephrology*. New York: Churchill Livingstone, 1982.

49. Wehrmann M, et al: Long-term prognosis of chronic idiopathic membranous glomerulonephritis. *Clin Nephrol* 31:67–76, 1989.

50. Davison AM, Cameron JS, and Kerr DNS: The natural history of renal function in untreated idiopathic membranous glomerulonephritis in adults. *Clin Nephrol* 22:61–67, 1984.
51. Porush JG and Faubert PF: Treatment of Idiopathic Membranous Glomerulopathy. In Avram MM (ed): *Proteinuria*, Vol 14. New York, Plenum Medical, 1983. Pp 175–193.
52. Collaborative Study of the Adult Idiopathic Nephrotic Syndrome: a controlled study of short term prednisone treatment in adults with membranous nephropathy. *N Engl J Med* 301:1301–1306, 1979.
53. Ponticelli C, et al: Controlled trial of methylprednisolone and chlorambucil in idiopathic membranous nephropathy. *N Engl J Med* 310:946–950, 1984.
54. Zucchelli P, et al: Clinical and morphologic evolution of membranous nephropathy. *Clin Nephrol* 25:282–288, 1986.
55. Ponticelli C, Zucchelli P, and Passerini P: A randomized trial of methylprednisolone and chlorambucil in idiopathic membranous nephropathy. *N Engl J Med* 320:8–13, 1989.
56. Garattini S, Berani T, and Remuzzi G: Steroids and cytotoxic drugs in the treatment of membranous glomerulopathy. *Nephron* 50:263–264, 1988.
57. Donadio JV Jr, et al: Idiopathic membranous nephropathy. The natural history of untreated patients. *Kidney Int* 33:708–715, 1988.
58. Catran DC, et al: A randomized controlled trial of prednisone in patients with idiopathic membranous nephropathy. *N Engl J Med* 320:210–215, 1989.
59. West ML, et al: A controlled trial of cyclophosphamide in patients with membranous glomerulonephritis. *Kidney Int* 32:579–584, 1987.
60. Heilman RL, et al: Crescentic glomerulonephritis (CGN): Multisystem involvement determining renal survival. *Clin Res* 33:84A, 1985.
61. Velosa JA: Idiopathic crescentic glomerulonephritis or systemic vasculitis? *Mayo Clin Proc* 62:145–147, 1987.
62. Beirne GJ, et al: Idiopathic crescentic glomerulonephritis. *Medicine* 56:349–381, 1977.
63. Stilmant MM, et al: Crescentic glomerulonephritis without immune deposits. Clinicopathologic features. *Kidney Int* 15:184–195, 1979.
64. Cohen AH, et al: Crescentic glomerulonephritis: Immune versus nonimmune mechanisms. *Am J Nephrol* 1:78–83, 1981.
65. Couser WG: Idiopathic rapidly progressive glomerulonephritis. *Am J Nephrol* 2:57–99, 1988.
66. Price RG and Wong M: Heterogeneity of Goodpasture's antigen. *J Pathol* 156:97–99, 1988.
67. Lewis EJ and Schwartz MM: Idiopathic crescentic glomerulonephritis. *Semin Nephrol* 2:193–213, 1982.
68. Groggel GC, et al: Role of the terminal complement pathway in the heterologous phase of antiglomerular basement membrane nephritis in the rabbit. *Kidney Int* 27:643–651, 1985.
69. Tucker BJ, et al: Effect of leucocyte depletion on glomerular dynamics during acute glomerular immune injury. *Kidney Int* 28:28–35, 1985.
70. Bonsib SM: Glomerular basement membrane necrosis and crescent organization. *Kidney Int* 33:966–974, 1988.
71. Germuth FG Jr, et al: Fatal immune complex glomerulonephritis. *Acta Pathol Microbiol Scand* 249 (Suppl) 20–28, 1974.
72. Olsen S, Peterson V, and Hansen H: Immunofluorescence studies of extracapillary glomerulonephritis. *Acta Pathol Microbiol Scand* 249 (Suppl) 20–28, 1974.

73. Wilson CB and Dixon FJ: Anti-glomerular basement membrane antibody-induced glomerulonephritis. *Kidney Int* 3:74–89, 1973.
74. Morrin PAF, et al: Rapidly progressive glomerulo-nephritis. *Am J Med* 65:446–460, 1978.
75. Simpson JJ, et al: Plasma exchange in Goodpasture's Syndrome. *Am J Nephrol* 2:301–311, 1982.
76. Flores JC, et al: Clinical and immunological evolution of oligoanuric anti-GBM nephritis treated by hemodialysis. *Lancet* 1:508, 1986.
77. Sonsino E, et al: Extra-capillary Proliferative Glomerulonephritis So-Called Malignant Glomerulonephritis. In Hamburger J, et al (eds): *Advances in Nephrology*, Vol 2. Chicago: Year Book, 1972. Pp 121–163.
78. O'Neill WM Jr, Etheridge WB, and Bloomer A: High dose corticosteroids. Their use in treating idiopathic rapidly progressive glomerulonephritis. *Arch Intern Med* 139:514–518, 1979.
79. Kline Bolton W and Couser WG: Intravenous pulse methylprednisolone therapy of acute crescentic rapidly progressive glomerulonephritis. *Am J Med* 66:495–502, 1979.
80. Oredugba O, et al: Pulse methylprednisolone therapy in idiopathic, rapidly progressive glomerulonephritis. *Ann Intern Med* 92:504–506, 1980.
81. Neild GH, et al: Rapidly progressive glomerulonephritis with extensive glomerular crescent formation. *Q J Med* 207:395–416, 1983.
82. Heilman RL, et al: Analysis of risk factors for patients and renal survival in crescentic glomerulonephritis. *Kidney Int* 29:189A, 1986.
83. Johnson JP, et al: Therapy of anti-glomerular basement membrane antibody disease: analysis of prognostic significance of clinical, pathologic and treatment factors. *Medicine* 64:219–227, 1985.
84. Niva T, et al: Beneficial effects of prostaglandin E$_1$ in rapidly progressive glomerulonephritis. *N Engl J Med* 308:969, 1983.
85. Gonzalo A, et al: Clinical significance of IgM mesangial deposits in the nephrotic syndrome. *Nephron* 41:246–249, 1985.
86. Lawer W, et al: IgM associated primary diffuse mesangial proliferative glomerulonephritis. *J Clin Pathol* 33:1029–1038, 1980.
87. Osakabe K and Matsumoto K: Concavalin A-induced suppressor cell activity in lipoid nephrosis. *Scand J Immunol* 14:161–166, 1981.
88. Schnaper HW and Aune TM: Identification of the lymphokine soluble immune response suppressor in urine of nephrotic children. *J Clin Invest* 76:341–349, 1985.
89. Levin M, et al: Steroid responsive nephrotic syndrome: A generalized disorder of membrane negative charge. *Lancet* 2:239–242, 1985.
90. Kreisberg JE, Wayne DB, and Karnovsky MJ: Rapid and focal loss of negative charge associated with mononuclear cell infiltration early in nephrotoxic serum nephritis. *Kidney Int* 16:290–300, 1979.
91. Lagrue G and Laurent J: Allergy and lipid nephrosis. *Adv Nephrol* 12:151–175, 1983.
92. Bohrer MP, et al: Mechanisms of the puromycin-induced defects in the transglomerular passage of water and macromolecules. *J Clin Invest* 60:152–161, 1971.
93. Bohman SD, et al: Foot process fusion and glomerular filtration rate in minimal change nephrotic syndrome. *Kidney Int* 25:696–700, 1984.
94. Bridges CR, et al: Glomerular charge alterations in human minimal change nephropathy. *Kidney Int* 22:677–684, 1982.
95. Carrie BJ, Salyer WR, and Myers BD: Minimal change nephropathy: An elec-

trochemical disorder of the glomerular membrane. *Am J Med* 70: 262–268, 1981.

96. Hooper J Jr, et al: Lipoid nephrosis in 31 adult patients: Renal biopsy study by light, electron and fluorescence microscopy with experience in treatment. *Medicine* 49:321–341, 1970.

97. Hayslett JP, et al: Clinicopathological correlations in the nephrotic syndrome due to primary renal disease. *Medicine* 52:93–120, 1973.

98. Cameron JS, et al: The nephrotic syndrome in adults with "minimal change" glomerular lesions. *Q J Med* 43:461–488, 1974.

99. Wang F, Looi LM, and Chua CT: Minimal change glomerular disease in Malaysian adults and use of alternate day steroid therapy. *Q J Med* 203:312–328, 1982.

100. Nolasco F, Cameron JS, and Heywood EF: Adult-onset minimal change nephrotic syndrome: A long term follow-up. *Kidney Int* 29:1215–1223, 1986.

101. Korbet SM, Schwartz MM, and Lewis EJ. Minimal-change glomerulopathy of adulthood. *Am J Nephrol* 8:291–297, 1988.

102. D'Amico G: Idiopathic IgA mesangial nephropathy. *Nephron* 41:1–13, 1985.

103. Power DA, et al: IgA nephropathy is not a rare disease in the United Kingdom. *Nephron* 40:180–184, 1985.

104. Cohen AH and Border WA: Mesangial proliferative glomerulonephritis. *Semin Nephrol* 2:228, 1982.

105. Habib R and Churg J: Minimal change disease, mesangial proliferative glomerulonephritis and focal sclerosis: Individual entities or a spectrum of disease? *Nephrology* 1:634–644, 1984. *Proceedings of the IXth International Congress of Nephrology* (Robinson RR [ed]).

106. Nicholls KM, et al: The clinical course of mesangial IgA associated nephropathy in adults. *Q J Med* 210:227–250, 1984.

107. Clarkson AR, et al: IgA nephropathy: A syndrome of uniform morphology, diverse clinical features and uncertain prognosis. *Clin Nephrol* 8:459–471, 1977.

108. Neela Kantappa K, Gallo GR, and Baldwin DS: Proteinuria in IgA nephropathy. *Kidney Int* 33:716–721, 1988.

109. Boyce NW, et al: Clinicopathological associations in mesangial IgA nephropathy. *Am J Nephrol* 6:246–252, 1986.

110. Sinniah R: IgA mesangial nephropathy: Berger's disease. *Am J Nephrol* 5:73–83, 1985.

111. Kobayashi Y, et al: IgA nephropathy: Prognostic significance of proteinuria and histological alterations. *Nephron* 34:146–153, 1983.

112. Yoskimura M, et al: Significance of IgA deposits on the glomerular capillary walls in IgA nephropathy. *Am J Kidney Dis* 9:404–409, 1987.

113. Emancipator SN, Gallo GR, and Lamm ME: IgA nephropathy: Perspective on pathogenesis and classification. *Clin Nephrol* 24:161–179, 1985.

114. Monteiro RC, et al: Charge and size of mesangial IgA in IgA nephropathy. *Kidney Int* 28:666–671, 1985.

115. Praga M, et al: Acute worsening of renal function during episodes of macroscopic hematuria in IgA nephropathy. *Kidney Int* 28:69–74, 1985.

116. Chida Y, Tomura S, and Takeuchi J: Renal survival rate of IgA nephropathy. *Nephron* 40:189–194, 1985.

117. Mustonen J, et al: Clinicopathologic correlations in a series of 143 patients with IgA glomerulonephritis. *Am J Nephrol* 5:150–157, 1985.

118. Lai KN, et al: Nephrotic range proteinuria—a good predictive index of disease in IgA nephropathy? *Q J Med* 222:677–688, 1985.
119. D'Amico G, et al: Prognostic indicators in idiopathic IgA mesangial nephropathy. *Q J Med* 228:363–378, 1986.
120. Clarkson AR, et al: Controlled trial of phenytoin therapy in IgA nephropathy. *Clin Nephrol* 13:215–218, 1980.
121. Egido J, et al: Phenytoin in IgA nephropathy: A long-term controlled trial. *Nephron* 38:30–39, 1984.
122. Coppo R, et al: Ineffectiveness of phenytoin treatment on IgA-containing circulating immune complexes in IgA nephropathy. *Nephron* 36:275–276, 1984.
123. Mustonen J, Pasternack A, and Rantala I: The nephrotic syndrome in IgA glomerulonephritis: Response to corticosteroid therapy. *Clin Nephrol* 20:172–176, 1983.
124. Kobayashi Y, et al: Steroid therapy in IgA nephropathy: A prospective pilot study in moderate proteinuric cases. *Q J Med* 61:935–943, 1986.
125. Brown EA, et al: The clinical course of mesangial proliferative glomerulonephritis. *Medicine* 58:295–303, 1979.
126. Coppo R, et al: Immunological monitorization of plasma exchange in primary IgA nephropathy. *Proceedings of the IX International Congress of Nephrology* 78A, 1984.
127. Genin C, et al: Efficiency of high dose steroids and plasma exchanges in severe mesangial IgA glomerulonephritis. *Proceedings of the IX International Congress of Nephrology* 89A, 1984.
128. Glassock RJ and Kurokawa K: IgA nephropathy in Japan. *Am J Nephrol* 5:127–137, 1985.
129. Lai KN, et al: Cyclosporin treatment of IgA nephropathy: A short-term controlled trial. *Br Med J* 295:1165–1168, 1987.
130. Cameron JS, et al: Idiopathic mesangiocapillary glomerulonephritis. Comparison of types I and II in children and adults and long-term prognosis. *Am J Med* 74:175–192, 1983.
131. Nuñez NJ, et al: Glomerular nephropathy in persons older than 50 years. *Kidney Int* 28:587A, 1985.
132. Abreo K and Moorthy AV: Type 3 membranoproliferative glomerulonephritis. Clinico-pathologic correlations and long term follow-up in nine patients. *Arch Pathol Lab Med* 106:413–417, 1982.
133. West CD: Pathogenesis and approaches to therapy of membranoproliferative glomerulonephritis. *Kidney Int* 9:1–7, 1976.
134. Davis CA, Marder H, and West CD: Circulating immune complexes in membranoproliferative glomerulonephritis. *Kidney Int* 20:728–732, 1981.
135. Ooi YM, Vallota EH, and West CD: Classical complement pathway activation in membranoproliferative glomerulonephritis. *Kidney Int* 9:46–53, 1976.
136. Whaley K, Ward D, and Ruddy S: Modulation of the properdin amplification loop in membranoproliferative and other forms of glomerulonephritis. *Clin Exp Immunol* 35:101–106, 1979.
137. Zimmerman SW, et al: Prospective trial of warfarin and dipyridamole in patients with membranoproliferative glomerulonephritis. *Am J Med* 75:920–927, 1983.
138. Donadio JV Jr, et al: Membranoproliferative glomerulonephritis. A prospective clinical trial of platelet-inhibitor therapy. *N Engl J Med* 310:1421–1426, 1984.

139. Velosa JA, Donadis JV Jr, and Holley KE: Focal sclerosing glomerulopathy. *Mayo Clin Proc* 50:121–132, 1975.

140. Bourgoignie JJ, Meneses R, and Pardo V: The nephropathy related to acquired immune deficiency syndrome. *Adv Nephrol* 17:113–126, 1988.

141. Torres VE, et al: The progression of vesicoureteral reflux nephropathy. *Ann Intern Med* 92:776–784, 1980.

142. Hoyer JR: Focal segmental glomerulosclerosis. *Semin Nephrol* 2:253–263,1982.

143. Matsumoto K, et al: Concavalin A-induced suppressor cell activity in focal glomerulosclerosis. *Nephron* 20:307–315, 1978.

144. Bolton WK, Westervelt FB, and Sturgill BC: Nephrotic syndrome and focal glomerular sclerosis in aging man. *Nephron* 20:307–315, 1978.

145. Winetz JA, et al: The nature of the glomerular injury in minimal change and focal sclerosing glomerulopathies. *Am J Kidney Dis* 2:91–98, 1981.

146. Newman WJ, et al: Focal glomerulosclerosis: Contrasting clinical patterns in children and adults. *Medicine* 55:67–87, 1976.

147. Velosa JA, et al: Significance of proteinuria on the outcome of renal function in patients with focal segmental glomerulosclerosis. *Mayo Clin Proc* 58:568–577, 1983.

148. Korbet SM, Schwartz MM, and Lewis EJ: The prognosis of focal segmental glomerulosclerosis of adulthood. *Medicine* 65:304–311, 1986.

149. Pei Y, et al: Evidence suggesting under-treatment in adults with idiopathic focal segmental glomerulosclerosis. *Am J Med* 82:938–944, 1987.

150. Cameron JS, et al: The long-term prognosis of patients with focal segmental glomerulosclerosis. *Clin Nephrol* 10:213–218, 1978.

151. Beaufils H, et al: Focal glomerulosclerosis: Natural history and treatment. *Nephron* 21:75–85, 1978.

152. Meyrier A and Simon P: Treatment of corticoresistant idiopathic nephrotic syndrome in the adult: Minimal change disease and focal segmental glomerulosclerosis. *Adv Nephrol* 17:127–150, 1988.

153. Velosa JA, et al: Treatment of severe nephrotic syndrome with meclofenamate: An uncontrolled pilot study. *Mayo Clin Proc* 60:586–592, 1985.

154. Anderson CF: Meclofenamate and the nephrotic syndrome: The use of the right drug in the right patient by the right physician. *Mayo Clin Proc* 59:206–207, 1984.

155. Montoliu J, et al: Acute and rapidly progressive forms of glomerulonephritis in the elderly. *J Am Geriatr Soc* 29:108–116, 1981.

156. Volpi A, et al: Postinfectious glomerulonephritis in the elderly. *Am J Nephrol* 8:431–432, 1988.

157. Rodriguez-Iturbe B, et al: Circulating immune complexes and serum immunoglobulins in acute poststreptococcal glomerulonephritis: Evidence for circulating immune complex pathogenesis. *Clin Nephrol* 13:1–5, 1980.

158. Van De Rijn I, Fillet H, and Brandeis WE: Serial studies on circulating immune complexes in poststreptococcal sequelae. *Clin Exp Immunol* 34:318–325, 1978.

159. Oite T, et al: Quantitative studies of in-situ immune complex glomerulonephritis in the rat induced by planted, cationized antigen. *J Exp Med* 155:4360–4374, 1982.

160. Batsford SR, Talamiya H, and Vogt: A model of in-situ immune complex glomerulonephritis in the rat employing cationized ferritin. *Clin Nephrol* 14:211–216, 1980.

161. McIntosh RM, et al: Evidence of autologous immune complex pathogenic mechanism in acute poststreptococcal glomerulonephritis. *Kidney Int* 14:501–510, 1978.

162. Abrams CK: Glomerulonephritis in the elderly. *Am J Nephrol* 5:409–418, 1985.
163. Samiy AH, Field RA, and Merrill JP: Acute glomerulonephritis in elderly patients. Report of seven cases over sixty years of age. *Ann Intern Med* 54:603–609, 1961.
164. Nesson R and Robbins SL: Glomerulonephritis in older age groups. *Arch Intern Med* 105:47–56, 1960.
165. Lee HA, Stirling G, and Sharpstone P: Acute glomerulonephritis in middle-aged and elderly patients. *Br Med J* 2:1361–1363, 1966.
166. Arieff A, Anderson RJ, and Massry SG: Acute glomerulonephritis in the elderly. *Geriatrics* 26:74–84, 1971.
167. Lien JWK, Matthew TH, and Meadows R: Acute post-streptococcal glomerulonephritis in adults: A long-term study. *Q J Med* 189:99–111, 1979.
168. Kaplan EL and Wanamaker LW: Suppression of the antistreptococcal response by cholesterol and by lipid extracts of rabbit skin. *J Exp Med* 144:754–767, 1976.
169. Montoliu J, et al: Primary acute glomerular disorders in the elderly. *Arch Intern Med* 140:755–756, 1980.
170. Sapir DG, Yardley JH, and Walker WG: Acute glomerulonephritis in older patients. *Johns Hopkins Med J* 132:145–152, 1968.
171. Vogel W, et al: Long-term prognosis for endocapillary glomerulonephritis of poststreptococcal type in children and adults. *Nephron* 44:58–65, 1986.
172. Coggins CH: Management of Nephrotic Syndrome. In Brenner BM and Stein J (eds): *Contemporary Issues in Nephrology*, Vol 9. New York, Churchill-Livingstone, 1982.
173. Inoue M, et al: Mechanism of furosemide resistance in analbuminemic rats and hypoalbuminemic patients. *Kidney Int* 32:198–203, 1987.
174. Golbetz H, et al: Mechanism of the antiproteinuric effect of indomethacin in nephrotic humans. *Am J Physiol* 256:F44–51, 1989.
175. Velosa JA and Torres VE: Benefits and risks of nonsteroidal anti-inflammatory drugs in steroid resistant nephrotic syndrome. *Am J Kidney Dis* 8:345–350, 1986.
176. Hutchinson FN, Schambelan M, and Kaysen GE: Modulation of albuminuria by dietary protein and converting enzyme inhibition. *Am J Physiol* 253:719–725, 1987.
177. Don B, Hutchinson E, and Kaysen G: Comparison of dietary protein restriction to angiotensin-converting enzyme inhibition in nephrosis: a randomized study. *Kidney Int* 33:188A, 1988.
178. Heeg JE, et al: Efficacy and variability of the antiproteinuric effect of ACE inhibition by linosinopril. *Kidney Int* 36:272–279, 1971.
179. Chopra JS, Mallick NP, and Stone MC: Hyperlipoproteinaemia in nephrotic syndrome. *Lancet* 1:317–320, 1971.
180. Appel GB, et al: The hyperlipidemia of the nephrotic syndrome. Relation to plasma albumin concentration, oncotic pressure and viscosity. *N Engl J Med* 312:1544–1548, 1985.
181. Newmark SR, Anderson CF, and Donadio JV Jr: Lipoprotein profiles in adult nephrotics. *Mayo Clin Proc* 50:359–364, 1975.
182. Short CP, et al: Serum and urinary high density lipoproteins in glomerular diseases with proteinuria. *Kidney Int* 29:1224–1228, 1986.
183. Warwick GL, et al: Low-density lipoprotein metabolism in the nephrotic syndrome. *Metabolism* 39:187–192, 1990.

184. Staprans J and Felts JM: The effect of alpha-acid glycoprotein (orosomucoid) on triglyceride metabolism in the nephrotic syndrome. *Biochem Biophys Res Comm* 79:1272–1278, 1977.

185. Felts JM and Mayerle JA: Urinary loss of plasma high density lipoprotein. A possible cause of the hyperlipidemia of the nephrotic syndrome. *Circulation* 263A (Suppl 3):49–50, 1974.

186. Saku K, et al: High-density lipoprotein apolipoprotein AI and AII turnover in moderate and severe proteinuria. *Nephron* 50:112–115, 1988.

187. Mallick NP and Short CD: The nephrotic syndrome and ischemic heart disease. *Nephron* 27:54–57, 1981.

188. Wass V and Cameron JS: Cardiovascular disease and the nephrotic syndrome: The other side of the coin. *Nephron* 27:58–61, 1981.

189. Levy RI: Current status of the cholesterol controversy. *Am J Med* 74 (Suppl): 1–4, 1983.

190. Lees RS and Lees AM: High-density lipoproteins and the risk of atherosclerosis. *N Engl J Med* 306:1546–1548, 1982.

191. Lipinska I and Gurewich V: The value of measuring percent high-density lipoprotein in assessing risk of cardiovascular disease. *Arch Intern Med* 142:469–472, 1982.

192. Grundy SM, et al: The place of HDL in cholesterol management. *Arch Intern Med* 149:505–510, 1989.

193. Grundy SM: Management of hyperlipidemia of kidney disease. *Kidney Int* 37:847–853, 1990.

194. Croggel GC, et al: Treatment of nephrotic hyperlipoproteinemia with gemfibrozil. *Kidney Int* 36:226–271, 1989.

195. Golper TA, et al: Lovastatin in the treatment of multifactorial hyperlipidemia associated with proteinuria. *Am J Kidney Dis* 13:312–329, 1989.

196. Vega GL and Grundy SM: Lovastatin therapy in nephrotic hyperlipidemia: Effects on lipoprotein metabolism. *Kidney Int* 33:1160–1168, 1988.

197. Rabelink AJ, et al: Effects of simvastatin and cholestyramine on lipoprotein profile in hyperlipidemia of nephrotic syndrome. *Lancet* 2:1335–1338, 1988.

198. Kasiske BL, et al: The effects of lovastatin in hyperlipidemic patients with the nephrotic syndrome. *Am J Kidney Dis* 15:8–15, 1990.

199. Goldstein DA, et al: Vitamin D metabolites and calcium metabolism in patients with nephrotic syndrome and normal renal function. *J Clin Endocrinol Metab* 52:116–121, 1981.

200. Goldstein DA, et al: Blood levels of 25-hydroxyvitamin D in nephrotic syndrome: Studies in 26 patients. *Ann Intern Med* 87:664–668, 1977.

201. Sato KA, Gray RW, and Lemann J Jr: Urinary excretion of 25-hydroxyvitamin D in health and the nephrotic syndrome. *J Lab Clin Med* 99:325–330, 1982.

202. Melluche HH, Goldstein DA, and Massry SG: Osteomalacia and hyperparathyroid bone disease in patients with nephrotic syndrome. *J Clin Invest* 63:494–500, 1979.

203. Malluche HH, et al: Bone histology in incipient and advanced renal failure. *Kidney Int* 9:355–362, 1976.

204. Klein RG, et al: Intestinal calcium absorption in exogenous hypercortisonism. Role of 25-hydroxyvitamin D and corticosteroid dose. *J Clin Invest* 60:253–259, 1977.

205. Lukert BP and Raisz LG: Glucocorticoid-induced osteoporosis: Pathogenesis and management. *Ann Intern Med* 112:352–364, 1990.

206. Lips P, et al: The effect of vitamin D supplementation on vitamin D status

and parathyroid function in elderly subjects. *J Clin Endocrinol Metab* 67:644–650, 1988.

207. Dykman TR, et al: Effect of oral 1,25-dihydroxyvitamin D and calcium on glucocorticoid-induced osteopenia in patients with rheumatic diseases. *Arth Rheum* 27:1336–1343, 1984.

208. Wagoner RD, et al: Renal vein thrombosis in idiopathic membranous glomerulopathy and nephrotic syndrome: Incidence and significance. *Kidney Int* 23:368–374, 1983.

209. Trew PA, et al: Renal vein thrombosis in membranous glomerulopathy: Incidence and association. *Medicine* 57:69–82, 1978.

210. Llach F, Papper S, and Massry SG: The clinical spectrum of renal vein thrombosis, acute and chronic. *Am J Med* 69:819–827, 1980.

211. Llach F, Arieff AL, and Massry SG: Renal vein thrombosis and nephrotic syndrome. A prospective study of 36 adult patients. *Ann Intern Med* 83:8–14, 1975.

212. Llach F: Hypercoagulability, renal vein thrombosis and other thrombotic complications of nephrotic syndrome. *Kidney Int* 28:429–439, 1985.

213. Cosio FG, et al: Plasma concentrations of the natural anticoagulants protein C and protein S in patients with proteinuria. *J Lab Clin Med* 106:218–222, 1985.

214. Manucci PM, et al: High plasma levels of protein C activity and antigen in the nephrotic syndrome. *Thromb Haemost* 55:31–33, 1986.

215. Allon M, et al: Protein S and C antigen levels in proteinuric patients, dependency on type of glomerular pathology. *Am J Hematol* 31:96–101, 1989.

216. Vigano-D'Angelo S, et al: Protein S deficiency occurs in the nephrotic syndrome. *Ann Intern Med* 107:42–47, 1987.

217. Du XH, et al: Nephrotic syndrome with renal vein thrombosis: Pathogenetic importance of a plasmin inhibitor (α_2-antiplasmin). *Clin Nephrol* 24:186–191, 1985.

218. Remuzzi G, et al: Platelet hyperaggregability and the nephrotic syndrome. *Thromb Res* 16:345–354, 1979.

219. Machleidt C, et al: Multifactorial genesis of enhanced platelet aggregability in patients with nephrotic syndrome. *Kidney Int* 36:1119–1124, 1989.

220. Rosenfield AT, et al: Ultrasound in experimental and clinical renal vein thrombosis. *Radiology* 137:735–741, 1980.

221. Braun B, Weilemann LS, and Weigand W: Ultrasonographic demonstration of renal vein thrombosis. *Radiology* 138:157–158, 1981.

222. Avasthi PS, et al: Noninvasive diagnosis of renal vein thrombosis by ultrasonic echo-Doppler flowmetry. *Kidney Int* 23:882–887, 1983.

223. Harrington JT and Kassirer JP: Renal vein thrombosis. *Ann Rev Med* 33:255–262, 1982.

224. Crowley JP, et al: Fibrinolytic therapy for bilateral renal vein thrombosis. *Arch Intern Med* 144:159–160, 1984.

225. Esparza AR, et al: Spectrum of acute renal failure in nephrotic syndrome with minimal (or minor) glomerular lesions. *Lab Invest* 45:510–521, 1981.

226. Chamberlain MJ, Pringle A, and Wrong OM: Oliguric renal failure in the nephrotic syndrome. *Q J Med* 138:215–235, 1966.

227. Conally ME, Wrong OM, and Jones NF: Reversible renal failure in idiopathic nephrotic syndrome with minimal glomerular changes. *Lancet* 1:665–668, 1968.

228. Raij L, et al: Irreversible acute renal failure in idiopathic nephrotic syndrome. *Am J Med* 61:207–214, 1976.

229. Lowenstein J, Schacht RG, and Baldwin DS: Renal failure in minimal change nephrotic syndrome. *Am J Med* 70:227–233, 1981.
230. Case records of the Massachusetts General Hospital. *N Engl J Med* 299: 136–145, 1978.
231. Hulter HN and Bonner EL Jr: Lipoid nephrosis appearing as acute oliguric renal failure. *Arch Intern Med* 140:403–405, 1980.
232. Imbasciati E, et al: Acute renal failure in idiopathic nephrotic syndrome. *Nephron* 28:186–191, 1981.
233. Sjoberg RJ, et al: Renal failure with minimal change nephrotic syndrome: Reversal with hemodialysis. *Clin Nephrol* 20:98–100, 1983.
234. Searle M, et al: Reversibility of acute renal failure in elderly patients with the nephrotic syndrome. *Postgrad Med* 61:741–744, 1985.
235. Thompson H and Odell M: Reversible uraemia in normotensive nephrotic syndrome. *Br Med J* 274:705–706, 1979.
236. Moorthy AV, et al: Association of crescentic glomerulonephritis with membranous glomerulopathy: A report of three cases. *Clin Nephrol* 6:319–325, 1976.
237. Hill GS, et al: An unusual variant of membranous nephropathy with abundant crescent formation and recurrence in the transplanted kidney. *Clin Nephrol* 10:114–120, 1978.
238. Bennett WM and Kincaid-Smith P: Macroscopic hematuria in mesangial IgA nephropathy: Correlation with glomerular crescents and renal dysfunction. *Kidney Int* 23:393–400, 1983.
239. Abrielo GJ, et al: Crescentic IgA nephropathy. *Medicine* 63:396–406, 1984.
240. Koethe JD, et al: Progression of membranous nephropathy to acute crescentic rapidly progressive glomerulonephritis and response to pulse methylprednisolone. *Am J Nephrol* 6:224–228, 1986.
241. Lee JC, Yamauchi H, and Hooper J Jr: The association of cancer and the nephrotic syndrome. *Ann Intern Med* 64:41–51, 1966.
242. Eagen JW and Lewis EJ: Glomerulopathies of neoplasia. *Kidney Int* 11:297–306, 1977.
243. Hooper J Jr, Trew PA, and Biava CG: Membranous nephropathy: Its relative benignity in women. *Nephron* 29:18–24, 1981.
244. Faubert PF and Porush JG: Unpublished observations, 1990.
245. Biava CG, et al: Crescentic glomerulonephritis associated with nonrenal malignancies. *Am J Nephrol* 4:208–214, 1984.
246. Haskell LP, et al: Crescentic glomerulonephritis associated with prostatic carcinoma: Evidence of immune-mediated glomerular injury. *Am J Med* 88:189–192, 1990.
247. Lund L, Jacobsen BA, and Schmidt EB: The occurrence of malignant disease in adult nephrotic syndrome. *J Intern Med* 226:201–203, 1989.

7 RENAL INVOLVEMENT IN SYSTEMIC DISEASE

DIABETIC NEPHROPATHY

INCIDENCE AND PREVALENCE

Diabetic nephropathy is the most common form of secondary glomerular disease in the elderly, and the problem is likely to grow because the prevalence of adult-onset diabetes mellitus has increased with age during the past three decades in the United States [1]. It should be noted that the incidence of renal disease is lower in type II diabetics (non-insulin-dependent) compared to type I (insulin-dependent) but appears earlier after the diagnosis of diabetes mellitus is made (5 to 10 years for type II compared to 10 to 15 years for type I) [2]. In one population study from Rochester (Minnesota), diabetic nephropathy was found to be present in 170 per 100,000 person-years in type I diabetics and in 133 per 100,000 in type II diabetics [3]. Since there are many more type II than type I diabetics, there are far more patients with type II diabetes who develop renal disease. As expected, the prevalence of nephropathy increases progressively with the duration of the diabetes [4, 5]. For example, heavy proteinuria (> 1 g per 24 hours) in the Pima Indians occurs in 15.7 per 1,000 persons per year after a 5- to 10-year history of type II diabetes mellitus, in 43.0 per 1,000 persons per year after a 10- to 15-year history, and in 77.0 per 1,000 persons per year after a 15-year or longer history [6].

PATHOLOGY

The early changes on light microscopy consist of widening of the glomerular mesangium and Bowman's capsule. As the disease progresses the capillary basement membranes thicken, and aneurysmal dilatation of capillaries occurs. Other findings include nodular glomerulosclerosis with a tendency toward a peripheral location and hyaline deposits in Bowman's capsule, the mesangium, or the lumens of dilated capillaries. Ultimately, the glomerulus becomes completely sclerosed. On electron microscopy there is thickening of the glomerular basement membrane, and thick strands of mesangial matrix are aggregated into nodules. With immunofluorescence microscopy, linear deposits of immunoglobulins (IgG), albumin, or fibrinogen can be found along the glomerular and tubular basement membranes.

PATHOGENESIS

Most of our knowledge concerning the pathogenesis of diabetic nephropathy derives from data obtained in young insulin-dependent subjects and from studies in the rat. In early insulin-dependent diabetes mellitus in both humans and the experimental animal there is an increase in the glomerular filtration rate (GFR) and nephromegaly. The increase in GFR seems to result from an elevation in glomerular capillary flow, in part due to a decrease in glomerular contractile responsiveness to angiotensin II (AII), suggested by the reduced AII receptor density seen in rats with streptozotocin-induced diabetes mellitus [7]. Glomerular capillary hypertension appears to play an important role in the pathogenesis of experimental diabetic nephropathy because its prevention with a converting enzyme inhibitor protects the animal against the subsequent development of glomerular structural injury and proteinuria despite persistent hyperglycemia [8]. In humans with type I diabetes mellitus, GFR can be reduced to essentially normal levels after euglycemia is achieved [9], but nephromegaly tends to persist, suggesting that other factors besides hyperperfusion and biochemical alterations are at play in the pathogenesis of diabetic nephropathy [10]. Supranormal GFR and glomerular hypertrophy are either absent [11–13] or less prominent in type II diabetics [14]. Since diabetes mellitus is associated with increased platelet activation [15], platelet-derived growth factor, which has the ability to bind to the mesangial cell, might well stimulate these cells to expand and subsequently become sclerotic [16].

CLINICAL MANIFESTATIONS

In the great majority of patients, diabetes has been present for at least several years, with the patient taking either an oral hypoglycemic agent or insulin. This diagnostic criterion will eliminate the occasional elderly patient with chronic renal insufficiency in whom fasting hyperglycemia is present as a consequence of the azotemic state [17].

Retinopathy

Since retinopathy and nephropathy are both manifestations of small vessel disease in diabetes mellitus, it is not surprising that they often occur together, even though their rate of progression and severity are often strikingly dissociated. For instance, of 106 patients receiving treatment for retinopathy, clinical evidence of renal disease was found in only 30 percent [18]. By contrast, between 80 and 90 percent of patients with renal failure have retinopathy [19]. Therefore, the absence of retinopathy (confirmed by fluorescein angiography) in a diabetic patient with significant proteinuria, with or without associated renal insufficiency, should alert the physician to the possibility of another glomerular disease.

Proteinuria With or Without Renal Insufficiency

Of 510 patients with maturity-onset diabetes mellitus, 48 percent had protein excretion above 150 mg per 24 hours, 81 (16 percent) had proteinuria in excess of 500 mg per 24 hours, and 18 (3.5 percent) had proteinuria greater than 3,000 mg per 24 hours [2]. In the same series, 83 percent of patients with protein excretion below 150 mg per 24 hours had normal kidney function compared to 65 percent of those with proteinuria above this value. Only 8.7 percent of the patients had a GFR below 60 ml per minute. The cumulative risk for chronic renal failure 10 years after the diagnosis of persistent proteinuria in type II diabetics is about 11 percent [3]. In a larger group of elderly patients with diabetic nephropathy referred to us during the past 10 years, the majority had diabetes mellitus for 5 to 10 years; proteinuria of greater than 3,000 mg per 24 hours was seen in more than 70 percent, and renal insufficiency of varying severity (serum creatinine 2 to 8 mg per dl) was almost a universal finding at the time of diagnosis. The proteinuria in such patients is, in general, nonselective and reflects a depletion of the fixed negative charges as well as an increasing impairment in barrier-size selectivity of the glomerular capillary wall [20–22]. The renal insufficiency most likely represents loss of ultrafiltration capacity of the glomerular capillaries [23, 24], a consequence of gradual mesangial expansion and vascular sclerosis [25].

Hematuria

In a prospective study of 30 patients of varying ages with a diagnosis of probable diabetic nephropathy, microscopic hematuria was found in 30 percent and red cell casts in 13 percent [26]. The incidence of hematuria in the elderly has been somewhat lower in our experience, closer to the 14 percent rate reported by Lopes de Faria et al [27]. In these patients the decision to undertake extensive urologic evaluation depends on the characteristics of the hematuria, which is suggestive of a glomerular origin in the majority of cases (see Chap. 6). For those with apparent nonglomerular bleeding, the incidence of a superimposed urologic disorder, other than benign prostatic hypertrophy in the male, has been low in our experience.

Hypertension

In the 510 patients reported by Fabre and associates [2], a diastolic BP of 110 mm Hg or more was twice as common in diabetics compared to the general population. The prevalence of hypertension in older diabetics is 58 percent in males and 72 percent in females aged 65 to 74 years, 55 percent in males and 71 percent in females aged 75 to 84 years, and 42 percent in males and 73 percent in females 85 years and older [28]. In a randomly selected group of 155 noninsulin-dependent patients attending a diabetic clinic, 39 percent were found to have hypertension compared to a prevalence of 16 percent in controls [29]. A positive correlation has been found between systolic BP and 24-hour urinary albumin excretion in these patients. This correlation, however, has not been found by others [30, 31]. More than 90 percent of our patients with proteinuria are also hypertensive. Those with a normal BP usually have significant cardiac dysfunction. Since the blood pressure rises progressively with decreasing renal function, the hypertension in patients with established diabetic glomerulosclerosis is probably largely a consequence of the kidney disease [32].

According to De Chatel and associates [33], at an early stage when the diabetic is still normotensive there is a significant increase in exchangeable sodium (Na), whereas plasma and blood volume are similar to those seen in normal controls. As hypertension sets in, however, both plasma and blood volume increase significantly. Even though basal levels of plasma renin, aldosterone, and catecholamines are identical in diabetics and normals, the pressor responsiveness of diabetes to norepinephrine (NE) and AII is exaggerated [34]. This increased sensitivity to AII must be selective and limited to the hypertensive diabetic because AII receptor density is reduced in platelets of insulin-dependent diabetics [35] and in the glomerular capillary [7]. The mechanism responsible for the sodium retention is not clear [36] but might be due in part to the endogenous hyperinsulinemia generally present in this condition (at least for the type II diabetic), since insulin has been shown to increase renal tubular sodium reabsorption [37, 38]. Intracellular sodium metabolism (estimated by Na/lithium [Li] countertransport and Na/potassium [K] cotransport) is similar in type II hypertensive diabetics and in type II normotensive diabetics [39]. Treatment with a thiazide diuretic often improves blood pressure and restores total body sodium to control levels and improves the cardiovascular responsiveness to NE and AII as well [40].

Based on an increased ratio of urinary kallikrein activity to supine plasma renin activity (a ratio that apparently correlates with renal blood flow), it has been suggested that abnormalities in the metabolism of these vasodilatory renal enzyme systems might play a pathogenetic role in the hypertension characteristic of type II diabetics [41]. The possible therapeutic implications of these findings remain to be determined. A marked defect in calcium [Ca]-ATPase activity has been found in the erythrocytes of hypertensive type II diabetics [42]. This defect is associated with an increase in intracellular Ca and appears to result partly from diabetes-induced alterations in calmodulin rather than from an intrinsic defect in pump function [43]. Until a similar observation is made in the vascular smooth muscle of type II hypertensive diabetics, the significance of this finding is highly speculative.

NATURAL HISTORY AND THERAPY

Microalbuminuria, defined as an albumin excretion of 30 to 140 μg per ml, is a good predictor of the subsequent development of renal impairment in type II diabetes, as it is in type I [5, 44, 45]. The prevalence rate of microalbuminuria in the former varies between 12 and 50 percent [44]. Clinical proteinuria (> 500 mg per 24 hours) will develop in 22 percent of patients with microalbuminuria compared to 5 percent of those with an albumin excretion of less than 30 μg per ml [44]. The mechanisms responsible for the transition from micro- to macroalbuminuria are not clear. The time course of the transition differs markedly among patients [45]. In general, once clinical proteinuria appears, the decline in GFR tends to be slower in type II diabetics compared with those with type I disease [46]. In our experience and that of others [47], however, elderly type II diabetic patients with proteinuria of greater than 500 mg per 24 hours developed end-stage kidney disease within 4 to 5 years, a rate similar to that reported for type I diabetics [48].

Strict glycemic control in insulin-dependent diabetics with established macroalbuminuria does not appear to have any effect on the rate of decline in the GFR [49]; therefore, to be successful, therapeutic intervention should start at the stage of microalbuminuria [50]. Whether aggressive glycemic control will be of help in such patients remains to be seen. Recently, Feldt-Rasmussen et al [51] have reported a significant decrease in kidney size after 12 months of strict glycemic control; however, the albuminuria could not be reversed. In a small group of type II diabetic patients with microalbuminuria, a specific thromboxane synthetase inhibitor was able to lower the albumin excretion after 2 months (independent of a change in glycosylated hemoglobin or mean blood glucose levels), suggesting that thromboxane, the synthesis of which is increased in diabetic nephropathy, plays a role in the proteinuria [52]. More recently, the administration of captopril, an angiotensin-converting enzyme inhibitor (37.5 mg thrice daily), was associated with a significant decrease in proteinuria as early as 2 weeks after treatment in 10 type I diabetics [53]. The mean protein excretion rate was 10.6 ± 2.2 g per 24 hours prior to therapy, which decreased to 4.9 ± 1.1 g per 24 hours after 8 weeks of therapy. Similar results have been reported in patients with lesser degrees of albuminuria [54, 55]. Serum creatinine, when elevated, did not change significantly. A decrease in proteinuria associated with either a calcium channel blocker or a converting enzyme inhibitor has been reported in type II diabetics with hypertension and microalbuminuria [56] but not in those with macroalbuminuria [57]. Before routinely adopting this approach further studies involving a larger number of patients are obviously needed and should be forthcoming. Besides captopril, dipyridamole (225 mg per day) and aspirin (975 mg per day), used over a long period of time, have been found to stabilize the progression of diabetic nephropathy in 24 percent of patients with insulin-dependent diabetic nephropathy [58, 59].

The therapy of hypertension in the diabetic patient is similar to that in the nondiabetic elderly (see Chap. 12). Early aggressive antihypertensive therapy has been associated with a reduction in the rate of loss of kidney function in a group of insulin-dependent young diabetics [60, 61], but similar findings are not available in the elderly. Since total exchangeable sodium is increased in the hypertensive diabetic, a low-sodium diet (2 to 3 g) [62], used alone or together with furosemide in a dose tailored to the patient's GFR and weight loss response, is part of our therapeutic strategy. Caloric reduction is necessary in the obese diabetic because weight loss per se may facilitate blood pressure control [63]. Given the preliminary data noted earlier, we presently favor the use of an angiotensin-converting enzyme inhibitor (ACEi) following this therapy, if necessary. We may also use an ACEi as the first drug after dietary restriction and reserve the diuretic for the second drug. Serum potassium must be monitored closely in these patients, particularly those with an elevated serum creatinine. We usually start with captopril, 12.5 mg bid, or enalapril, 5 mg daily. If an ACEi cannot be used, a calcium channel blocker or any other agent (beta blocker, sympatholytic, vasodilator) can be added to the diuretic. In a group of 20 elderly hypertensive diabetics treated by us recently, the average systolic and diastolic pressures prior to control were 190 mm Hg and 110 mm Hg, respectively. We were able to bring the systolic below 150 mm Hg and diastolic below 95 mm Hg in all patients with minimal side effects. Occasionally, an elderly diabetic hypertensive is seen with supine hypertension and symptomatic orthostatic hypotension. These patients can be managed with a combination of antihypertensives and 9-alpha-fluorohydrocortisone, 0.05 to 0.3 mg per day. Volume status must be carefully monitored to prevent fluid overload [64].

DIFFERENTIAL DIAGNOSIS
The diagnosis of diabetic nephropathy is most often made on clinical grounds when the triad of retinopathy, proteinuria, and hypertension is present in a patient with long-standing diabetes mellitus; however, the development of proteinuria or the nephrotic syndrome in long-standing diabetes does not necessarily imply diabetic glomerulopathy.

In biopsies of 47 patients with long-standing diabetes mellitus performed by Hatch et al [65], six (13 percent) showed histologic findings other than diabetic glomerulosclerosis. Two had chronic glomerulonephritis, two had nephrosclerosis, one had membranous glomerulopathy, and one had acute endoproliferative glomerulonephritis. Chihara and associates [66] found a glomerular disease other than diabetic glomerulosclerosis in 36 (22 percent) of 164 diabetic patients. The reason for the biopsy in these 164 diabetic patients is not stated by the authors.

They noted that those patients with superimposed glomerular disease were older and had had their diabetes mellitus for a shorter period of time, and 70 percent of them had hematuria (compared to 28 percent of those with diabetic glomerulosclerosis). Retinopathy was detected in 82 percent of patients with diabetic glomerulosclerosis and in 41 percent of those with superimposed glomerular disease. The glomerular diseases most commonly found in 56 diabetics in whom biopsies were done and reported in the literature were mesangial proliferative (30 percent), membranous nephropathy (23 percent), and acute endoproliferative glomerulonephritis (20 percent) [65–73]. In the majority of these patients there were several factors that raised the suspicion of a diagnosis other than diabetic nephropathy including rapid onset of proteinuria and microscopic hematuria in a patient without retinopathy or with normal blood pressure, rapid deterioration of kidney function in an otherwise stable patient, gross hematuria, difficulty in controlling the blood pressure in a patient in whom it was previously under control, and the absence of neuropathy [74].

Immune complex glomerular disease superimposed on pre-existing diabetic glomerulosclerosis has also been reported [75–76]. Given the poor prognosis associated with diabetic nephropathy at the present time, we do not think that any attempt to treat the superimposed glomerulonephritis will significantly alter the outcome in these patients unless it is rapidly progressive glomerulonephritis (crescentic disease).

In our experience, the natural history of a given glomerular disease does not differ in the diabetic patient. It is our opinion (even though reliable data are not available) that once the diagnosis of a glomerulopathy other than diabetic glomerulosclerosis is made in a diabetic, therapy should be the same as that for the nondiabetic (see Chapter 6).

KIDNEY DISEASES ASSOCIATED WITH DYSPROTEINEMIA AND PARAPROTEINEMIA

As seen in Table 7-1, which represents the combined experience of three studies [77–79] plus our own and includes only patients in whom biopsies were performed, after diabetes dysglobulinemias account for the majority of renal disorders due to systemic diseases in the elderly. This group of diseases includes amyloidosis, "myeloma kidney," light chain nephropathy, essential mixed cryoglobulinemia, and macroglobulinemia.

AMYLOIDOSIS
Amyloidosis encompasses a group of diseases characterized by the deposition of a proteinaceous material in a variety of tissues, with the classification based on the biochemical composition of the protein subunit

TABLE 7-1. Incidence of renal involvement
other than diabetes mellitus in the elderly*

Disease	No. patients (%)
Dysproteinemia and paraproteinemia	52 (49)
Amyloidosis	
Multiple myeloma	
Cast nephropathy	
Light chain nephropathy	
Cryoglobulinemia	
Waldenström's macroglobulinemia	
Vasculitis	26 (25)
Wegener's granulomatosis	
Periarteritis nodosa	
Giant cell arteritis	
Henoch-Schönlein purpura	
Others	
Collagen vascular diseases	19 (18)
Systemic lupus erythematosus	
Scleroderma	
Others	9 (8)
Hemolytic uremic syndrome	
Thrombotic thrombocytopenic purpura	
Rheumatoid arthritis	
Sjögren's syndrome	
Drug-induced glomerular disease	
Infections and glomerular disease	
Sarcoidosis	

*Includes only biopsy-proven cases.

deposited [80, 81] (Table 7-2). Since renal amyloidosis in the elderly is almost entirely limited to AL and AA protein, this discussion will involve these two entities only.

Incidence

Primary amyloidosis (AL, amyloid light chain protein) is relatively common in the elderly and should be considered in the differential diagnosis of any elderly patient presenting with the nephrotic syndrome. Of 229 patients with amyloidosis reported by Kyle and Greipp [82], 145 (63 percent) were over the age of 60. The elderly made up 60 to 63 percent of the reported cases with renal involvement [83].

The reported incidence of secondary amyloidosis (AA, amyloid A protein) in the elderly has been quite variable. In 32 patients reported by Triger and Joekes [84], three (10 percent) were over 60 years, whereas in the series reported by Browning et al [85], 36 of 75 patients (48 percent) were over 60 years of age. The most common diseases associated with

TABLE 7-2. Classification of amyloidosis

Type of amyloidosis	Associated diseases	Designation
Primary (light chain kappa, lambda)	Myeloma, macroglobulinemia, related plasma cell neoplasms	AL
Secondary (amyloid A protein)	Chronic infections, inflammatory diseases, malignancies	AA
Familial (prealbumin)	Many familial types	AF
Senile cardiac (prealbumin)	—	SSA
Dialysis amyloid (beta-2 micro-globulin)	—	$A\beta_2M$
Localized (calcitonin)	Medullary carcinoma of thyroid	AE
Cerebral (alpha-4 or beta)	Senile dementia, Down's syndrome	CAA

SOURCE: Adapted from Franklin EC: Immunopathology of the amyloid diseases. *Hosp Pract* 15:70–77, 1980; and Gertz MA and Kyle RA: Primary systemic amyloidosis— A diagnostic primer. *Mayo Clin Proc* 64:1505–1519, 1989.

AA amyloidosis in the elderly are rheumatoid arthritis, bronchiectasis, chronic osteomyelitis, tuberculosis, Hodgkin's disease, carcinoma of the kidney, and inflammatory bowel diseases.

Pathology
The diagnosis of amyloidosis depends on the demonstration of amyloid deposits in the kidney, using appropriate staining procedures, such as Congo red, crystal violet, or thioflavin T. On light microscopy, deposits of amyloid are found in the mesangium and in the capillary walls. In the former, they form nodules of various sizes or diffuse infiltrates that expand the intercapillary space and compress the lumina. In the latter, the deposits are present in the basement membrane and appear in a pattern of perpendicular projections on the epithelial side, referred to as spicules. These spicules are of prognostic significance because they are associated morphologically with accelerated amyloid deposition and clinically with a fulminant clinical course [86]. The severity of the proteinuria has also been found to correlate with the presence of spicules [86]. Under electron microscopy the deposits take the form of fine, nonbranching fibrils arranged in bundles. With immunofluorescence microscopy, kappa or lambda light chain deposits are found in AL amyloidosis, whereas A protein deposits are present in AA amyloidosis.

Pathogenesis

In AL amyloidosis, a clone of plasma cells secretes an excessive amount of light chains, some of which are incompletely digested by phagocytes whereas others escape degradation. The amyloid fibrils result from incorporation of light chain fragments alone or with whole light chains that have bypassed degradation. Fibrils, singly and in aggregates, may then be deposited in the kidneys [80].

The A protein in AA amyloidosis results from cleavage by monocytes of serum AA (SAA), a substance secreted by hepatocytes. The A protein in turn aggregates into fibrils and is deposited between renal cells. The concentration of SAA has been found to be markedly increased in some patients with rheumatoid arthritis and Crohn's disease. The level appears to correspond to the incidence of systemic amyloidosis in these patients [87]. Besides the increased serum level of AA protein, decreased activity of a serum factor capable of degrading AA fibrils has also been described [88]. It thus appears that both primary and secondary amyloidosis occurs in situations in which the immune system becomes overwhelmed by an antigenic load or has undergone neoplastic transformation. The specific immunologic defect remains to be unraveled.

Clinical Manifestations

Since amyloid proteins can be deposited in several organs, the initial manifestations associated with the syndrome are quite variable [89]. Proteinuria is the most common renal manifestation associated with both AL and AA amyloidosis. In AL amyloidosis, proteinuria is found in 29 to 86 percent of the reported cases [77–79, 82, 83, 85]. Nephrotic syndrome is present in 35 percent of these patients, 90 percent at the time of diagnosis. Sixty-six percent of patients without myeloma-associated AL have monoclonal light chains in their urine noted by immunoelectrophoresis, whereas the incidence is 93 percent for those with myeloma. The proteinuria is usually nonselective. The urine sediment is usually benign, although macroscopic or microscopic hematuria has occasionally been described [82, 83]. Renal insufficiency (serum creatinine > 2 mg per dl) is found in 25 to 43 percent of patients at initial diagnosis. Hypertension is found in 42 percent of patients, whereas orthostatic hypotension is present in 10 to 20 percent. As might be expected, a larger number of patients with myeloma (11 percent) have associated hypercalcemia (Ca > 11 mg per dl) compared to only 2 percent of those without myeloma. Kidney size varies considerably among patients at the time of diagnosis.

In patients with AA amyloidosis, proteinuria occurs in 57 percent, half of whom have the nephrotic syndrome [84, 85].

Natural History and Treatment
Renal disease due to amyloidosis is usually progressive, virtually all patients reaching end stage or dying from other complications within a relatively short period of time (1 to 3 years). The prognosis appears to be better in those with AA amyloidosis, in whom survival up to 11 years has been reported [85]. A precipitous and irreversible decrease in renal function, also noted by others [86], has been observed in some of our patients with AL amyloidosis without a morphologic or hemodynamic explanation. Specifically, renal vein thrombosis was ruled out in our patients.

Several forms of therapy have been tried in patients with amyloidosis, with little success in general. There are a few case reports describing disappearance of the amyloid deposits (in patients with the AA form) after treatment of the chronic infection or removal of a renal cell carcinoma [90–93]. Based on these reports, every attempt should be made either to treat or correct the underlying condition judged responsible for the amyloidosis. D-Penicillamine, alone or in combination with chlorambucil, has been tried in patients with rheumatoid arthritis and AA amyloidosis with varied success [94]. Colchicine has been shown to prevent amyloidosis in high-risk patients with familial Mediterranean fever and also prevents additional deterioration of renal function in patients with amyloidosis who have proteinuria, but not the nephrotic syndrome [95]. Whether this drug will benefit other patients with AA amyloidosis is worth investigating.

In a recent prospective randomized study, the combination of prednisone and melphalan was found to be superior to colchicine in patients with AL amyloidosis [96]. Proteinuria decreased more than 50 percent in 21 of 39 patients with the nephrotic syndrome. No such response was noted in patients treated with colchicine. Four patients in the melphalan and prednisone group developed acute nonlymphocytic leukemia. The dose of melphalan was 0.15 mg per kg given in two divided doses; that of prednisone was 0.8 mg per kg given in four divided doses daily. The treatment schedule in the study was 7 days of treatment repeated every 6 weeks.

In patients who do not tolerate this regimen we use colchicine (0.6 mg once or twice a day) because there have been some data suggesting that this approach is better than no therapy at all, even in patients with AL protein [97]. Dimethyl sulfoxide (DMSO), an agent that theoretically can accelerate the destruction of the amyloid fibril, has also been tried with some success [98, 99].

Besides the amyloid fibrils, which consist of nonglycosylated polypeptide chains, amyloid deposits may also contain a nonfibrillar glycoprotein called amyloid P component (AP). It has been postulated that AP forms a protective coating over the amyloid fibrils; if so, methyl 4,6-0-(1-carboxyethylidene)-B-D-galactopyranoside (MOBDG), a substance capable of dissociating AP from amyloid fibrils, may open some new therapeutic avenues in managing patients with amyloidosis [100].

MULTIPLE MYELOMA

The renal lesions associated with multiple myeloma can be divided into two broad categories, as discussed by Hill et al [101]: (1) cast nephropathy (also called myeloma kidney), and (2) tissue deposition of paraproteins, either amyloid (discussed earlier) or light chains (rarely, heavy chains). The latter condition is also referred to as light chain nephropathy. As shown by these authors, cast and light chain nephropathy tend to be mutually exclusive, since few or no myeloma casts are seen in patients with diffuse tissue deposition of light chains and, in patients with cast nephropathy, mild mesangial lesions, focal interstitial and vascular deposits of amyloid, or light chains are seen only occasionally. The reason a given patient develops one form or the other is not clear. The nature and characteristics of the monoclonal protein (or M component) being produced surely play an important role, however [102].

CAST NEPHROPATHY (MYELOMA KIDNEY)
Incidence
The elderly account for 62 percent of reported cases of multiple myeloma [103]. The incidence of renal failure in patients of all age groups with multiple myeloma is 40 to 50 percent. The incidence in the elderly is 58 percent, suggesting that age per se constitutes only a minor risk factor for developing renal insufficiency [103]. The elderly male-to-female ratio is 3:2.

Pathology
The pathologic hallmark of the myeloma kidney is the presence of intratubular protein casts on light microscopy. These casts have a granular appearance with a characteristic "fracture line." Multinucleated giant cells can be seen engulfing those casts. Marked tubular atrophy and degeneration are found in advanced cases with renal insufficiency and are associated with a poor outcome [104]. In general, the amount of interstitial fibrosis present parallels the amount of tubular atrophy. Flecks of calcium in tubular casts or the interstitium have occasionally been reported [105]. On immunofluorescent studies, the casts can contain all classes of immunoglobulins and kappa and lambda light chains. Albumin, Tamm-Horsfall protein, and complement components are also found occasionally. On electron microscopy, the casts are composed of

homogeneous, finely granular material. Tears in the tubular basement membrane and intracytoplasmic inclusions may be seen. The glomeruli rarely may show finely granular electron-dense amorphous deposits in a mesangial, subendothelial, or intramembranous location [106].

Pathogenesis
A strong association exists between the presence of light chain proteinuria and the development of renal insufficiency in the myeloma patient [107]. Light chains, because of their molecular weight, are easily filtered and reabsorbed by the tubular cells through a saturable process [108]. In multiple myeloma, the amount of light chains produced frequently exceeds the reabsorptive capacity of the tubular cells. As a consequence, these unreabsorbed free proteins may precipitate in the lumen, particularly in the presence of volume contraction, ischemia produced by hypercalcemia, sepsis, or exposure to iodinated contrast agents. Also, light chains may be directly toxic to tubule cells, as evidenced by the presence on histologic examination of varying degrees of proximal tubule damage such as cell desquamation, vacuolation, and coagulation necrosis [109]. In studies by DeFronzo et al [110], creatinine clearance and PAH clearance (renal plasma flow) were statistically lower in myeloma patients with Bence Jones proteinuria compared to those without. Urinary pH, after ammonium chloride loading, was higher, and urinary osmolality, after an overnight fast and antidiuretic hormone (ADH) administration, was lower in the patients with Bence Jones proteinuria. It should be emphasized that the typical myeloma cast is not a universal finding in the myeloma patient with renal insufficiency; thus, factors other than the presence of light chains are involved in the pathogenesis of the renal disease. Patients with abundant light chain proteinuria have been followed for years without developing any renal functional abnormality [111], and in patients with renal insufficiency GFR can improve despite the persistence of light chain proteinuria [112].

Besides the intrinsic structure of monoclonal proteins, their isoelectric point (pI) may also be a determinant of pathogenicity. A negative correlation between the level of the pI and creatinine clearance has been found in patients studied by Coward et al [113]. Acute reversible renal failure has been associated with light chains of low pI and chronic irreversible renal failure with light chains of high pI [114]; however, this has not been a consistent finding [104, 115]. Further studies are obviously needed to clarify the exact role of pI in the pathogenesis of cast nephropathy.

Clinical Manifestations
Renal involvement in cast nephropathy in the majority of patients (90 to 93 percent) is insidious and usually progresses over a period of several

months to years. In the remaining 7 to 10 percent the disease presents abruptly with acute renal failure. In up to 40 to 50 percent of these cases the diagnosis of both myeloma and acute renal failure is made simultaneously, making it mandatory that multiple myeloma be considered in the elderly with unexplained acute renal failure [116, 117]. In some of these patients nonsteroidal anti-inflammatory drugs, dehydration, sepsis, hypercalcemia, or contrast agents have been the precipitating factor [104, 118]. Oliguria is present in 50 percent of the patients with acute renal failure. Bence Jones proteinuria, 850 to 2,000 mg per 24 hours, is found in patients with either the chronic or acute form of the disease. The presence of a low anion gap in a patient with renal failure and proteinuria should raise the suspicion of multiple myeloma [119, 120]. The low gap is due to the presence of cationic paraproteins.

Fanconi syndrome (glycosuria, aminoaciduria, phosphaturia, renal tubular acidosis) and hyporeninemic hypoaldosteronism have been reported in association with multiple myeloma. Their exact incidence in the elderly is not known [121].

Natural History and Treatment
An attempt should be made to uncover the presence of a precipitating factor leading to acute renal failure in patients with myeloma. Aggressive treatment of hypercalcemia has been found to reverse the renal failure in 67 percent of the patients reported by Bernstein and Humes [122]. Volume should be replaced in the dehydrated patient and sepsis treated with the appropriate antibiotics. Alkalinization of the urine without any attempt to characterize the pI of the light chain has been found to have a marginal benefit [112].

The primary therapy for the renal disease is that recommended for the multiple myeloma, and these patients should be followed in concert with an oncologist. A discussion of the currently used cytotoxic agents is beyond the scope of this chapter. The addition of plasma exchange to cytotoxic agents has been found to be more effective than chemotherapy alone in reversing renal failure in patients with rapidly deteriorating kidney function [123]. Five recent reports have provided additional evidence of the possible benefits of plasma exchange added to chemotherapy [124–128]. In the Italian Collaborative Study, patients who received plasma exchange in addition to chemotherapy recovered renal function more frequently (61 percent) than those treated with chemotherapy alone (27 percent) [124]. Thirty-seven of the 50 reported patients were 60 years or older. Twenty-five received chemotherapy and plasma exchange (group I), whereas 12 received chemotherapy alone (group II). The average time of follow-up was 11.0 ± 3.9 months for group II and 13.0 ± 2.7 months for group I. Forty-two percent of the patients in group II and 32 percent of those in group I were alive at the end of the follow-up period.

It appears that despite its beneficial effect on recovery of kidney function, plasma exchange did not prolong the survival of myeloma patients. Zucchelli et al [125], however, noted a 1-year survival rate of 66 percent in patients treated with plasmapheresis compared to 28 percent in untreated patients. Further studies are needed before this approach can be routinely recommended. We suggest that a kidney biopsy be performed before considering plasma exchange, since the presence of large numbers of tubular casts and chronic tubulointerstitial changes were associated with a rather poor response [124].

The use of plasmapheresis in patients with cast nephropathy has not been standardized. We use the approach outlined by Zucchelli et al [125]. Initially, therapy consists of intravenous pulse steroids (the equivalent of 20 mg per kg per day of methylprednisolone) given on 3 consecutive days followed by oral prednisone (20 to 30 mg per m^2 per day) for 7 days. Cyclophosphamide (200 mg per m^2 per day) is simultaneously administered parenterally for 5 days. Daily plasma exchange (3 to 4 liters) is performed for 5 consecutive days. Maintenance therapy consists of prednisone (60 mg per m^2 per day) and cyclophosphamide (100 mg per m^2 per day) given orally for 4 days at 4- to 6-week intervals. In general, patients who respond do so within the first month after therapy is initiated. We usually discontinue therapy in patients who do not respond after a 6-month trial.

Dialysis should not be withheld in the patient with multiple myeloma and associated end-stage renal failure [128–130]. The 1-year survival rate for this group is similar to that in the general myeloma population [131]. Cytotoxic therapy for the myeloma should be continued or initiated in such patients because occasionally patients may recover enough kidney function to survive without dialysis [132, 133]. The response of the tumor to chemotherapy is independent of the recovery of renal function and clearly remains the critical feature in these patients.

LIGHT CHAIN NEPHROPATHY
Incidence
The true incidence of the disease is not known. Of a total of 46 patients, including those reported in the literature of whom age was given plus our personal experience, 16 (35 percent) were over the age of 60. In the elderly, the ratio of males to females is 3:2 [134–144]. Sixty to seventy percent of patients with light chain nephropathy have multiple myeloma. The remaining 30 to 40 percent either have other myelomatous monoclonal gammopathies or do not have any associated condition [145].

Pathology
The pathology of light chain nephropathy, like that of amyloidosis, is mainly glomerular rather than tubulointerstitial as in cast nephropathy.

On light microscopy, the most common finding is nodular accumulation in the mesangium of PAS-positive material, which may be indistinguishable from the intercapillary nodule of diabetic glomerulosclerosis [137, 139]. The tubular basement membranes have a thickened refractile appearance and are outlined on their external aspect by ribbonlike continuous deposits, mainly along the distal tubules and loops of Henle. Occasional tubular casts are found. On immunofluorescence, either kappa or lambda light chains may be found in a linear pattern along glomerular and tubular basement membranes or as granular to nodular deposits in the mesangium. In some patients immunofluorescence microscopy is entirely negative. On electron microscopy, continuous granular deposits may be found in the subendothelial space and the lamina rara interna of the glomerular basement membrane. In others, the electron-dense material tends to accumulate in the area between the lamina densa and the lamina rara interna. Mesangial and paramesangial nodules of granular electron-dense material continuous with those in the subendothelial space may also be noted. Aneurysmal dilatation of the capillaries secondary to loss of the endothelial cell lining and disruption of mesangial anchoring points of the basement membrane are frequently found [146].

Pathogenesis
The deposits in light chain nephropathy, as in amyloidosis, are extracellular and present in multiple organs. The precise mechanism of tissue precipitation is not known. In five of six patients studied by Ganeval et al [144], abnormal immunoglobulin chains were produced. The authors postulated that such structural immunoglobulin abnormalities might possibly trigger their visceral deposition.

Clinical Manifestations
Clinical features of chronic renal disease constitute the initial manifestation in the majority of patients [134–145]. In others the disease is discovered during the course of established multiple myeloma. Renal insufficiency of varying severity and a nonselective proteinuria are found in all patients. Microhematuria is also a universal finding. Nephrotic syndrome is found in 20 to 30 percent of patients. The extrarenal manifestations of the disease may be present during the initial investigation of the renal disease or may appear later; these include involvement of the liver and heart, with hepatic or cardiac failure a consequence.

Natural History and Treatment
Renal disease associated with light chain nephropathy is usually rapidly progressive; therefore, chemotherapy with prednisone and melphalan is recommended for all patients and should be initiated early. One patient treated while on maintenance hemodialysis showed a remarkable im-

provement in renal function [142]. The dosage and regimen are the same as those used for patients with amyloidosis.

CRYOGLOBULINEMIA

Cryoglobulinemias can occur in association with a variety of disorders [147]. The presence of the cryoglobulins per se does not significantly alter the clinical course of the underlying disease, and renal involvement is rare. By contrast, in patients with so-called mixed essential cryoglobulinemia, a syndrome characterized by the presence of arthralgia, purpura, liver involvement, and Raynaud's phenomenon, renal disease often dominates the clinical picture and plays a major role in the prognosis [148]. It should be emphasized that cryoimmunoglobulins are commonly found in low concentrations (less than 20 mg per dl) in patients with various forms of primary glomerular diseases and appear to have neither diagnostic nor prognostic significance [149].

Incidence
In more than 218 patients with essential mixed cryoglobulinemia reported in the literature, 44 (20 percent) were 60 years or older [150–157]. The overall incidence of kidney involvement varied between 50 and 60 percent, and 20 percent of patients were 60 years and older, suggesting that age per se is not a risk factor for developing renal disease in essential mixed cryoglobulinemia. The female-to-male ratio was 3 : 1.

Pathology
The light microscopic appearance of this disorder is that of mesangiocapillary glomerulonephritis. The glomeruli have a lobular appearance with increased mesangial matrix and cellularity. Endothelial cell swelling and focal areas of necrosis with extensive "splitting" of the glomerular basement membranes are usually seen. In 18 percent of patients an acute necrotizing vasculitis involving medium-sized arteries and small arterioles with polymorphonuclear white blood cell infiltration is found. On immunofluorescence microscopy, granular IgM, IgG, and C3 deposits are found along the glomerular capillary loops and in the mesangium. Less common are IgA, C1a, and C4 deposits. On electron microscopy, the capillary lumen is obliterated by swollen endothelial cells and by cells with the characteristics of macrophages. Large crystalloid deposits are seen in the subendothelial areas [158].

Pathogenesis
Cryoimmunoglobulins result from the reaction of an IgM monoclonal rheumatoid factor with the Fc portion of a polyclonal IgG. The resulting immune complexes deposit in the glomeruli, initiating glomerular inflammation and damage [157]. Indeed, patients with the more severe

histologic changes and greater renal functional impairment display anti-globulin activity [155]. Neither the mechanism involved in the glomerular deposition of these immune complexes nor the basis for the glomerular injury are well understood. A decrease in the clearance of immune complexes by the mononuclear phagocytic system of patients with essential mixed cryoglobulinemia has been found. In such a situation more of the complexes could theoretically reach the kidneys, thereby increasing the likelihood of being entrapped and causing injury [159]. It is also possible that the mononuclear macrophages found on histologic examination in these patients are responsible in part for the glomerular injury and proteinuria, as postulated for other glomerulonephritides [160]. Finally, the complement system probably plays a role in the pathogenesis of the renal disease.

Clinical Manifestations

The diagnosis of essential mixed cryoglobulinemia should be suspected in any elderly patient presenting with weakness, purpura, arthralgia, and renal disease. An analysis of 30 elderly patients with these symptoms revealed that proteinuria (present in 63 percent) and renal insufficiency (present in 68 percent) were the most common manifestations [150–157]. Nephrotic syndrome was found in 17 percent. Microscopic hematuria is a universal finding, and red blood cell casts are frequently found. At the time of diagnosis 80 percent of the patients are hypertensive. C4 or C3 (or both) is depressed in 80 percent of patients. Acute renal failure has been reported as the initial manifestation of kidney involvement [158].

Natural History and Treatment

The development of kidney disease in patients with essential mixed cryoglobulinemia is associated with a poor prognosis. Of 20 patients followed by Gorevic et al [148] for an average of 5.6 years, 70 percent with renal failure died versus 31 percent with normal kidney function. Generally, the causes of death were extrarenal complications such as systemic vasculitis and cardiovascular and cerebrovascular accidents. Several therapeutic modalities have been tried with some success [156, 161–164]. The major problem with these studies, however, is that none were controlled, and the number of patients involved has been rather small. Nevertheless, for the patient with rapid deterioration in kidney function or rapidly increasing proteinuria, we recommend a 3-day course of 1 g intravenous "pulse" methylprednisolone followed by a maintenance dose of 0.4 mg per kg per day of prednisone together with 1 to 2 mg per kg per day of cyclophosphamide (or chlorambucil 0.1 mg per kg per day). In addition, plasmapheresis is used simultaneously 10 to 15 times, depending on changes in cryocrit, serum creatinine, and proteinuria.

In patients with stable renal disease, the long-term course is quite variable with spontaneous remissions, either partial or complete, occurring in as many as 33 percent of patients. End-stage disease will develop in 10 percent [165]. Since the natural history of the renal disease in those with stable kidney function is so unpredictable, therapy as outlined earlier should probably be reserved only for control of the extrarenal manifestations of the disease. The optimal length of therapy is not clear. Some authors have stopped it once a response occurs, whereas others have continued for a total of 12 months [156, 161–164].

WALDENSTRÖM'S MACROGLOBULINEMIA

Waldenström's macroglobulinemia most likely represents a spectrum of malignant disorders identified as separate from other malignant diseases by the presence of an increase in the IgM protein [166]. Even though diffuse interstitial infiltrate with lymphoid cells similar to those found in the bone marrow has been seen commonly in the kidney on autopsy, overt renal disease does not usually accompany the syndrome [167]. The majority of reported patients with renal disease were 60 years or older. The most specific histologic lesions found in Waldenström's macroglobulinemia are large eosinophilic hyaline thrombi within the capillary loops. On immunofluorescence, the thrombi stain strongly with IgM. The latter has a fibrillar structure on electron microscopy [168].

The renal disease can become manifest either as acute renal failure or as a more chronic form with either moderate to severe renal insufficiency or proteinuria, hematuria, and hypertension. In 15 elderly patients with proteinuria or chronic renal disease, five had the characteristic large glomerular thrombi described above; no detectable glomerular lesion was found in four, amyloidosis was seen in three, and there was one case each of mesangiocapillary glomerulonephritis, intercapillary glomerulosclerosis (light chain nephropathy), and crescentic glomerulonephritis [168–170]. It should be noted that crescentic glomerulonephritis can be seen as the initial manifestation of other plasma cell dyscrasias. Several such elderly patients have been reported [170, 171]. In two patients reported with acute renal failure, one had mesangiocapillary glomerulonephritis and the other the characteristic thrombi [172].

There is not enough information about the renal response to specific forms of therapy for the disease. Since the physical characteristics of the IgM protein are frequently responsible for a great majority of the patient's clinical manifestations (hyperviscosity syndrome), therapy should be directed toward reducing the serum concentration of IgM by plasmapheresis. Drugs such as busulfan or cyclophosphamide can be added to plasma exchange. Whereas such a regimen might benefit the patient with the characteristic lesion, other forms of therapy (e.g., melphalan and prednisone for those with amyloidosis, pulse steroids for those with crescentic disease) may be needed as well.

GLOMERULAR INJURY IN THE ELDERLY WITH NEOPLASIA

In the previous chapter, we discussed the probable association between membranous nephropathy, extracapillary glomerulonephritis, and solid tumors as well as between minimal change disease (lipoid nephrosis) and lymphomas. Recently, an increasing number of patients with glomerular disease associated with chronic lymphocytic leukemia (CLL) have been reported [173]. In most of these patients the CLL was diagnosed simultaneously with or prior to the kidney disease. Ten of the reported patients were over 60 years old. Kidney biopsy revealed mesangiocapillary glomerulonephritis in five, membranous nephropathy in two, focal glomerulosclerosis in one, minimal change disease in one, and focal nephritis in one [174–181]. A preponderance of mesangio-capillary glomerulonephritis has also been noted in younger patients with CLL [180]. The reason for this association is not clear; however, because of the putative role of immune complexes in the generation of the idiopathic form of mesangiocapillary glomerulonephritis, immune complexes should be considered the prime pathogenetic candidate in patients with CLL-associated glomerulonephritis [180, 181]. Remission of the renal disease has been reported following chemotherapy-induced remission of the CLL [181].

VASCULITIS

The term vasculitis refers to a heterogeneous group of disorders that have in common inflammatory destruction of blood vessel walls occurring de novo (in contrast to the vasculitis that occurs as a secondary feature of such diseases as, for example, systemic lupus erythematosus and rheumatoid arthritis) [182]. Several forms of classification have been proposed. Even though enough clinical and laboratory information [185, 186] is usually available to classify a given patient into one disease group or the other (periarteritis nodosa versus Wegener's granulomatosis), overlap is common [183, 184]. Since the renal histologic lesions associated with this group of disorders, known as systemic necrotizing arteritis, are in general rather strikingly homogeneous, we will discuss them as a group, emphasizing at times the specific points that might help in the differential diagnosis [182].

INCIDENCE

The incidence of renal involvement in the elderly with systemic vasculitis is not known; however, in patients with vasculitis and renal disease, 28 to 37 percent are 60 years or older [187, 188].

PATHOLOGY

As noted by Serra et al [187], it is difficult on histologic examination of the renal tissue alone to categorize a given patient into a specific classification of vasculitis. That is, the histologic changes described subsequently could correspond to one or various vasculitic diseases that present with renal involvement.

Both vascular and glomerular structures can be affected either alone or in combination on light microscopy. The vascular involvement is characterized by fibrinoid necrosis of the vessel wall with polymorphonuclear, eosinophilic, and mononuclear cell infiltration. In Wegener's granulomatosis the infiltrating cells are mainly lymphocytes and monocytes [189]. In Wegener's granulomatosis one sees segmental necrotizing glomerulitis with crescent formation, and in periarteritis nonspecific ischemic shrinkage of the capillary tuft is evident. When there are numerous crescents, pathologic differentiation from idiopathic rapidly progressive crescentic glomerulonephritis may be difficult. On immunofluorescence, various patterns of immunoglobulins, albumin, complement, or fibrinogen in the vessel wall have been reported. In cases of necrotizing glomerulitis, immunofluorescence studies are usually negative. The presence of IgA and C3 should raise the suspicion of Henoch-Schönlein purpura, and evidence of IgG, IgA, IgM, C3, and C4 of systemic lupus erythematosus (see later sections in this chapter on these disorders).

With electron microscopy, fibrin and poorly defined electron-dense deposits may be seen, and in patients with segmental necrotizing glomerulitis degeneration, swelling, and hypertrophy of endothelial and mesangial cells are common. Localized subepithelial or subendothelial deposits have also been described [187]. It should be noted that bacterial endocarditis, rheumatoid vasculitis, and Goodpasture's syndrome may also show necrotizing glomerulitis on kidney biopsy [190, 191]. The problem becomes even more difficult when autoantibodies to glomerular basement membrane, the hallmark of Goodpasture's syndrome, and antineutrophil cytoplasm antibodies, the hallmark of systemic vasculitis, are both present in the same patient [192]. The diagnosis may remain uncertain even after autopsy. The different diseases that can potentially present with both renal disease and pulmonary hemorrhage in the elderly are Wegener's granulomatosis, periarteritis nodosa, essential mixed cryoglobulinemia, Goodpasture's syndrome, systemic lupus erythematosus, and idiopathic crescentic glomerulonephritis. The incidence of combined pulmonary and renal disease in the elderly is not known, however.

PATHOGENESIS

The pathogenesis of the tissue inflammation and resulting damage to the vessel wall in the various forms of vasculitis is not known. Immune complexes probably play an important role, since these complexes have been found to be present in a large number of patients using different methods of measurement [193]. Moreover, a close association between active disease and circulating immune complexes has been reported in patients with Wegener's granulomatosis and kidney disease [194]. The nature of the antigenic challenge could be chemical (e.g., allopurinol, phenytoin), bacterial, viral, or tumoral; the individual immune response of the host ultimately determines the type and extent of the vasculitic process [195]. The absence of detectable vascular electron-dense deposits (except in patients with Henoch-Schönlein purpura) [196], however, raises important questions about this hypothesis. This discrepancy has been explained by two theories: (1) rapid removal of these deposits by phagocytic or other means of circulating immune complexes, or (2) the binding of complement or activation of coagulation mechanisms by circulating immune complexes locally at the level of the vascular lumen, thereby causing endothelial injury without intramural deposits [197]. This process includes chemotaxis and attraction of polymorphonuclear leukocytes, which release lysosomal enzymes with generation of H_2O_2. The latter is converted into hydroxyl radicals [198]. The end point is vascular injury and necrosis. Platelets, monocytes, and basophils may also release vasoactive amines that increase the permeability of the vessel wall, thereby contributing to the inflammatory response [199, 200]. Another pathogenic possibility is direct cytopathic effects of certain infectious agents on the arterial endothelium, resulting in injury independent of circulating immune complexes [201].

CLINICAL MANIFESTATIONS, NATURAL HISTORY, AND TREATMENT

The diagnosis of vasculitis should be suspected in any elderly patient with a multiple systemic disease presenting with microscopic hematuria and proteinuria. Kidney function may be normal in about half of these patients, the remainder presenting with varying degrees of renal failure. The overall prognosis is generally worse for patients over the age of 50 [202]. In some patients complete loss of kidney function can develop in a relatively short period of time.

WEGENER'S GRANULOMATOSIS

Renal involvement occurs in 70 to 85 percent of patients with Wegener's granulomatosis [203]. In an analysis of 44 elderly patients, the lung was involved in 94 percent, the upper airway in 78 percent, and both in 72 percent; these signs preceded clinical manifestations of renal disease by weeks or months. In some patients, rapidly progressive glomerulonephritis may antedate the extrarenal manifestations by months or even years [204]. Hematuria was a universal finding, as were red blood cell casts (found in 11 of 11 cases when mentioned). Proteinuria, 500 to 1,800 mg per 24 hours, was present in 56 percent of patients and the nephrotic syndrome in an additional 6 percent. Renal insufficiency was initially present in 70 percent of the patients. In some patients the progression to end-stage kidney disease was rather rapid, crescentic disease being found on histologic examination [205–217].

All these patients were treated with cyclophosphamide with or without the addition of steroids. Plasmapheresis was also attempted in some. Among the 20 patients with renal insufficiency, follow-up in 44 percent showed that half responded to therapy with improved kidney function, whereas the remaining half either died while still in renal failure or were started on dialysis. In general, patients who are treated prior to the onset of severe renal damage do better [218]. The regimen we have adopted consists of cyclophosphamide 2 mg per kg per day and prednisone 1 mg per kg administered daily for 2 to 4 weeks and then gradually converted to an alternate-day regimen over a 1- to-2-month period. Cyclophosphamide is usually continued for a full year and then decreased by 25 mg per day every 2 to 3 months. Such therapy is well tolerated by the elderly [217]. In patients with fulminant and rapidly progressive disease, a higher dose of cyclophosphamide, 4 to 5 mg per kg (using the WBC count to guide dosage adjustment), together with oral or parenteral steroids, 2 mg per kg per day, is recommended [203]. We have used pulse steroid therapy successfully in patients with lung hemorrhage. As noted earlier, plasmapheresis has also been used, but its usefulness has yet to be determined [219]. Finally, some groups have reported a beneficial effect from trimethoprim-sulfamethoxazole, 1 or 2 double-strength tablets daily, used either alone or in combination with immunosuppressive therapy [216, 220]. It is not clear how long such therapy should be continued.

PERIARTERITIS NODOSA
The elderly patient with periarteritis nodosa usually presents with fever, weight loss, fatigue, and involvement of the musculoskeletal and neurologic (peripheral neuropathy) systems. The kidneys are involved in 60 to 70 percent of patients and always in association with other system involvement. Hematuria is present in 40 to 80 percent of patients, with red cell casts found in 40 percent. Seventy-five to 90 percent of the patients have proteinuria; nephrotic syndrome is, however, rare. Renal insufficiency is present in approximately 50 percent of patients and hypertension in 30 to 70 percent. Crescentic disease with angiitis and ischemic glomerular lesions are usually found on histologic examination of the kidney [188, 221]. Patients with periarteritis nodosa and renal in-

volvement should probably be treated with steroids and cytotoxic agents, since this regimen is associated with a better outcome than steroids alone, as reported by Lieb and associates [222]. It should be noted, however, that others have not found any difference in the outcome between patients treated with corticosteroids alone and those treated with a combination of corticosteroids and a cytotoxic agent (either azathioprine or cyclophosphamide) [223]. Of these two immunosuppressive agents we prefer cyclophosphamide. The regimen we use is identical to the one outlined previously for patients with Wegener's granulomatosis [224]. If azathioprine is used, the dose is 2 mg per kg per day. The efficacy of intermittent pulse therapy with methylprednisolone or of plasma exchange cannot yet be assessed. There are virtually no data available on the duration of therapy or on its effect on the natural history of the kidney disease in the elderly.

GIANT CELL ARTERITIS
The incidence of renal involvement in patients with giant cell arteritis is not known. Klein et al [225] found red cell casts in 10 of 86 patients (12 percent). Of eight patients with renal disease, hematuria was present in seven (four had red cell casts) and proteinuria in six (two had nephrotic syndrome) [210, 225–230]. Four had normal kidney function, and four had renal failure (three chronic, one acute). Histology varied from interstitial mononuclear cell infiltration with increased cellularity in the glomerular tuft to necrotizing glomerulonephritis. One patient had membranous nephropathy, which might have been coincidental. Therapy with glucocorticoids is usually effective even in patients with advanced renal failure.

Whether a kidney biopsy should be performed in all elderly patients with proven giant cell arteritis and kidney involvement is not clear. A legitimate approach might be to treat with steroids and monitor kidney function or the urinary sediment. If the patient fails to respond, a biopsy is necessary to rule out other renal disease such as amyloidosis, which can occur with giant cell arteritis [231]. The recommended treatment for giant cell arteritis is prednisone, 40 to 60 mg per day, since the alternate-day regimen is ineffective in controlling symptoms [232]. When control of the disease has been achieved, as monitored by the erythrocyte sedimentation rate (ESR), the prednisone is tapered to a maintenance dose, generally 7.5 to 10 mg per day. Therapy should be continued for a period of 1 to 2 years [233].

HENOCH-SCHÖNLEIN NEPHRITIS
This disease is not rare in the elderly, which comprise 20 to 30 percent of the cases reported in the adult population [234]. In a total of 13 elderly patients with renal involvement reported in the literature [210, 235–

239], including one seen by us, cutaneous vasculitis (purpura) was found in the lower extremities in 11, joint pains in four, and vague abdominal complaints in three. Seven were taking medication at the time of diagnosis: antibiotics in two, analgesics in two, a diuretic in two, and an antiarrhythmic drug in one. All patients had hematuria (red cell casts were seen in five) with mild to moderate proteinuria in 11 (five had nephrotic range proteinuria). Kidney function was abnormal at the time of diagnosis in six patients. Hypertension was present in four. The disease was transient and self-limiting with complete recovery in all patients who had normal kidney function. In general, the kidney biopsy revealed only focal proliferative glomerulonephritis with IgA and C3 deposits. The patients with renal insufficiency had diffuse proliferative glomerulonephritis with crescents. Three of the six had partial recovery of kidney function; not enough follow-up information is available in the other three. Cyclophosphamide and plasmapheresis have been used in patients in whom the disease persists or progresses [239]; however, this treatment should be considered experimental at this time.

OTHER VASCULITIDES
Renal involvement has been described in other vasculitides such as hypocomplementemic urticarial vasculitis [240] and Churg-Strauss syndrome [241]. At the present time the incidence of these diseases in the elderly is not known. Some patients have clinical and pathologic features characteristic of two different vasculitides, such as periarteritis nodosa and allergic granulomatous angiitis or periarteritis nodosa and Wegener's granulomatosis, but do not fit precisely into either category. This situation has been labeled the "overlap syndrome." In such cases therapeutic considerations should be similar to those outlined for periarteritis nodosa.

SYSTEMIC LUPUS ERYTHEMATOSUS

INCIDENCE
Systemic lupus erythematosus (SLE) is not uncommon in the elderly, with a reported incidence of 7 to 17 percent in large series of patients [242, 243]. Most authors agree that, in general, the disease tends to follow a more benign course in the elderly [244]; however, there is disagreement about the incidence of clinically evident renal disease in this group. In some reports, renal disease was less common in the elderly compared with younger patients (12 percent versus 29 percent) [245]. Others have found a significant positive correlation between age and prevalence of nephritis [246]. In a 10-year period (1978 to 1987) we have

seen 80 patients with SLE with evidence of kidney disease (defined as the presence of RBC casts, proteinuria of greater than 1 g per 24 hours, serum creatinine of greater than 1.5 mg per dl, or biopsy-proven disease), ten (13 percent) of whom were 55 years or older (eight females and two males). It should be noted that the vast majority of these patients had biopsy-proven lupus nephritis.

PATHOLOGY

The glomerulonephritis of lupus has been classified into six different types (WHO classification) [247]:

Type I. Normal or minimal changes.

Type II. Pure mesangial alteration with mild to moderate mesangial widening or proliferation. On immunofluorescence the deposits are usually limited to the mesangium.

Type III. Focal segmental glomerulonephritis with one or multiple segmental necrotizing lesions in a given glomerulus. Deposits are localized to the affected areas.

Type IV. Diffuse proliferative glomerulonephritis in which at least 80 percent of the glomeruli are involved with mesangial and endothelial cell proliferation. Areas of necrosis may be found as well as epithelial cell proliferation (crescents). Deposits are usually diffuse.

Type V. Membranous glomerulonephritis constitutes the most common histologic form found in our elderly group (60 percent). Mesangial cellularity with deposits or focal segmental or diffuse proliferative changes may be seen also. These latter changes should help differentiate membranous lupus from idiopathic membranous nephropathy.

Type VI. Mixed patterns: An interstitial nephritis, characterized by plasma cells, histiocytes, lymphocytes, and polymorphonuclear cells, may be seen with or without glomerular changes. Deposits are seen along the tubular basement membrane [248].

Acute necrotizing arteritis, consisting of focal areas of necrosis and infiltration of the vessel wall by inflammatory cells, may occur in lupus and may affect the kidney.

PATHOGENESIS

The renal disease developed by patients with SLE is the consequence of glomerular (or tubular basement membrane) deposits of immune complexes with subsequent inflammation and tissue damage. These complexes are mainly composed of DNA (either double- or single-stranded) and anti-DNA or, to a lesser extent, ribonucleoprotein and immunoglobulins (IgG, IgM) and their respective antibodies. The factors responsible for the deposition of these immune complexes in the glomerulus and for the various histologic patterns are not completely understood. The two major theories are that the complexes are derived from the circulation or are formed in situ as a result of the combination of circulating antibodies with glomerular antigens (either structural components of the glomerulus or "planted" antigens). It is also possible that an immunologic mechanism other than immune complex formation such as delayed hypersensitivity contributes to glomerular injury [249].

CLINICAL MANIFESTATIONS

The nonrenal clinical features in our 10 patients with lupus nephritis were similar to those characteristic of younger patients, a fact noted by others as well [250, 251]. There were eight females and two males. Renal insufficiency in varying degrees of severity was present in every patient, as was proteinuria (range 2 to 5.5 g per 24 hours). Complement (C3, C4) was decreased in seven patients. Hypertension was a universal finding. Membranous nephritis histology (type V) was found on kidney biopsy in six patients, diffuse proliferative disease (type IV) in three, and vasculitis in one. The decrease in GFR noted in this disease is probably secondary to a curtailment of the filtration surface area due to glomerular obliteration by either mesangial matrix expansion or glomerular cell swelling, proliferation, or infiltration [252]. The proteinuria results from the presence of a subpopulation of large protein-permeable pores not present in normals [252]. Those changes may be reversed by immunosuppressive therapy.

As noted earlier, interstitial nephritis may be seen in patients with lupus glomerulonephritis, but it may also occur in the absence of glomerular disease [253–255]. This histologic variation also seems to be immunologically mediated because granular deposits may be found along the tubular basement membrane on immunofluorescence microscopy. In the patients reported, acute or chronic renal insufficiency was present. Proteinuria was usually less than 1 g per 24 hours, and the urinary sediment was generally benign [254]. Tubular abnormalities as evidenced by the increased excretion of beta-2 microglobulin are common in these patients [256], and hyperkalemia due to a defect in the distal nephron's ability to secrete potassium maximally or due to hyporenin-hypoaldosteronism has also been reported [257, 258]. The incidence and course of lupus interstitial nephritis in the elderly are not known.

NATURAL HISTORY AND TREATMENT

Our approach to the treatment of lupus nephritis in the elderly is similar to that in younger patients, since in our experience the natural history of a given histologic form is similar in all age groups. In patients with acute and rapid worsening in kidney function, we recommend "pulse therapy," consisting of 1 g of methylprednisolone (or its equivalent) given intravenously over 30 minutes for 3 successive days, followed by maintenance oral therapy (60–80 mg prednisone) [259]. Other patients are started on oral prednisone, 60 to 80 mg per day. If the patient responds, after a period of 6 to 12 weeks we switch to alternate-day therapy and then gradually reduce the dose. We reserve the use of cyclophosphamide or azathioprine therapy for patients who cannot tolerate prednisone (difficult-to-control hypertension being the most common problem in our experience) or who do not respond well to steroids. It should be noted that this approach is not universally accepted, as there is some evidence that cytotoxic drugs added to steroids reduce the risk of renal scarring [260]. It remains to be determined whether the long-term toxicity of cyclophosphamide can be avoided by using intravenous pulses of cyclophosphamide (up to 1.0 g per m^2 body surface area every 3 months). Plasma exchange added to immunosuppressive therapy has not been shown to improve the outcome significantly in patients with severe diffuse proliferative lupus nephritis [262, 263].

All of the elderly patients in our series, except for one with membranous nephropathy who presented with severe renal failure, were treated with long-term steroids. The one patient with vasculitis expired from sepsis due to a perforated viscous. Of the three with diffuse proliferative diseases, one died from a surgical complication (removal of a hypernephroma) after being treated with steroids for 3 months. At the time of death, creatinine clearance was 15 ml per minute and prorenin excretion was 5 g per 24 hours, unchanged from the time of diagnosis. In the remaining two patients, proteinuria disappeared, and C3 and C4 increased to normal; these results were sustained up to 2 years during follow-up with prednisone continued at a lower dose for nonrenal manifestations of the disease. Two patients with membranous lupus nephritis showed moderate improvement in kidney function even though proteinuria remained unchanged. The other three did not respond to therapy given for at least 1 year, and are now lost to follow-up. C3 and C4 increased in all five patients with membranous glomerulonephritis. The two patients who showed improvement in kidney function are presently off steroids after 5 and 6 years of follow-up and are stable.

Patients with interstitial nephritis should be treated as outlined in this section. Hyperkalemia, when present, may respond to steroids or can be treated as described in Chap. 3.

SCLERODERMA

INCIDENCE

Scleroderma (progressive systemic sclerosis) is a syndrome characterized by excessive collagen deposition and vascular changes in multiple organ systems; the skin (Raynaud's phenomenon), gastrointestinal tract, lungs, heart, and kidneys are most frequently involved. The incidence of renal involvement in scleroderma (15 to 58 percent) does not vary much among various age groups [264–267].

PATHOLOGY
Light microscopy reveals a mild to moderate nonspecific increase in the mesangial matrix. Areas of patchy interstitial fibrosis with associated tubular atrophy can be seen. The major changes involve the vessel wall, with intimal fibrosis in the arcuate and interlobular arteries. Fibrinoid degeneration or thrombi are seen in arterioles. Fibrinoid necrosis of afferent arterioles and glomerular loops have been reported. Immunofluorescence microscopy may show immune deposits of C3 and immunoglobulins (usually IgM) in the intima of arcuate and intralobular arteries. On electron microscopy, the most common finding is wrinkling of the glomerular basement membrane. Electron-dense deposits are not usually found.

PATHOGENESIS
The mechanisms underlying the vascular changes seen in the kidneys (and elsewhere) in scleroderma are not known. Studies by Kahaleh and colleagues [268] have shown the presence of a serum factor specifically toxic to endothelial cells. The response to such a substance is either periadventitial fibrosis with subsequent obliteration of capillaries and lymphatics or endothelial cell migration into the media. Once there, these cells proliferate and produce excessive amounts of connective tissue components. The source of this serum factor is not clear but could be lymphocytes responding to an immunologic, infectious, endocrine, or other insult. Whatever the pathogenesis, the end point is repeated vascular insults with a proliferative vascular response, luminal narrowing, reduced blood flow, and local ischemia.

CLINICAL MANIFESTATIONS
Involvement of the kidneys in scleroderma can take the form of chronic renal insufficiency or scleroderma renal crisis. The incidence of these and their possible interrelationships in the elderly are not known.

In elderly patients with chronic renal insufficiency the serum creatinine varied from 1.7 mg per dl to 11.0 mg per dl at the time of diagnosis [269, 271]. Proteinuria, usually less than 2 g per 24 hours, was present in more than 80 percent of patients. Hypertension of varying degree was present in all patients with renal insufficiency and in 20 percent of those with normal kidney function. The relationship between the histologic findings in the kidney and the presence of renal insufficiency or hypertension is not clear, since these changes may also be present in patients with normal kidney function and normotension [272]. Furthermore, improvement in kidney function may take place despite persistence of the same histologic findings [271].

Scleroderma renal crisis is characterized by a sudden rise in blood pressure, hypertensive retinopathy, and rapid deterioration of renal function. This complication occurs in 8 percent of patients with scleroderma and generally tends to occur relatively early in the course of the disease [273]. The rise in the blood pressure may be modest. The pathogenesis of this complication is not clear. It seems to occur more commonly during the winter months and is associated with a marked elevation of plasma renin activity (PRA), suggesting the following course of events. Most patients with scleroderma have a compromised renal cortical blood flow, as demonstrated by Cannon et al [264]. Given an appropriate stimulus (e.g., cold weather), the renal vasculature may undergo further vasoconstriction (the equivalent of a Raynaud's phenomenon) and the juxtaglomerular apparatus may be stimulated, resulting in excessive renin release and leading to further vasoconstriction, worsening kidney function, and uncontrolled hypertension.

It has not been possible on clinical or laboratory grounds to predict which patients will develop this complication. Several markers have been found; however, their application in individual patients is not clear. Nevertheless, it is important to note that an unexplained increase in PRA in an otherwise stable patient [274], a greater than 2.0 ng per ml per hour rise in PRA in response to the cold pressor test [272], or rapidly progressive skin thickening [275] associated with the development of anemia, pericardial effusion, or congestive heart failure [276] all point to the possible development of scleroderma renal crisis.

NATURAL HISTORY AND TREATMENT

In a study of 358 hospitalized male veterans with scleroderma, the 17 patients with renal insufficiency died within 10 months [277]. Preliminary data using D-penicillamine, 500 to 1500 mg per day for at least 6 months, have revealed a reduction in the rate of new visceral organ involvement, especially the kidney [275]. Further studies with a larger number of patients are obviously needed. The drug acts by inhibiting the synthesis and accelerating the turnover of collagen, the overproduction of which, together with glycosaminoglycan, seems to be responsible for the fibrosis associated with this disease. Plasmapheresis together with prednisone and cyclophosphamide has been tried but should be considered only experimental at the present time [278, 279].

Up to a decade ago, scleroderma renal crisis was invariably fatal because the hypertension was usually refractory to therapy and the majority of patients succumbed within 2 to 3 months after onset of the crisis. In some instances it was necessary to perform bilateral nephrectomy to bring the blood pressure down. In the past 8 years several reports have shown a beneficial effect of the ACEi captopril on the natural history of both the kidney disease and the hypertension in patients with scleroderma [270–271, 273, 280]. Since recovery of renal function with an ACEi may take place even after months of dialysis, nephrectomy should not be performed in these patients [281]. ACEis should be considered the drugs of choice in the therapy of scleroderma patients with hypertension, with or without renal insufficiency [271]. It should be noted, however, that renal insufficiency may not improve or may even progress despite control of the blood pressure [282]. If the GFR is above 30 ml per minute, both captopril and enalapril can be used at the maximum recommended dose. For enalapril, a starting dose of 2.5 mg is recommended for patients with a GFR of less than 30 ml per minute, adjusting it upward depending on the results of titration. For captopril, Beckett and associates [271] have recommended a maximum dose of 100 mg if the GFR is 20 to 30 ml per minute, 75 mg for a GFR of 10 to 20 ml per minute, and 50 mg for a GFR of less than 10 ml per minute. In some patients, even a maximum dose of the ACEi may not adequately control the blood pressure. In these instances a calcium channel blocker can be used because the effect of AII on the renal vasculature is critically dependent on transmembrane calcium ion transport [283, 284].

HEMOLYTIC UREMIC SYNDROME AND THROMBOTIC THROMBOCYTOPENIC PURPURA

Hemolytic uremic syndrome (HUS) and thrombotic thrombocytopenic purpura (TTP) most likely are part of the spectrum of a single syndrome; HUS occurring mainly in children and involving predominantly the kidneys, and TTP occurring in adults (20 years or older) and involving other organ systems as well. The diagnosis of HUS should be considered in any elderly patient presenting with hemolytic anemia, thrombocytopenia, and acute renal failure, whereas TTP should be considered if fever and neurologic disease are apparent in addition. The syndrome is rare in the elderly, comprising approximately 6 percent of the reported cases; however, renal involvement is seen in 77 percent of elderly with HUS/TTP [286]. Damage to the kidneys and other organs is a direct consequence of intravascular coagulation followed by lysis of fibrin and release of fibrin degradation products. A deficiency of the immunoglobulins that normally inhibit platelet-aggregating factors or large multimers of factor VIII (von Willebrand factor) may be the cause of the abnormal platelet agglutination seen in TTP [287]. The triggering factors have not been characterized, but may be facilitated by bacterial endotoxins, vasoactive amines, anticancer drug therapy, or metastatic disease [288, 289]. They can either initiate the clotting cascade directly with resulting disseminated intravascular coagulation, or, by damaging the endothelium, start a process of localized coagulation leading to microthrombosis [290]. Alteration in the metabolism of prostacyclin has also been suggested [291].

Moderate to marked thickening of the glomerular capillary wall with luminal obliteration is usually seen on biopsy. Arteries and arterioles with intimal thickening of varying severity may be of prognostic significance, since patients with less intimal thickening have a better chance of recovering kidney function [292]. Interstitial fibrosis and tubular atrophy may be seen. Immunofluorescence studies reveal the presence of fibrinogen in vessels and in glomerular capillary loops, sometimes accompanied by C3. Immunoglobulins usually are not seen. On electron microscopy the intima of the arterial wall shows cellular proliferation, granular material containing red cells, red cell fragments, and degenerative thrombotic material. The glomerular capillary walls reveal wrinkling and irregular thickening of the basement membrane.

The most common renal manifestation is hematuria with or without RBC casts. Proteinuria is seen in 70 to 80 percent of patients, occasionally in the nephrotic range. Elevated BUN and serum creatinine values are seen in more than 80 percent of patients. The renal disease may progress rapidly to end stage but may follow a more variable course or may even reverse [293]. In some patients factors such as volume depletion superimposed on hemolysis may contribute to the genesis of the renal failure.

Several forms of therapy have been tried in patients with HUS/TTP, including platelet function inhibitors [293], high doses of prednisone, and splenectomy, with variable degrees of success [286]. Recently, vincristine has been advocated for the form of disease caused by mitomycin [288]. At present, plasmapheresis with replacement by fresh frozen plasma seems to be the therapy of choice; it is associated with a survival rate similar to that seen in younger patients. Approximately one plasma volume (40 ml per kg) is exchanged during each session. It is not clear whether prednisone or antiplatelet agents (aspirin and dipyridamole) can potentiate the therapeutic benefits of plasmapheresis [285–286, 291, 294–295]. High-dose intravenous gamma-immunoglobulin infusion can be tried in patients who fail to respond to plasmapheresis [287].

RHEUMATOID ARTHRITIS

The percentage of elderly patients with rheumatoid arthritis who develop kidney disease (manifested by either proteinuria or an elevated serum creatinine) is not known. Of those who ultimately develop renal disease, a wide variety of histologic pictures may be seen. In 43 patients reported in the literature, ten had AA amyloidosis, ten had membranous nephropathy, seven had chronic interstitial nephritis, two had nephrosclerosis, one had arteritis, and one had end-stage kidney disease. Various other glomerulopathies were found in the remaining 12 patients [79, 297]. It appears that there is no specific renal lesion characteristic of rheumatoid arthritis, although the incidence of membranous nephropathy and other glomerulopathies (55 percent) was higher than that found in a general population of patients with renal disease. This finding may be partially explained by the presence of penicillamine- and gold-induced membranous nephropathy in these patients [298]. Also, circulating immune complexes containing rheumatoid factor may play a role. Management of these varied renal lesions is the same as that in patients without rheumatoid arthritis.

Systemic vasculitis complicates the course of long-standing rheumatoid arthritis in a small percentage of patients. The lesion can involve blood vessels of all sizes, with a predilection for the small digital arteries. Renal involvement is present in 24 to 40 percent of these patients [299, 300]. Glomerular changes are minimal, since the lesion is mainly localized to the arcuate arteries and includes both acute necrotizing injury and intimal scarring with organized thrombi [301, 302]. A kidney biopsy is needed to differentiate between patients with vasculitis and those with the histologic findings described earlier. For instance, of the 12 patients with evidence of vasculitis reported by Scott et al [300], four had amyloidosis and two had chronic nonspecific changes on renal biopsy. Mortality is higher in patients with renal involvement, particularly in older patients [300]. A regimen consisting of intravenous methylprednisolone (500 mg) and cyclophosphamide (500 mg) used on days 1, 8, 29, and 50, followed by an oral maintenance dose of cyclophosphamide (1.5 mg per kg per day) or azathioprine (2 mg per kg per day) appears to be the best form of therapy available [300, 302].

RELAPSING POLYCHONDRITIS

Relapsing polychondritis is diagnosed when three or more of the following clinical features are present: (1) bilateral auricular chondritis; (2) nonerosive seronegative inflammatory polyarthritis; (3) nasal chondritis; (4) ocular inflammation; (5) respiratory tract chondritis; and (6) audiovestibular damage. Thirteen percent of reported patients were 60 years or older when the diagnosis was made [303].

Renal involvement is quite rare but has been reported with a higher frequency in the elderly [304]. When present, it takes the form of acute renal failure with hematuria and proteinuria. Histologic examination of the kidney reveals the presence of glomerulonephritis with segmental

fibrinoid necrosis and abundant crescents or segmental glomerulosclerosis [304–306]. Interstitial cellular infiltrates and fibrosis are also commonly seen. On immunofluorescence microscopy, immunoglobulins
(IgG, IgM) and complement (C3) are frequently found, predominantly
in the mesangium. Electron-dense deposits have been noted in the basement membrane and mesangium. Prednisone (60–100 mg per day) constitutes the treatment of choice. Cyclophosphamide may also be tried if
prednisone fails or if the patient is intolerant of steroids. The combination of 4,4'-diaminodiphenylsulfone (Dapsone) and prednisone has also
been tried [306]. The prognosis is, in general, worse in patients with renal involvement.

SJÖGREN'S SYNDROME

Sjögren's syndrome is a chronic inflammatory disorder that may occur as
a primary disease (sicca syndrome) or in association with other autoimmune diseases, particularly rheumatoid arthritis, systemic lupus erythematosus, primary biliary cirrhosis, or scleroderma. The disease
primarily affects postmenopausal women. In series in which age is given,
patients over the age of 60 make up 21 percent of the cases [307, 308].
Renal involvement can take the form of tubulointerstitial disease or a
glomerulonephritis.

Tubulointerstitial disease may present as a urine-concentrating defect,
most likely due to impaired water permeability of the cortical collecting
tubule [309]. A distal renal tubular acidosis (type I) may also be seen
[310, 311]. Kidney function is usually normal in these patients, and proteinuria is uncommon. On kidney biopsy diffuse interstitial inflammatory cell infiltration, composed predominantly of plasma cells and
lymphocytes, with relatively well preserved glomerular morphology has
been found. The contribution of the infiltrates to the pathogenesis of the
tubular dysfunction is not clear. It is interesting to note, however, that in
a repeat kidney biopsy in one such patient after treatment with steroids
and remission of the renal tubular acidosis, the interstitial inflammation
had also disappeared [312]. Moderate renal insufficiency with mild proteinuria (< 1 g per 24 hours) is occasionally found in patients with
chronic interstitial nephritis [313]. Both cyclophosphamide and low-
dose prednisone (30 mg qod) have been used with some success in these
patients.

Glomerulonephritis as a complication of Sjögren's syndrome is rare.
The patients usually present with hematuria, renal insufficiency of varying severity, and proteinuria, occasionally in the nephrotic range. Circulating immune complexes have been found in such patients. Their
presence seems to be of pathogenetic significance, since their level

decreases concomitantly with drug-induced improvement in kidney function [314].

A picture of mesangiocapillary glomerulonephritis (with low C3), membranous nephropathy with endocapillary hypercellularity, or even necrotizing arteriolitis may be found on histologic examination of kidney tissue. The response to moderate doses of prednisone (20–30 mg per day) in two of our elderly patients with Sjögren's syndrome and mesangiocapillary glomerulonephritis has not been as good as that described by Motsopoulos and colleagues [314]. In one patient kidney function acutely worsened, and she died from septic shock. The other died from GI bleeding with renal insufficiency (serum creatinine 4 mg per dl). She had been previously treated with cyclophosphamide and prednisone.

DRUG-INDUCED GLOMERULAR DISEASE

NONSTEROIDAL ANTI-INFLAMMATORY DRUGS
The adverse effects of nonsteroidal anti-inflammatory drugs (NSAIDs) in the kidney are multiple and will be dealt with under separate headings according to the specific complication. In this section we will discuss the problem of nephrotic syndrome, usually associated with acute interstitial nephritis.

Incidence
Nephrotic syndrome is seen mainly in the elderly, the ratio of females to males being 2:1 [315–319]. The reason for the higher incidence in the elderly is not clear. It is not simply because the use of these agents increases with age because the incidence of all side effects of NSAIDs increases disproportionately with age [320]. The drugs most commonly associated with the nephrotic syndrome are fenoprofen, ibuprofen, and naproxen. Zomepirac, sulindac, phenylbutazone, indomethacin, and tolmetin sodium have also been implicated.

Pathology
On light microscopy, the glomeruli are normal. Most of the abnormalities are located in the interstitium with edema and cellular infiltrates made up mainly of lymphocytes, histiocytes, and eosinophils. Granulomatous interstitial changes have also been reported [321]. Tubular degeneration and atrophy have been described on occasion. Immunofluorescent studies are normal in most patients. Variable staining for IgG, IgA, IgM, and C3 can be seen in the interstitium or in the tubular basement membrane. On electron microscopy, fusion of foot processes is the major finding. In

general, it is not possible to separate patients with renal failure from those without on histologic findings alone.

Pathogenesis
The pathogenesis of the renal injury associated with use of NSAIDs is not clear and is most likely multifactoral. These factors include direct glomerular and tubular toxicity, delayed hypersensitivity reaction, and specific facilitation of lymphocytic interstitial infiltration through augmentation of polyenoic acid synthesis from arachidonic acid [315, 319].

Clinical Manifestations
Duration of exposure to the drug before the apparent onset of nephropathy may vary from days to years. The hypersensitivity response of fever, skin rash, eosinophilia, or eosinophiluria that is so commonly associated with allergic interstitial nephritis is unusual with NSAID use, occurring in only 20 percent of patients. Renal insufficiency is present in 87 percent of patients, with approximately one-third requiring dialysis. Edema is the most common presenting complaint followed by oliguria or anuria and malaise. Besides proteinuria, microscopic hematuria and granular casts are present in half the patients [315–319, 322].

Natural History
Following discontinuation of the offending agent, almost all patients eventually recover, although renal insufficiency may persist occasionally. The period of time required for complete recovery is quite variable, and therefore therapeutic benefit from steroids has been difficult to assess. It is recommended that such therapy be reserved for patients with severe disease (e.g., those requiring dialysis) or those who fail to improve after the offending agent has been removed [315–319, 322].

A clinical picture identical to that associated with NSAID use has been reported in an elderly man during therapy with rifampin [323].

PENICILLAMINE
Proteinuria occurs in 16 percent of elderly patients with rheumatoid arthritis who are treated with this drug [324]. This complication seems to be related, in part, to the rate at which the dose is increased and can appear at any time during therapy. It should be remembered that oral iron inhibits penicillamine absorption by chelation in the gut. If the iron is stopped, a larger amount of the maintenance dose of penicillamine will be reabsorbed, making drug toxicity more likely. Such was the case in 4 of 16 patients reported by Harkness and Blake [325]. The proteinuria is usually in the nephrotic range. Kidney function is generally well preserved. On biopsy the findings are those of membranous nephropathy,

making an immune pathogenesis quite likely. Minimal change disease and mesangial proliferation with electron-dense deposits on electron microscopy have also been reported [326]. The proteinuria and histologic changes remit after discontinuation of the drug; however, remission may take up to 16 months. Other modalities of therapy for the rheumatoid arthritis should then be considered, since a recrudescence of proteinuria has been observed on restarting penicillamine [327]. Rapidly progressive glomerulonephritis with a renal histologic picture identical to that of Goodpasture's syndrome has also been reported with penicillamine use. Treatment with plasmapheresis and immunosuppressives is worth trying [328–331].

GOLD
Nephropathy occurs in 5 to 25 percent of patients treated with the parenteral form of the drug and in 3 percent of those who receive the oral form [332]. The majority of patients (42 percent) present with moderate proteinuria (1–3.5 g per day). Mild proteinuria (< 1 g per day) develops in 37 percent, and the remaining 21 percent have nephrotic syndrome. As with penicillamine use, kidney function is generally well preserved, and the renal histology is predominantly that of membranous nephropathy. Other histologic forms such as minimal change disease and mesangial nephritis have also been reported [333, 334]. The development of renal disease does not appear to be dose related. The pathogenesis is not clear but most likely is immune related. Patients with rheumatoid arthritis with beta-lymphocyte alloantigens HLA-DRW3 or B8 are at increased risk of developing proteinuria with parenteral gold therapy [335, 336]. The level of circulating metallothioneine may also be involved in the relationship between chrysotherapy and nephrotoxicity [337]. The proteinuria usually disappears on discontinuing the gold. It is recommended that these patients not be rechallenged with the drug.

CAPTOPRIL
The use of captopril has been associated with membranous nephropathy and proteinuria in the elderly. This rather rare complication has been seen in patients taking large doses (400–600 mg per day) or patients with underlying renal disease [338, 339]. Generally, the proteinuria will disappear (or decrease to predrug levels in those with underlying disease) on discontinuation of the drug; however, persistent proteinuria long after discontinuing captopril has been reported [340].

OTHER DRUGS
Besides the two patterns of glomerular injury discussed earlier (minimal change disease and membranous glomerulopathy), proliferative glomer-

ulonephritis associated with systemic vasculitis has been reported in association with a variety of drugs [341]. No data are available, however, as to how often these disorders occur in the elderly.

INFECTIONS AND GLOMERULAR DISEASE

Glomerulonephritis can occur as a complication of infections. This complication appears to be rare in the elderly, although the true incidence is not known.

BACTERIAL ENDOCARDITIS
Both subacute and acute bacterial endocarditis can be complicated by a renal lesion. The latter, seen in about 1 percent of elderly persons with endocarditis [342], is usually manifested by acute renal failure, proteinuria, and hematuria. The renal failure can be progressive, with some patients requiring dialysis. Serum complement (C3, C4) is decreased in most patients. In patients with subacute bacterial endocarditis kidney biopsy reveals the presence of diffuse mesangial proliferation, which may be accompanied by epithelial crescents. Mesangial and subendothelial electron-dense deposits may be found on electron microscopy, and diffuse granular deposits of IgG (less commonly of IgM or IgA) and C3 may be evident in subendothelial and mesangial areas on immunofluorescence. In patients with acute bacterial endocarditis the renal lesion resembles that of acute poststreptococcal glomerulonephritis (see Chap. 6). The association of severe renal failure and diffuse glomerulonephritis heralds a poor prognosis as far as recovery of kidney function is concerned [343]. Also, patients with diffuse glomerulonephritis may have persistent hematuria or proteinuria despite bacteriologic cure of the endocarditis, although clinical recovery from the primary disease is usually associated with complete resolution of the glomerulonephritis [344]. The treatment is that of the underlying infection.

VISCERAL SUPPURATION
Glomerulonephritis can complicate other organ infections without cardiac involvement. In the elderly these infections have been seen in the lungs or retroperitoneal space (arterial graft). The clinical manifestations and laboratory data are identical to those characteristic of bacterial endocarditis. The serum complement (C3, C4), however, is usually normal. The prognosis is closely related to the course of the infection. In three patients reported by Forrest et al [345], capsular antigen for the organism was localized in the glomeruli of all the patients. Other investigators have reported a high intraglomerular monocytic infiltration [346], a

finding that may provide a clue to the diagnosis of visceral infection in patients in whom the diagnosis is not apparent [347, 348].

VIRAL INFECTIONS

Hepatitis B virus infection and complexes of hepatitis B antigen and antibody may be associated with polyarteritis nodosa, essential mixed cryoglobulinemia, or membranous nephropathy. The incidence of these complications in the elderly is not known. In fact, it is not at all clear that membranous nephropathy as a complication of hepatitis B infection occurs in older patients [349–351].

Several mechanisms have been proposed by which infections induce glomerular damage: (1) circulating immune complexes of microorganism antigen-antibody may become trapped in the glomerular capillary with subsequent inflammatory reaction; (2) there may be direct glomerular toxicity of microorganism products; (3) other pathogenic mechanisms may be triggered by the infectious process.

SARCOIDOSIS

Glomerulonephritis (membranous, focal glomerulosclerosis, mesangio-capillary) has been reported in association with sarcoidosis. The frequency of the problem in the elderly is not known. It is not clear whether therapy should be directed toward the sarcoidosis alone (steroids) or also toward the specific glomerulopathy, when appropriate.

REFERENCES

1. Wilson PWF, Anderson KM, and Kannel WB: Epidemiology of diabetes mellitus in the elderly. *Am J Med* 80 [Suppl 5A]:3–9, 1986.
2. Fabre J, et al: The kidney in maturity-onset diabetes mellitus: A clinical study of 510 patients. *Kidney Int* 21:730–738, 1982.
3. Humphrey LL, et al: Chronic renal failure in non-insulin-dependent diabetes mellitus. A population-based study in Rochester, Minnesota. *Ann Intern Med* 111:788–796, 1989.
4. Greene DA: Acute and chronic complications of diabetes mellitus in older patients. *Am J Med* 80 [Suppl 5A]:39–53, 1986.
5. Schmitz A and Vaeth M: Microalbuminemia: A major risk factor in non-insulin-dependent diabetes. A 10-year follow-up study of 503 patients. *Diabetic Med* 5:126–134, 1988.
6. Keinzelman CL, et al: Incidence of proteinuria in type 2 diabetes mellitus in the Pima Indians. *Kidney Int* 35:681–687, 1989.
7. Ballerman BJ, Skorecki KL, and Brenner BM: Reduced glomerular angiotensin II receptor density in early untreated diabetes mellitus in the rat. *Am J Physiol* 247:F110–F116, 1984.

8. Zatz R, et al: Prevention of diabetic glomerulopathy by pharmacological amelioration of glomerular capillary hypertension. *J Clin Invest* 77:1925–1930, 1986.
9. Wiseman MJ, et al: Effect of blood glucose control on increased glomerular filtration rate and kidney size in insulin-dependent diabetes. *N Engl J Med* 312:617–621, 1985.
10. Hostetter TH: Diabetic nephropathy. *N Engl J Med* 312:642–643, 1985.
11. Friedman EA, et al: No supranormal glomerular filtration (GFR) in type II (non-insulin dependent) diabetics. *Am Soc Nephrol* 14:102A, 1981.
12. Damsgaard EM and Mogensen CE: Microalbuminuria in elderly hyperglycemic patients and controls. *Diabetic Med* 3:430–435, 1986.
13. Schmitz A, Gundersen HJG, and Osterby R: Glomerular morphology by light microscopy in non-insulin-dependent diabetes mellitus. Lack of glomerular hypertrophy. *Diabetes* 37:38–43, 1988.
14. Schmitz A, Hansen HH, and Christensen T: Kidney function in newly diagnosed type 2 (non-insulin-dependent) diabetic patients, before and during treatment. *Diabetologia* 32:434–439, 1989.
15. Nath KA: Platelets, antiplatelet therapy, and diabetic nephropathy. *Mayo Clin Proc* 63:80–85, 1988.
16. Mene P, et al: Platelet-derived growth factor (PDGF) modulates contraction and cytosolic free calcium (Ca^{++}) in cultured rat mesangial cells. *Kidney Int* 31:175A, 1987.
17. Bagdade JD: Disorders of glucose metabolism in uremia. *Adv Nephrol* 8:87–100, 1979.
18. Chahal PS and Kohner EM: The relationship between diabetic retinopathy and diabetic nephropathy. *Diabetic Nephrop* 2:4–5, 1983.
19. Pirart J: Diabetes mellitus and its degenerative complications: a prospective study of 4,400 patients observed between 1947 and 1973. *Diabetes Care* 1:168–188, 1978.
20. Aronoff SL, et al: Urinary excretion and renal clearance of specific plasma proteins in diabetes of short and long duration. *Diabetes* 30:656–663, 1981.
21. Winetz JA, et al: Glomerular function in advanced human diabetic nephropathy. *Kidney Int* 21:750–756, 1982.
22. Ala-Houhala I and Pasternack A: Fractional dextran and protein clearances in glomerulonephritis and in diabetic nephropathy. *Clin Sci* 72:289–296, 1987.
23. Tomlanovich S, et al: Functional nature of glomerular injury in progressive diabetic glomerulopathy. *Diabetes* 36:556–565, 1987.
24. Osterby R, et al: A strong correlation between glomerular filtration rate and filtration surface in diabetic nephropathy. *Diabetologia* 31:265–270, 1988.
25. Mauer SM, et al: Structural-functional relationships in diabetic nephropathy. *J Clin Invest* 74:1143–1155, 1984.
26. O'Neill WM Jr, Wallin JD, and Walker PD: Hematuria and red cell casts in typical diabetic nephropathy. *Am J Med* 74:389–395, 1983.
27. Lopes de Faria JB, et al: Glomerular hematuria in diabetics. *Clin Nephrol* 30:117–121, 1988.
28. Klein R, et al: Blood pressure and hypertension in diabetes. *Am J Epidemiol* 122:75–89, 1985.
29. Ferriss JB, et al: Blood pressure in diabetic patients: Relationships with exchangeable sodium and renin activity. *Diabetic Nephrop* 5:27–30, 1986.
30. Jerumus G, et al: Spectrum of proteinuria in type I and type II diabetes. *Diabetes Care* 10:419–427, 1987.

31. Jarrett RJ, et al: Microalbuminemia predicts mortality in non-insulin dependent diabetes. *Diabetic Med* 1:17–19, 1984.
32. Reubi FC, Franz KA, and Horber F: Hypertension as related to renal function in diabetes mellitus. *Hypertension* [Suppl II]7:II21–II28, 1985.
33. De Chatel R, et al: Sodium, renin, aldosterone, catecholamines and blood pressure in diabetes mellitus. *Kidney Int* 12:412–421, 1977.
34. Weidmann P, Beretta-Piccoli C, and Trost BN: Pressor factors and responsiveness in hypertension accompanying diabetes mellitus. *Hypertension* [Suppl II]7:II33–II42, 1985.
35. Connell JMC, et al: Reduced number of angiotensin II receptors on platelets in insulin-dependent diabetes. *Clin Sci* 71:217–220, 1986.
36. Trujillo A, et al: Renin regulation in type II diabetes mellitus: Influence of dietary sodium. *Hypertension* 13:200–205, 1989.
37. DeFronzo RA, et al: The effect of insulin on renal handling of sodium, potassium, calcium and phosphate in man. *J Clin Invest* 55:845–855, 1975.
38. DeFronzo RA, Goldberg M, and Agus Z: The effects of glucose and insulin on renal electrolyte transport. *J Clin Invest* 58:83–90, 1976.
39. Trevison M, et al: Hypertension, non-insulin dependent diabetes and intracellular sodium metabolism. *Hypertension* 11:264–268, 1988.
40. Weidmann P, et al: Sodium-volume factor, cardiovascular reactivity and hypotensive mechanisms of diuretic therapy in hypertension associated with diabetes mellitus. *Am J Med* 67:779–784, 1979.
41. Oshan AR, et al: Hypertension in adult onset diabetes mellitus: Abnormal renal hemodynamics and endogenous vasoregulatory factors. *Am J Kidney Dis* 2:271–279, 1982.
42. Zemel MB, et al: Altered cation transport in diabetic hypertension. *Clin Res* 35:853A, 1987.
43. Zemel MB, et al: Role of impaired calcium (Ca^{++}) transport in obesity-associated hypertension. *Federation of American Society for Experimental Biology Journal* 2:A502, 1988.
44. Mogensen CE, et al: Microalbuminuria in elderly hyperglycemic patients and controls. *Diabetic Med* 3:430–435, 1986.
45. Parving HH, et al: Early detection of patients at risk of developing diabetic nephropathy: A longitudinal study of urinary albumin excretion. *Acta Endocrinol* 100:550–555, 1982.
46. Andersen AR, et al: Diabetic nephropathy in type I (insulin-dependent): An epidemiological study. *Diabetologia* 25:4496–501, 1983.
47. Ordonez JD and Hiatt RA: Comparison of type II and type I diabetics treated for end-stage renal disease in a large prepaid health plan population. *Nephron* 51:524–529, 1989.
48. M'Crary RF, Pitts TO, and Puschett JB: Diabetic nephropathy: Natural course, survivorship and therapy. *Am J Nephrol* 1:206–218, 1981.
49. Viberti GC, et al: Long-term correction of hyperglycemia and progression of renal failure in insulin-dependent diabetes. *Br Med J* 286:598–602, 1983.
50. Mohamed A, et al: Response of urinary albumin to submaximal exercise in newly diagnosed non-insulin dependent diabetes. *Br Med J* 288:1342–1343, 1984.
51. Feldt-Rasmussen B, et al: Kidney function during 12 months of strict metabolic control in insulin-dependent diabetic patients with incipient nephropathy. *N Engl J Med* 314:665–670, 1986.
52. Barnett AH, et al: Specific thromboxane synthetase inhibition and albumin excretion rate in insulin-dependent diabetes. *Lancet* 1:1322–1325, 1984.

53. Taguma T, et al: Effect of captopril on heavy proteinuria in azotemic diabetics. *N Engl J Med* 313:1617–1620, 1985.
54. Hommel E, et al: Effect of captopril on kidney function in insulin-dependent diabetic patients with nephropathy. *Br Med J* 293:467–471, 1986.
55. Bjorck S, et al: Beneficial effects of angiotensin converting enzyme inhibition on renal function in patients with diabetic nephropathy. *Br Med J* 293:471–474, 1986.
56. Baba T, Murabayashi S, and Takeke K: Comparison of the renal effects of angiotensin converting enzyme inhibitor and calcium antagonist in hypertensive type 2 (non-insulin dependent) diabetic patients with microalbuminuria: A randomized clinical trial. *Diabetologia* 32:40–44, 1989.
57. Valvo E, et al: Captopril in patients with type II diabetes and renal insufficiency: Systemic and renal hemodynamic alterations. *Am J Med* 85:344–348, 1988.
58. Donadio JV Jr, et al: Platelet-inhibitor treatment of diabetic nephropathy: A 10-year prospective study. *Mayo Clin Proc* 63:3–15, 1988.
59. Christopher TG and Edmonds KS: A study of aspirin and dipyridamole in slowing the progression of diabetic glomerulosclerosis. *Am Soc Nephrol*, 19th Annual Meeting, 37A, 1986.
60. Parving HN, et al: Early aggressive antihypertensive treatment reduces rate of decline in kidney function in diabetic nephropathy. *Lancet* 1:1175–1178, 1983.
61. Mogensen CE: Long term antihypertensive treatment inhibiting progression of diabetic nephropathy. *Br Med J* 285:685–688, 1982.
62. Dodson PM, et al: Sodium restriction and blood pressure in hypertensive type II diabetics: Randomized blind controlled and crossover studies of moderate sodium restriction and sodium supplementation. *Br Med J* 298:227–230, 1989.
63. Tuck ML, et al: Reductions in plasma catecholamines and blood pressure during weight loss in obese subjects. *Acta Endocrinol* 102:252–257, 1983.
64. Working group on hypertension in diabetes: Statement on hypertension in diabetes mellitus. *Arch Intern Med* 147:830–842, 1987.
65. Hatch FE, et al: Diabetic glomerulosclerosis. A long term follow-up study based on renal biopsies. *Am J Med* 31:216–230, 1961.
66. Chihara J, et al: Glomerulonephritis in diabetic patients and its effects on the prognosis. *Nephron* 43:45–49, 1986.
67. Gellman DD, et al: Diabetic nephropathy: A clinical and pathologic study based on renal biopsies. *Medicine* 38:321–367, 1959.
68. Murphy WM, et al: Immunopathologic studies in glomerular diseases with membranous lesions. *Am J Clin Path* 60:364–376, 1973.
69. Warms PC, et al: Idiopathic membranous glomerulonephritis occurring with diabetes mellitus. *Arch Intern Med* 132:735–738, 1973.
70. Sharma HM, Yum MN, and Kleit S: Acute glomerulonephritis with diabetes mellitus. Report of a case. *Arch Pathol* 97:152–154, 1974.
71. Olivero J and Suki WN: Acute glomerulonephritis complicating diabetic nephropathy. *Arch Intern Med* 137:732–734, 1977.
72. Wass JAH, et al: Renal failure, glomerular disease and diabetes mellitus. *Nephron* 21:289–296, 1978.
73. Rao KV and Crosson JT: Idiopathic membranous glomerulonephritis in diabetic patients. Report of three cases and review of the literature. *Arch Intern Med* 140:624–627, 1980.
74. Amoak E, et al: Clinical identification of non-diabetic renal disease in dia-

betic patients with type I and type II disease presenting with renal dysfunction. *Am J Nephrol* 8:204–211, 1988.

75. Cavallo T, Pinto JA, and Rajaraman S: Immune complex disease complicating diabetic glomerulosclerosis. *Am J Nephrol* 4:347–354, 1984.

76. Bertani T, et al: Superimposed nephritis: A separate entity among glomerular diseases? *Am J Kidney Dis* 7:205–212, 1986.

77. Moorthy AV and Zimmerman SW: Renal disease in the elderly: Clinicopathologic analysis of renal disease in 115 elderly patients. *Clin Nephrol* 14:223–229, 1980.

78. Zech P, et al: The nephrotic syndrome in adults aged over 60: Etiology, evolution and treatment of 76 cases. *Clin Nephrol* 18:232–236, 1982.

79. Kingswood JC, et al: Renal biopsy in the elderly: Clinicopathological correlations in 143 patients. *Clin Nephrol* 22:183–187, 1984.

80. Franklin EC: Immunopathology of the amyloid diseases. *Hosp Pract* 15:70–77, 1980.

81. Gertz MA and Kyle RA: Primary systemic amyloidosis—A diagnostic primer. *Mayo Clin Proc* 64:1505–1519, 1989.

82. Kyle RA and Greipp PR: Amyloidosis (AL). Clinical and laboratory features in 229 cases. *Mayo Clin Proc* 58:665–683, 1983.

83. Ogg CS, et al: Presentation and course of primary amyloidosis of the kidney. *Clin Nephrol* 15:9–13, 1981.

84. Triger DR and Joekes AM: Renal amyloidosis. A fourteen-year follow-up. *Q J Med* 165:15–40, 1973.

85. Browning MJ, et al: Ten years' experience of an amyloid clinic—a clinicopathological survey. *Q J Med* 215:213–227, 1985.

86. Dikman SH, Churg J, and Kahn T: Morphologic and clinical correlates in renal amyloidosis. *Hum Pathol* 12:160–169, 1981.

87. DeBeer FC, et al: Serum amyloid-A protein concentrations in inflammatory diseases and its relationship to the incidence of reactive systemic amyloidosis. *Lancet* 2:231–234, 1982.

88. Maury CPJ and Teppo AM: Mechanism of reduced amyloid A degrading activity in serum of patients with secondary amyloidosis. *Lancet* 2:234–237, 1982.

89. Kyle RA and Bayrd ED: Amyloidosis: Review of 236 cases. *Medicine* 54:271–299, 1975.

90. Parkins RA and Bywaters EGL: Regression of amyloidosis secondary to rheumatoid arthritis. *Br Med J* 50:536–540, 1959.

91. Lowenstein J and Gallo G: Remission of the nephrotic syndrome in renal amyloidosis. *N Engl J Med* 282:128–131, 1970.

92. Dikman SH, et al: Resolution of renal amyloidosis. *Am J Med* 63:430–433, 1977.

93. Karenty G, et al: Clinical and histological resolution of systemic amyloidosis after renal cell carcinoma removal. *Nephron* 40:232–234, 1985.

94. Bacon PA, et al: Rheumatoid disease, amyloidosis and its treatment with penicillamine. *Eur J Rheumatol Inflamm* 3:70–74, 1979.

95. Zemer D, et al: Colchicine in the prevention and treatment of the amyloidosis of familial Mediterranean fever. *N Engl J Med* 314:1001–1005, 1986.

96. Kyle RA, et al: Primary systemic amyloidosis. Comparison of melphalan/prednisone versus colchicine. *Am J Med* 79:708–716, 1985.

97. Cohen AS, et al: Survival of patients with primary (AL) amyloidosis colchicine-treated cases from 1976–1983 compared with cases seen in previous years (1961–1973). *Am J Med* 82:1182–1190, 1987.

98. Scheinberg MA, Pernambuco JC, and Benson MD: DMSO and colchicine therapy in amyloid disease. *Ann Rheum Dis* 43:421–423, 1984.
99. Glenner GG: Amyloid deposits and amyloidosis. *N Engl J Med* 302:1283–1292, 1980.
100. Hind CRK, et al: Specific chemical dissociation of fibrillar and non-fibrillar components of amyloid deposits. *Lancet* 2:376–379, 1984.
101. Hill GS, et al: Renal lesions in multiple myeloma: Their relationship to associated protein abnormalities. *Am J Kidney Dis* 2:423–438, 1983.
102. Ganeval D, et al: Visceral deposition of monoclonal light chains and immunoglobulins: A study of renal and immunopathologic abnormalities. *Adv Nephrol* 11:25–63, 1982.
103. Kyle RA: Multiple myeloma. Review of 869 cases. *Mayo Clin Proc* 50:29–40, 1975.
104. Rofa S, et al: Multiple myeloma and severe renal failure: A clinicopathologic study of outcome and prognosis in 34 patients. *Medicine* 66:126–137, 1987.
105. Hill GS, et al: Renal lesions in multiple myeloma: Their relationship to associated protein abnormalities. *Am J Kidney Dis* 2:423–438, 1983.
106. Pirani CL, et al: Renal lesions in plasma cell dyscrasias: Ultrastructural observations. *Am J Kidney Dis* 10:208–211, 1987.
107. Coward RA, Mallick NP, and Delamore IW: Tubular function in multiple myeloma. *Clin Nephrol* 24:180–185, 1985.
108. Beaufils M and Morel-Maroger L: Pathogenesis of renal disease in monoclonal gammopathies: Current concepts. *Nephron* 20:125–131, 1978.
109. Sanders PW, et al: Morphologic alterations of the proximal tubules in light chain related disease. *Kidney Int* 33:881–889, 1988.
110. DeFronzo RA, et al: Renal function in patients with multiple myeloma. *Medicine* 57:151–166, 1978.
111. Perry MC and Kyle RA: The clinical significance of Bence Jones proteinuria. *Mayo Clin Proc* 50:234–238, 1975.
112. MRC working party on leukemia in adults: Analysis and management of renal failure in fourth MRC myelomatosis trial. *Br Med J* 288:1411–1415, 1984.
113. Coward RA, et al: The importance of urinary immunoglobulin light chain isoelectric point (pI) in nephrotoxicity in multiple myeloma. *Clin Sci* 66:229–232, 1984.
114. Melcion C, et al: Renal failure in myeloma: Relationship with isoelectric point of immunoglobulin light chains. *Clin Nephrol* 22:138–143, 1984.
115. Norden AGW, et al: Renal impairment in myeloma: Negative association with isoelectric point of excreted Bence-Jones protein. *J Clin Pathol* 42:59–62, 1989.
116. DeFronzo RA, et al: Acute renal failure in multiple myeloma. *Medicine* 54:209–223, 1975.
117. Cohen DJ, et al: Acute renal failure in patients with multiple myeloma. *Am J Med* 76:247–256, 1984.
118. Olmer M, Berland Y, and Schutz G: Acute renal failure (ARF) and multiple myeloma. *Min Electrol Metab* 12:268A, 1986.
119. Murray T, Long W, and Narins RG: Multiple myeloma and the anion gap. *N Engl J Med* 292:574–575, 1975.
120. Flanagan NG, Ridway JC, and Irving AG: The anion gap as a screening procedure for occult myeloma in the elderly. *J R Soc Med* 81:27–28, 1988.

121. Mehta BR, et al: Hyporeninemic hypoaldosteronism in a patient with multiple myeloma. *Am J Kidney Dis* 4:175–178, 1984.
122. Bernstein SP and Humes HD: Reversible renal insufficiency in multiple myeloma. *Arch Intern Med* 142:2083–2086, 1982.
123. Pasquali S, et al: Rapidly progressive renal failure (RPRF) in patients with multiple myeloma. *Min Electrol Metab* 12:268A, 1986.
124. Pozzi C, et al: Prognostic factors and effectiveness of treatment in acute renal failure due to multiple myeloma: A review of 50 cases. *Clin Nephrol* 28:1–9, 1987.
125. Zucchelli P, et al: Controlled plasma exchange trial in acute renal failure due to multiple myeloma. *Kidney Int* 33:1175–1180, 1988.
126. Johnson WJ, et al: Plasmapheresis, hemodialysis and chemotherapy in the treatment of renal failure associated with multiple myeloma. *Am Soc Nephrol* 88A, 1989.
127. Misiani R, et al: Plasmapheresis in the treatment of acute renal failure in multiple myeloma. *Am J Med* 66:684–688, 1979.
128. Wahlin A, Lofvenberg E, and Holm J: Improved survival in multiple myeloma with renal failure. *Acta Med Scand* 221:205–209, 1987.
129. Cosio FG, et al: Severe renal failure in multiple myeloma. *Clin Nephrol* 15:206–210, 1981.
130. Iggo N, et al: Chronic dialysis in patients with multiple myeloma and renal failure. *Q J Med* 270:903–910, 1989.
131. Lazarus HM, et al: Long-term survival of patients with multiple myeloma and acute renal failure at presentation. *Am J Kidney Dis* 2:521–525, 1983.
132. Brown WW, et al: Reversal of chronic end-stage renal failure due to myeloma kidney. *Ann Intern Med* 90:793–794, 1979.
133. Dahlberg PJ, et al: Myeloma kidney: Improved renal function following long-term chemotherapy and hemodialysis. *Am J Nephrol* 3:2422–243, 1983.
134. Randall RE, et al: Manifestations of systemic light chain deposition. *Am J Med* 60:293–299, 1976.
135. Rao TKS, et al: Membranoproliferative glomerulonephritis (MPGN), an unusual manifestation of multiple myeloma. *Kidney Int* 14:659A, 1978.
136. Herf S, et al: An evaluation of diabetic and pseudo-diabetic glomerulosclerosis. *Am J Med* 66:1040–1045, 1979.
137. Gallo GR, et al: Nodular glomerulopathy associated with nonamyloidotic kappa light chain deposits and excess immunoglobulin light chain synthesis. *Am J Pathol* 99:621–644, 1980.
138. Solling K, et al: Nonsecretory myeloma associated with nodular glomerulosclerosis. *Acta Med Scand* 207:137–143, 1980.
139. Tubbs RR, et al: Light chain nephropathy. *Am J Med* 71:263–269, 1981.
140. Glassock RJ and Goldstein DA: Nephrotic syndrome in a 52 year old woman with monoclonal gammopathy. *Am J Nephrol* 1:199–205, 1981.
141. Cohen JR and Colvin R: Plasma cell dyscrasia, with systemic light-chain deposition, kappa type, widespread with renal failure. (Case records of Massachussetts General Hospital.) *N Engl J Med* 304:33–43, 1981.
142. Gipstein RM, et al: Kappa light chain nephropathy without evidence of myeloma cells. Response to chemotherapy with cessation of maintenance hemodialysis. *Am J Nephrol* 2:276–281, 1982.
143. Nakamoto Y, et al: IgM monoclonal gammopathy accompanied by nodular glomerulosclerosis, urine concentrating defect and hyporeninemic hypoaldosteronism. *Am J Nephrol* 5:53–58, 1985.

144. Ganeval D, et al: Visceral deposition of monoclonal light chains and immunoglobulins: A study of renal and immunopathologic abnormalities. *Adv Nephrol* 11:25–63, 1982.

145. Confaloniere R, et al: Light chain nephropathy: Histological and clinical aspects in 15 cases. *Nephrol Dial Transplant* 2:150–156, 1988.

146. Sinniah R and Cohen AH: Glomerular capillary aneurysms in light-chain nephropathy. An ultrastructural proposal of pathogenesis. *Am J Pathol* 118:298–305, 1985.

147. Brouet JC, et al: Biologic and clinical significance of cryoglobulins: A report of 86 cases. *Am J Med* 57:775–788, 1987.

148. Gorevic PH, et al: Mixed cryoglobulinemia: Clinical aspects and long-term follow-up of 40 patients. *Am J Med* 69:287–308, 1980.

149. Agrafiotis A, et al: Is cryoglobulin detection of clinical significance in chronic glomerulonephritis not related to systemic diseases? *Clin Nephrol* 16:146–150, 1981.

150. Meltzer M, et al: Cryoglobulinemia. A clinical and laboratory study. II. Cryoglobulins with rheumatoid factor activity. *Am J Med* 40:837–856, 1966.

151. Invernizzi F, et al: A long term follow-up in essential cryoglobulinemia. *Acta Haematol* 61:93–99, 1979.

152. Popp JW, et al: Essential mixed cryoglobulinemia without evidence for hepatitis B virus infection. *Ann Intern Med* 92:379–383, 1980.

153. Migliorini P, et al: HLA antigens in essential mixed cryoglobulinemia. *Arth Rheum* 24:932–936, 1981.

154. Tarantino A, et al. Renal disease in essential mixed cryoglobulinemia. Long-term follow-up of 44 patients. *Q J Med* 197:1–30, 1981.

155. Maggiore Q, et al: Glomerular localization of circulating antiglobulin activity in essential mixed cryoglobulinemia with glomerulonephritis. *Kidney Int* 21:387–394, 1982.

156. Cordonnier D, et al: Renal diseases in 18 patients with mixed type II IgM-IgG cryoglobulinemia: Monoclonal lymphoid infiltration (2 cases) and membranoproliferative glomerulonephritis. *Adv Nephrol* 12:177–204, 1983.

157. Sinico RA, et al: Identification of glomerular immune deposits in cryoglobulinemia glomerulonephritis. *Kidney Int* 34:109–116, 1988.

158. D'Amico G, et al: Renal involvement in essential mixed cryoglobulinemia. *Kidney Int* 35:1004–1014, 1989.

159. Hamburger MI, et al: Mixed cryoglobulinemia: Association of glomerulonephritis with defective reticuloendothelial system Fc receptor function. *Trans Assoc Am Phys* 92:104–112, 1979.

160. Monga G, et al: The presence and possible role of monocyte infiltration in human chronic proliferative glomerulonephritides. *Am J Pathol* 94:271–81, 1979.

161. Gettner D, et al: The effect of combination therapy (steroids, immunosuppressives and plasmapheresis) on 5 mixed cryoglobulinemia patients with renal, neurologic and vascular involvement. *Arth Rheum* 24:1124–1127, 1981.

162. Germain MJ, Anderson RW, and Keane WF: Renal disease in cryoglobulinemia type II: Response to therapy. A case report and review of the literature. *Am J Nephrol* 2:221–226, 1982.

163. DeVecchi A, et al: Intravenous methylprednisolone pulse therapy in essential cryoglobulinemia nephropathy. *Clin Nephrol* 19:221–227, 1983.

164. Delaney VB, et al: Plasmapheresis as sole therapy in a patient with essential mixed cryoglobulinemia. *Am J Kidney Dis* 4:75–77, 1984.

165. D'Amico G, et al: Renal involvement in essential mixed cryoglobulinemia: A peculiar type of immune mediated renal disease. *Adv Nephrol* 17:219–240, 1988.
166. MacKenzie MR and Fudenberg HH: Macroglobulinemia: An analysis of forty patients. *Blood* 39:874–889, 1972.
167. Dutcher TF and Fahey JL: The histopathology of the macroglobulinemia of Waldenström. *J Nat Cancer Inst* 22:887–917, 1959.
168. Morel-Maroger L, et al: Pathology of the kidney in Waldenström's macroglobulinemia. Study of sixteen cases. *N Engl J Med* 283:123–129, 1970.
169. Lin JH, et al: Waldenström's macroglobulinemia, mesangiocapillary glomerulonephritis angiitis and myositis. *Nephron* 10:262–270, 1973.
170. Meyrier A, et al: Rapidly progressive ("crescentic") glomerulonephritis and monoclonal gammopathies. *Nephron* 38:156–162, 1984.
171. Biava CG, et al: Crescentic glomerulonephritis associated with nonrenal malignancies. *Am J Nephrol* 4:208–214, 1984.
172. Argani I and Kipli GF: Macroglobulinemic nephropathy. Acute renal failure in macroglobulinemia of Waldenström. *Am J Med* 36:151–157, 1964.
173. Alpers CE and Cotran RS: Neoplasia and glomerular injury. *Kidney Int* 30:465–473, 1986.
174. Dathan JRE, Heyworth MF, and Maciver AG: Nephrotic syndrome in chronic lymphocytic leukaemia. *Br Med J* 3:655–657, 1974.
175. Cameron S and Ogg CS: Nephrotic syndrome in chronic lymphocytic leukaemia. *Br Med J* 4:164, 1974.
176. Gilboa N, et al: Immune deposit nephritis and single-component cryoglobulinemia associated with chronic lymphocyte leukemia. *Nephrol* 24:223–231, 1979.
177. Feehally J, et al: Recurrent proteinuria in chronic lymphocytic leukemia. *Clin Nephrol* 16:51–64, 1981.
178. Stalnikowica R, et al: Hyporeninemic hypoaldosteronism associated with focal glomerular sclerosis in a patient with chronic lymphocytic leukemia. *Nephron* 31:277–278, 1982.
179. White CA, Dillman RO, and Royston I: Membranous nephropathy associated with an unusual phenotype of chronic lymphocytic leukemia. *Cancer* 52:2253–2255, 1983.
180. Seney FD Jr., et al: A review of nephrotic syndrome associated with chronic lymphocytic leukemia. *Arch Intern Med* 146:137–141, 1986.
181. Touchard G, et al: Nephrotic syndrome associated with chronic lymphocytic leukemia: An immunological and physiological study. *Clin Nephrol* 31:107–116, 1989.
182. Editorial. Systemic vasculitis. *Lancet* 1:1252–1254, 1985.
183. Alarcon-Segovia D: The necrotizing vasculitides. A new pathogenetic classification. *Med Clin North Am* 61:241–260, 1977.
184. Fauci AS, Haynes BF, and Katz P: The spectrum of vasculitis. Clinical, pathologic, immunologic and therapeutic implications. *Ann Intern Med* 89:660–676, 1978.
185. Cohen Tervaert JW, van der Woude FJ, and Fauci AS: Association between active Wegener's granulomatosis and anticytoplasmic antibodies. *Arch Intern Med* 149:2461–2465, 1989.
186. Savage COS and Lockwood CM: Antineutrophil antibodies in vasculitis. *Adv Nephrol* 19:225–236, 1990.
187. Serra A, et al: Vasculitis affecting the kidney: presentation, histopathology and long-term outcome. *Q J Med* 210:181–207, 1984.

188. Adu D, et al: Polyarteritis and the kidney. *Q J Med* 239:221–237, 1987.
189. Gerhardt GM, Ahmad M, and Tubbs RR: Pulmonary vasculitis (Wegener's granulomatosis): Immunohistochemical study of T and B cell markers. *Am J Med* 74:700–704, 1983.
190. Parfrey PS, et al: The spectrum of diseases associated with necrotizing glomerulonephritis and its prognosis. *Am J Kidney Dis* 6:387–396, 1985.
191. Furlong TJ, Ibels LS, and Eckstein RP: The clinical spectrum of necrotizing glomerulonephritis. *Medicine* 66:192–201, 1987.
192. Jayne DRW, et al: Autoantibodies to GBM and neutrophil cytoplasm in rapidly progressive glomerulonephritis. *Kidney Int* 37:965–970, 1990.
193. Ronco P, et al: Immunopathological studies of polyarteritis nodosa and Wegener's granulomatosis: A report of 43 patients with 51 renal biopsies. *Q J Med* 206:212–223, 1983.
194. Pinching AJ, et al: Wegener's granulomatosis: observations on 18 patients with severe renal disease. *Q J Med* 208:435–460, 1983.
195. Fauci AS: Vasculitis: New insights amid old enigmas. *Am J Med* 67:916–918, 1979.
196. Kauffman RH, et al: Circulating IgA-immune complexes in Henoch-Schönlein purpura. A longitudinal study of their relationship to disease activity and vascular deposition of IgA. *Am J Med* 69:859–866, 1980.
197. D'Agati V, et al: Idiopathic microscopic polyarteritis nodosa: Ultrastructural observations on the renal vascular and glomerular lesions. *Am J Kidney Dis* 7:95–110, 1986.
198. Fligiel SEG, et al: Evidence for a role of hydroxyl radical in immune-complex-induced vasculitis. *Am J Pathol* 115:375–382, 1984.
199. Patrick GB: An approach to vasculitis syndromes. *Hosp Pract* 17:47–65, 1982.
200. Bacon PA: Evolving concepts in vasculitis. *Q J Med* 222:609–610, 1985.
201. Hart MN, et al: Autoimmune vasculitis resulting from in vitro immunization of lymphocytes to smooth muscle. *Am J Pathol* 119:448–455, 1985.
202. Wilkowski MJ, et al: Risk factors in idiopathic renal vasculitis and glomerulonephritis. *Kidney Int* 36:1133–1141, 1989.
203. Fauci AS, et al: Wegener's granulomatosis: Prospective clinical and therapeutic experience with 85 patients for 21 years. *Ann Intern Med* 98:76–85, 1983.
204. Woodworth TG, et al: Severe glomerulonephritis with late emergence of classic Wegener's granulomatosis. Report of 4 cases and review of the literature. *Medicine* 66:181–191, 1987.
205. Fauci AS and Wolf SM: Wegener's granulomatosis. Studies in eighteen patients and a review of the literature. *Medicine* 52:535–562, 1973.
206. Shillitoe EJ, Lehner T, and Lessop MH: Immunological features of Wegener's granulomatosis. *Lancet* 1:281–284, 1974.
207. Landman S and Burgener F: Pulmonary manifestations in Wegener's granulomatosis. *AJR* 122:750–757, 1975.
208. Conn DL, et al: Raised serum immunoglobulin E in Wegener's granulomatosis. *Ann Rheum Dis* 35:377–380, 1976.
209. Baker SB and Robinson DR: Unusual renal manifestations of Wegener's granulomatosis: Report of 2 cases. *Am J Med* 64:885–889, 1978.
210. Droz D, et al: Glomerulonephritis and necrotizing angiitis. *Adv Nephrol* 8:343–363, 1979.
211. Stoker TC, et al: Acute fulminating intrapulmonary haemmorhage in Wegener's granulomatosis. *Thorax* 37:315–316, 1982.
212. Novak RF, Christiansen RG, and Sorensen ET: The acute vasculitis of

Wegener's granulomatosis in renal biopsies. *Am J Clin Pathol* 78:367–372, 1982.
213. Pinching AJ, et al: Wegener's granulomatosis: observations in 18 patients with severe renal disease. *Q J Med* 208:435–460, 1983.
214. Brandwein S, et al: Wegener's granulomatosis. Clinical features and outcome in 13 patients. *Arch Intern Med* 143:476–479, 1983.
215. tenBerge IJM, et al: Clinical and immunological follow-up of patients with severe renal disease in Wegener's granulomatosis. *Am J Nephrol* 5:21–29, 1985.
216. DeRemee RA, McDonald TJ, and Weiland LH: Wegener's granulomatosis. Observations and treatment with antimicrobial agents. *Mayo Clin Proc* 60:27–32, 1985.
217. Weiner SR, Paulus HE, and Weisbart RH: Wegener's granulomatosis in the elderly. *Arth Rheum* 29:1157–1159, 1986.
218. Appel GB, et al: Wegener's granulomatosis. Clinical-pathologic correlations and long-term course. *Am J Kidney Dis* 1:27–37, 1981.
219. Hind CK, et al: Prognosis after immunosuppression of patients with crescentic nephritis requiring dialysis. *Lancet* 1:263–265, 1983.
220. Israel HL: Sulfamethoxazole-trimethoprim therapy for Wegener's granulomatosis. *Arch Intern Med* 148:2293–2295, 1988.
221. D'Agati V, et al: Idiopathic microscopic polyarteritis nodosa: Ultrastructural observations in the renal vascular and glomerular lesions. *Am J Kidney Dis* 7:95–110, 1986.
222. Lieb ES, Restivo C, and Paulus HE: Immunosuppressive and corticosteroid therapy of polyarteritis nodosa. *Am J Med* 67:941–945, 1979.
223. Cohen RD, Conn DL, and Ilstrup DM: Clinical features, prognosis and response to treatment in polyarteritis. *Mayo Clin Proc* 55:146–155, 1980.
224. Fauci AS, et al: Cyclophosphamide therapy of severe systemic necrotizing vasculitis. *N Engl J Med* 301:235–238, 1979.
225. Klein RG, et al: Large artery involvement in giant cell (temporal) arteritis. *Ann Intern Med* 83:806–812, 1975.
226. Balmforth GV: Temporal arteritis and renal failure. *Arch Intern Med* 113:230–234, 1964.
227. Von Knorring J, Erma M, and Lindstrom D: The clinical manifestations of temporal arteritis. *Acta Med Scand* 179:691–702, 1966.
228. Tallgren LG and von Knorring J: Renal vascular involvement in a case of polymyalgia rheumatica with temporal arteritis. A study of successive biopsies. *Acta Med Scand* 185:421–425, 1969.
229. Miller LM and Galdabini JJ: Case records of Massachusetts General Hospital. *N Engl J Med* 289:628–634, 1973.
230. Truong L, et al: Temporal arteritis and renal disease. Case report and review of the literature. *Am J Med* 78:171–175, 1985.
231. Hamilton CR Jr, Shelley WM, and Tumulty PA: Giant cell arteritis: Including temporal arteritis and polymyalgia rheumatica. *Medicine* 50:1–27, 1971.
232. Hunder GG, et al: Daily and alternate-day corticosteroid regimens in treatment of giant cell arteritis: Comparison in a prospective study. *Ann Intern Med* 82:613–618, 1975.
233. Bowers DG, Harpur JE, and Turks KAD: Giant cell arteritis—the need for prolonged treatment. *J Chron Dis* 26:571–573, 1973.
234. Cream JJ, Gumpel JM, and Peachey RDG: Schönlein-Henoch purpura in the adult. A study of 77 adults with anaphylactoid or Schönlein-Henoch purpura. *Q J Med* 39:461–484, 1970.

235. Ballard HS, Eisinger RP, and Gallo G: Renal manifestations of the Schöenlein-Henoch syndrome in adults. *Am J Med* 49:328–335, 1970.
236. Bar-On H and Rosenmann E: Schöenlein-Henoch syndrome in adults. A clinical and histological study of renal involvement. *Isr J Med Sci* 8:1702–1715, 1972.
237. Harrington JT and McCluskey R: Case records of Massachusetts General Hospital. *N Engl J Med* 308:267–273, 1983.
238. Roth DA, Wilz DR, and Theil GB: Schöenlein-Henoch syndrome in adults. *Q J Med* 217:145–152, 1985.
239. McKenzie PE, et al: Plasmapheresis in glomerulonephritis. *Clin Nephrol* 12:97–108, 1979.
240. Schwartz HR, et al: Hypocomplementemic urticarial vasculitis: Association with chronic obstructive pulmonary disease. *Mayo Clin Proc* 57:231–238, 1982.
241. Chumbley LC, Harrison EG, and DeRemee RA: Allergic granulomatosis and angiitis (Churg-Strauss syndrome). Report and analysis of 30 cases. *Mayo Clin Proc* 52:477–484, 1977.
242. Kellim RE and Haserick JR: Systemic lupus erythematosus. A statistical evaluation of mortality based on a consecutive series of 299 patients. *Arch Intern Med* 113:200–207, 1964.
243. DiMant J, et al: Systemic lupus erythematosus in the older age group: Computer analysis. *J Am Geriatr Soc* 27:58–61, 1979.
244. Hochberg MC, et al: Systemic lupus erythematosus: A review of clinicolaboratory features and immunogenetic markers in 150 patients with emphasis on demographic subsets. *Medicine* 64:285–295, 1985.
245. Wilson AH, et al: Age influences the clinical and serologic expression of systemic lupus erythematosus. *Arth Rheum* 24:1230–1235, 1981.
246. Morowitz MB, Stevens MB, and Shulman LE: The influence of age on the clinical pattern of systemic lupus erythematosus. *Arth Rheum* 10:319–320A, 1967.
247. Grishman E, Gerber MA, and Churg J: Patterns of renal injury in systemic lupus erythematosus: Light and immunofluorescence microscopic observations. *Am J Kidney Dis* 2:[Suppl 1] 135–141, 1982.
248. Brentjens JR, et al: Interstitial immune complex nephritis in patients with systemic lupus erythematosus. *Kidney Int* 7:342–350, 1975.
249. McCluskey RT: Evidence for an immune complex disorder in systemic lupus erythematosus (SLE). *Am J Kidney Dis* 2:[Suppl 1] 119–125, 1982.
250. Baker SB, et al: Late onset systemic lupus erythematosus. *Am J Med* 66:727–732, 1979.
251. Cohen AS, Fries J, and Masi AT: The 1982 revised criteria for the classification of systemic lupus erythematosus. *Arth Rheum* 25:1271–1277, 1982.
252. Friedman S, et al: Glomerular capillary wall function in human lupus nephritis. *Am J Physiol* 246:F580–F591, 1984.
253. Tron F, Ganeval D, and Droz D: Immunologically-mediated acute renal failure of non-glomerular origin in the course of systemic lupus erythematosus (SLE). Report of two cases. *Am J Med* 67:529–532, 1979.
254. Epstein FH and McCluskey RT: Case records of Massachusetts General Hospital. *N Engl J Med* 294:100–105, 1976.
255. Clinicopathologic Conference: Interstitial nephritis in a patient with systemic lupus erythematosus. *Am J Med* 69:775–781, 1980.
256. Yeung CK, et al: Tubular dysfunction in systemic lupus erythematosus. *Nephron* 36:84–88, 1984.

257. DeFronzo RA, Cooke CR, and Goldberg M: Impaired renal tubular K secretion in systemic lupus erythematosus. *Ann Intern Med* 86:268–271, 1977.
258. Kiley J and Zager P: Hyporeninemic hypoaldosteronism in two patients with systemic lupus erythematosus. *Am J Kidney Dis* 4:39–43, 1984.
259. Kimberly RP, et al: High-dose intravenous methylprednisone pulse therapy in systemic lupus erythematosus. *Am J Med* 70:817–824, 1981.
260. Balow JE, et al: Effect of treatment on the evaluation of renal abnormalities in lupus nephritis. *N Engl J Med* 311:491–495, 1984.
261. Austin HA III, et al: Therapy of lupus nephritis. Controlled trial of prednisone and cytotoxic drugs. *N Engl J Med* 314:614–619, 1986.
262. Lewis EJ: Plasmapheresis for the treatment of severe lupus nephritis. Uncontrolled observations. *Am J Nephrol* 2:182–187, 1982.
263. Lewis EJ and Lachin J: Primary outcomes in the controlled trial of plasmapheresis therapy (PTT) in severe lupus nephritis. *Kidney Int* 31:208A, 1987.
264. Cannon PJ, et al: The relationship of hypertension and renal failure in scleroderma (progressive systemic sclerosis) to structural and functional abnormalities of the renal cortical circulation. *Medicine* 53:1–46, 1974.
265. Clements PJ, et al: The relationship of arrythmias and conduction disturbances to other manifestations of cardiopulmonary disease in progressive systemic sclerosis (PSS). *Am J Med* 71:38–46, 1981.
266. D'Angelo WA, et al: Pathologic observations in systemic sclerosis. *Am J Med* 46:428–440, 1969.
267. Campbell PM and Le Roy EC: Pathogenesis of systemic sclerosis: A vascular hypothesis. *Semin Arth Rheum* 4:351–368, 1975.
268. Kahaleh MB, Sherer GK, and Le Roy EC: Endothelial injury in scleroderma. *J Exp Med* 149:1326–1335, 1979.
269. Oliver JA, et al: Renal vasoactive hormones in scleroderma (progressive systemic sclerosis). *Nephron* 29:110–116, 1981.
270. Thurm RH and Alexander JC: Captopril in the treatment of scleroderma renal crisis. *Arch Intern Med* 144:733–735, 1984.
271. Beckett VL, et al: Use of captopril as early therapy for renal scleroderma: A prospective study. *Mayo Clin Proc* 60:736–771, 1985.
272. Kovalchik MT, et al: The kidney in progressive systemic sclerosis. A prospective study. *Ann Intern Med* 89:881–887, 1978.
273. Traub YM, et al: Hypertension and renal failure (scleroderma renal crisis) in progressive systemic sclerosis. Review of a 25-year experience with 68 cases. *Medicine* 62:335–352, 1983.
274. Gavras H, et al: Is elevated plasma renin activity of prognostic importance in progressive systemic sclerosis. *Arch Intern Med* 137:1554–1558, 1977.
275. Steen VD, Medsger TA, and Rodman GP: D-Penicillamine therapy in progressive systemic sclerosis (scleroderma). *Ann Intern Med* 97:652–659, 1982.
276. Steen VD, et al: Factors predicting development of renal involvement in progressive systemic sclerosis. *Am J Med* 76:779–786, 1984.
277. Medsger TA and Masi AT: Survival with scleroderma II. A life-table analysis of clinical and demographic factors in 358 male U.S. veteran patients. *J Chron Dis* 26:647–660, 1973.
278. Dau PC, Kahalek MB, and Sagebiel RW: Plasmapheresis and immunosuppressive drug therapy in scleroderma. *Arth Rheum* 24:1128–1136, 1981.
279. Mascaro G, et al: Plasma exchange in the treatment of nonadvanced stages of progressive systemic sclerosis. *J Clin Apheresis* 3:219–225, 1987.
280. Whitman HH III and Case DB: New developments in the treatment of scleroderma. *Drug Ther* 12:85–97, 1981.

281. Simon NM, et al: Resolution of renal failure with malignant hypertension in scleroderma. Case report and review of the literature. *Am J Med* 67:533–539, 1979.
282. Whitman HH III, et al: Variable response to oral angiotensin-converting-enzyme blockade in hypertensive scleroderma patients. *Arth Rheum* 25:241–248, 1982.
283. Ichikawa I, Miele JF, and Brenner BM: Reversal of renal cortical actions of angiotensin II by verapamil and manganese. *Kidney Int* 16:137–147, 1979.
284. Cases A, et al: Captopril vs nifedipine. *Clin Nephrol* 27:269, 1987.
285. Ridolfi RL and Bell WR: Thrombotic thrombocytopenic purpura. Report of 25 cases and review of the literature. *Medicine* 60:413–428, 1981.
286. Knupp CL: Thrombotic thrombocytopenic purpura in older patients. *J Am Geriatr Soc* 36:331–338, 1988.
287. Schmidt JL: Thrombotic thrombocytopenic purpura: Successful treatment unlocks etiologic secrets. *Mayo Clin Proc* 64:956–961, 1989.
288. Grem JL, Merritt JA, and Carbone PP: Treatment of mytocin-associated microangiopathic hemolytic anemia with vincristine. *Arch Intern Med* 146:566–568, 1986.
289. Hostetter AL, et al: Chronic glomerular microangiopathy complicating metastatic carcinoma. *Hum Pathol* 18:342–348, 1987.
290. Editorial: Hemolytic uraemic syndrome. *Lancet* 2:1078–1079, 1984.
291. Neild G: The haemolytic uraemic syndrome: A review. *Q J Med* 241:367–376, 1987.
292. Morel-Maroger L, et al: Prognostic importance of vascular lesions in acute renal failure with microangiopathic hemolytic anemia (hemolytic-uremic syndrome): Clinicopathologic study in 20 adults. *Kidney Int* 15:548–558, 1979.
293. Eknoyan G and Riggs SA: Renal involvement in patients with thrombotic thrombocytopenic purpura. *Am J Nephrol* 6:117–131, 1986.
294. Thorsen CA, et al: The treatment of the hemolytic uremic syndrome with inhibitors of platelet function. *Am J Med* 66:711–716, 1979.
295. Hakim RM, et al: Successful management of thrombocytopenia, micro-angiopathic anemia and acute renal failure by plasmapheresis. *Am J Kidney Dis* 5:170–176, 1985.
296. Myers TJ, et al: Thrombotic thrombocytopenic purpura: Combined treatment with plasmapheresis and antiplatelet agents. *Ann Intern Med* 92:149–155, 1980.
297. Brun C, et al: Renal biopsy in rheumatoid arthritis. *Nephron* 2:65–81, 1965.
298. Samuels B, et al: Membranous nephropathy in patients with rheumatoid arthritis: Relationship to gold therapy. *Medicine* 57:319–327, 1977.
299. Schmid FR, et al: Arteritis in rheumatoid arthritis. *Am J Med* 30:56–83, 1961.
300. Scott DGI, Bacon PA, and Tribe CR: Systemic rheumatoid vasculitis. A clinical and laboratory study of 50 cases. *Medicine* 60:288–297, 1981.
301. Meriwether JH Jr, Weinberger HJ, and Gleason IO: The renal vascular lesion in rheumatoid disease. *Arth Rheum* 10:298A, 1967.
302. Kuznetsky KA, et al: Necrotizing glomerulonephritis in rheumatoid arthritis. *Clin Nephrol* 26:257–264, 1986.
303. McAdam LP, et al: Relapsing polychondritis: Prospective study of 23 patients and a review of the literature. *Medicine* 55:193–215, 1976.
304. Chang-Miller A, et al: Renal involvement in relapsing polychondritis. *Medicine* 66:202–217, 1987.
305. Neild GH, et al: Relapsing polychondritis with crescentic glomerulonephritis. *Br Med J* 1:743–745, 1978.

306. Espinoza LR, et al: Immune-complex-mediated renal involvement in relapsing polychondritis. *Am J Med* 71:181–183, 1981.
307. Bloch KJ, et al: Sjögren's syndrome. A clinical, pathological and serological study of sixty-two cases. *Medicine* 44:187–231, 1965.
308. Pavlidis NA, Karsh J, and Motsopoulos HM: The clinical picture of primary Sjögren's syndrome: a retrospective study. *J Rheumatol* 9:685–690, 1982.
309. Kahn M, et al: Renal concentrating defect in Sjögren's syndrome. *Ann Intern Med* 56:883–895, 1962.
310. Whaley K, et al: Sjögren's syndrome. *Q J Med* 167:513–548, 1973.
311. Talal N, Zisman E, and Schur PH: Renal tubular acidosis, glomerulonephritis and immunologic factors in Sjögren's syndrome. *Arth Rheum* 11:774–786, 1968.
312. El-Mallakh RS, et al: Long-term low-dose glucocorticoid therapy associated with remission of overt renal tubular acidosis in Sjögren's syndrome. *Am J Med* 79:509–514, 1985.
313. Tu WH, et al: Interstitial nephritis in Sjögren's syndrome. *Ann Intern Med* 69:1163–1170, 1968.
314. Motsopoulos HM, et al: Immune complex glomerulonephritis in sicca syndrome. *Am J Med* 64:955–960, 1978.
315. Abraham PA and Keane WF: Glomerular and interstitial disease induced by nonsteroidal anti-inflammatory drugs. *Am J Nephrol* 4:1–6, 1984.
316. Garella S and Matarese RA: Renal effects of prostaglandins and clinical adverse effects of non-steroidal anti-inflammatory agents. *Medicine* 63:165–181, 1984.
317. Clive DM and Stoff JS: Renal syndromes associated with non-steroidal anti-inflammatory drugs. *N Engl J Med* 310:563–572, 1984.
318. Carmichael T and Shankel SW: Effects of non-steroidal anti-inflammatory drugs on prostaglandins and renal function. *Am J Med* 78:992–1000, 1985.
319. Cameron JS: Immunologically mediated interstitial nephritis: Primary and secondary. *Adv Nephrol* 18:207–248, 1989.
320. Lamy PP: Renal effects of non-steroidal anti-inflammatory drugs. Heightened risk in the elderly? *J Am Geriatr Soc* 34:361–367, 1986.
321. Mignon F, et al: Granulomatous interstitial nephritis. *Adv Nephrol* 13:219–245, 1984.
322. Warren GV, et al: Minimal change glomerulopathy associated with non-steroidal anti-inflammatory drugs. *Am J Kidney Dis* 13:127–130, 1989.
323. Neugarten J, Gallo GR, and Baldwin DS: Rifampin-induced nephrotic syndrome and acute interstitial nephritis. *Am J Nephrol* 3:38–42, 1983.
324. Kean WF, et al: Efficacy and toxicity of D-penicillamine for rheumatoid disease in the elderly. *J Am Geriatr Soc* 30:94–100, 1982.
325. Harkness JAL and Blake DR: Penicillamine nephropathy and iron. *Lancet* 2:1368–1369, 1982.
326. Hall CL, et al: Natural course of penicillamine nephropathy: A long-term study of 33 patients. *Br Med J* 296:1083–1086, 1988.
327. Walshe JM: Management of penicillamine nephropathy in Wilson's disease: A new chelating agent. *Lancet* 2:1401–1403, 1969.
328. Sternlieb I, Bennett B, and Scheinberg HI: D-Penicillamine induced Goodpasture's syndrome in Wilson's disease. *Ann Intern Med* 82:673–676, 1975.
329. Gibson T, Burry HC, and Ogg C: Goodpasture's syndrome and D-penicillamine. *Ann Intern Med* 84:100, 1976.
330. Matloff DS and Kaplan MM: D-Penicillamine-induced Goodpasture's like syndrome in primary biliary cirrhosis: Successful treatment with plasmapheresis and immunosuppressives. *Gastroenterology* 78:1046–1049, 1980.

331. Ntoso KA, et al: Penicillamine-induced rapidly progressive glomerulo-nephritis in patients with progressive systemic sclerosis: Successful treatment of two patients and a review of the literature. *Am J Kidney Dis* 8:159–163, 1986.
332. Katz WA, Blodgett RC Jr, and Pietrusko RG: Proteinuria in gold-treated rheumatoid arthritis. *Ann Intern Med* 101:176–179, 1984.
333. Hall CL: Gold nephropathy. *Nephron* 50:265–272, 1988.
334. Silverberg DS, et al: Gold nephropathy. A clinical and pathologic study. *Arth Rheum* 13:812–825, 1970.
335. Wooley PH, et al: HLA-DR antigens and toxic reaction to sodium auro-thiomalate and D-penicillamine in patients with rheumatoid arthritis. *N Engl J Med* 303:300–302, 1980.
336. Grant JT, Husby G, and Thorsby E: HLA-DR antigens and gold toxicity. *Ann Rheum Dis* 42:63–66, 1983.
337. Shaw CF: The biochemistry and subcellular distribution of gold in kidney tissue: Implications of chrysotherapy and nephrotoxicity. *Agents Actions* 8 (Suppl):509–528, 1981.
338. Case DB, et al: Proteinuria during long-term captopril therapy. *JAMA* 244:346–349, 1980.
339. Lewis EJ: Angiotensin-converting enzyme inhibitors: Considerations regarding proteinuria. *Am J Kidney Dis* 10:30–38, 1987.
340. Textor SC, et al: Membranous glomerulopathy associated with captopril therapy. *Am J Med* 74:705–712, 1983.
341. Adler SG, Cohen AH, and Border WA: Hypersensitivity phenomena and the kidney. Role of drugs and environmental agents. *Am J Kidney Dis* 5:75–96, 1985.
342. Terpenning MS, Buggy BP, and Kauffman CA: Infective endocarditis. Clinical features in young and elderly patients. *Am J Med* 83:626–634, 1987.
343. Neugarten J, Gallo GR, and Baldwin DS: Glomerulonephritis in bacterial endocarditis. *Am J Kidney Dis* 3:371–379, 1984.
344. Beaufils M, et al: Glomerulonephritis in severe bacterial infections with or without endocarditis. *Adv Nephrol* 7:217–234, 1978.
345. Forrest JW Jr, et al: Immune complex glomerulonephritis associated with *Klebsiella pneumoniae* infection. *Clin Nephrol* 7:76–80, 1977.
346. Magil AB: Monocytes and glomerulonephritis associated with remote visceral infection. *Clin Nephrol* 22:169–175, 1984.
347. Beaufils M, et al: Acute renal failure of glomerular origin during visceral abscesses. *N Engl J Med* 295:185–189, 1976.
348. Coleman M, et al: Glomerulonephritis associated with chronic bacterial infection of a dacron arterial prosthesis. *Clin Nephrol* 20:315–320, 1983.
349. Shusterman N and London WR: Hepatitis B and immune-complex disease. *N Engl J Med* 310:43–45, 1984.
350. Hirose H, et al: Deposition of hepatitis B antigen in membranous glomerulonephritis: Identification by F(ab')2 fragments of monoclonal antibody. *Kidney Int* 26:338–341, 1984.
351. Sergent JS, et al: Vasculitis with hepatitis B antigenemia: Long-term observations in nine patients. *Medicine* 55:1–18, 1976.

8 UROLITHIASIS AND OBSTRUCTIVE UROPATHY

UROLITHIASIS

INCIDENCE AND PREVALENCE

Patients 60 years and over made up 19 percent of those seen in a community practice for their first symptomatic kidney stone [1, 2]. Sixty-three percent were between the ages of 30 and 60 years, and 18 percent below the age of 30 [1–3]. Sixty-five to 70 percent of our elderly patients with renal colic have had a past history of stone disease, and only 30 to 35 percent were "new" symptomatic stone formers. So it would appear that new onset of clinical stone disease occurs less frequently in the elderly. The prevalence of renal calculi in the elderly varies geographically, affecting 5.7 to 5.9 percent of elderly males and 3.2 to 5 percent of elderly females in the United States, and 17.2 to 18.2 percent of elderly males and 7.3 to 8.1 percent of elderly females in Denmark [4]. In both countries the male-to-female ratio in the elderly is approximately 2:1.

ETIOLOGY

No systematic studies in a large number of elderly have been carried out to determine the distribution of the different forms of urolithiasis. Based on stone analysis in a relatively small number (20) of well-studied patients, we found calcium oxalate stones in 80 percent, uric acid (pure or mixed) in 5 percent, struvite in 10 percent, and phosphate in the remainder. In 40 percent of patients neither metabolic nor structural abnormalities could be found. Hypercalciuria was present in 30 percent, with hyperuricosuria in 10 percent, chronic infection in 10 percent, hyperoxaluria in 5 percent, and hypocitraturia in 5 percent.

PATHOGENESIS

General

Stones form when salts present in the urine (e.g., calcium oxalate, calcium phosphate) crystallize in the renal tubule and collecting system. The different mechanisms responsible for this phenomenon include (1) supersaturation, because a solubilizer for the constituent substances is excreted at a low rate (e.g., citrate for calcium oxalate) [5], or the volume of distribution of the constituents (in this case urine) is low, or an appropriate milieu facilitating insolubility or precipitation (e.g., low urine pH for uric acid stones) is present; (2) formation of alternative nuclei such as cell debris, uric acid, or a calcium phosphate crystal nidus that promote crystallization [6] (a process referred to as heterogeneous nucleation); or (3) deficiency of naturally occurring inhibitors such as nephrocalcin or glycosaminoglycans (glycoproteins capable of inhibiting the growth of calcium oxalate crystals by adsorption on the surface) [7, 8].

The 40 percent of patients with no "detectable abnormality" that we found in the elderly is higher than the 10 to 25 percent of such patients found in the general population [9, 10]. These patients form calcium oxalate stones, and it is not clear exactly what mechanism triggers the process of stone formation. The possibilities include (1) an imbalance between urinary calcium and citrate in favor of the former (the so-called calcium-citrate index) [11]; (2) an anomalous cellular transport of oxalate [12]; (3) a mild degree of hyperoxaluria [13]; and (4) the formation of a qualitatively defective glycoprotein inhibitor [14]. It is to be noted that these studies suggesting mechanisms for stone formation were performed in younger patients and may not be applicable in the elderly.

Hypercalciuria

Hypercalciuria is defined as the urinary excretion of calcium greater than 140 mg per g of urinary creatinine. Hypercalciuria is divided into hypercalcemic and normocalcemic varieties. In our experience, hypercalcemic hypercalciuria with stone formation occurs almost exclusively in elderly persons with hyperparathyroidism and sarcoidosis. In these situations the high urinary calcium level is a function of an increase in the filtered load (see Hypercalcemia in Chap. 5). Stone formers with normocalcemic hypercalciuria either have renal tubular acidosis (RTA), are immobilized, or have idiopathic hypercalciuria. Distal renal tubular acidosis (type I) as a cause of lithiasis is rare in the elderly. In these patients the hypercalciuria reflects a decrease in tubular reabsorption of calcium due to the acidosis per se [15]. During acidosis there is an increase in citrate oxidation by renal cortical cell mitochondria that lowers the urinary concentration of citrate [16]. Since citrate normally binds about half of the urine calcium, more free calcium is available for crystallization with PO_4, resulting in stone formation. The high urinary concentration of PO_4 is a result of the persistently alkaline urine characteristic of this form of RTA.

Prolonged immobilization with its resulting resorptive hypercalciuria has been associated with calcium oxalate or mixed stones in younger patients and, less frequently, in the elderly [17–19].

The "idiopathic" variety is by far the most common form of hypercalciuria found in the elderly stone former, the renal type being present in 80 percent and the absorptive type seen in the remaining 20 percent

[20]. Patients with hypercalciuria most likely are a heterogeneous group in whom either one or more of the following abnormalities are operative [21]: (1) a decrease in distal tubular calcium reabsorption induced by phosphate depletion; the primary defect in such patients may be an intrinsic defect in the reabsorption of phosphate in the proximal tubule through a non-parathyroid hormone (PTH)–dependent mechanism [22]; (2) accelerated intestinal calcium absorption, resulting in an increase in serum postprandial calcium followed by suppression of PTH; the increase in jejunal calcium absorption may be secondary to an increase in the mucosal cell sensitivity to normal levels of $1,25(OH)_2$ vitamin D_3 or to an increase in sensitivity of renal 1 alpha-hydroxylase to circulating PTH (see Chap. 5) for those with elevated $1,25(OH)_2$ vitamin D_3 [23, 24]; or (3) both an elevation of intestinal calcium absorption and a defect in renal calcium reabsorption [25, 26].

The percentage of elderly patients with hypercalciuria who will form stones is not clear. For those who do, in addition to the hypercalciuria, abnormalities of the different crystal growth inhibitors are probably playing a significant role [27–29].

Hyperuricosuria

Hyperuricosuria is defined as the urine excretion of uric acid of more than 800 mg per day. Patients with hyperuricosuria may form pure uric acid stones, pure calcium oxalate stones, or stones containing both calcium oxalate and uric acid. Patients in the last group are referred to as mixed-stone formers and usually are hypercalciuric [30]. Pure uric acid stones are the most common in the elderly with hyperuricosuria, followed by mixed and calcium oxalate stones in that order.

Uric acid stones form when the urinary concentration of undissociated uric acid exceeds its solubility limit, which in humans is approximately 96 mg per liter at 37°C [31]. Because the dissociation of uric acid is pH dependent, the lower the urinary pH the higher the concentration of undissociated uric acid. In the presence of a low urine pH (5.5) the urine becomes supersaturated with free uric acid, thereby increasing the risk of stone formation [32]. The impact of a change in urine pH on uric acid stone formation is greater than a change in the amount of uric acid excreted. Dietary purine excess from meat is largely responsible for the hyperuricosuria and low urinary pH. When such patients are placed on a purine-free diet, urinary uric acid decreases dramatically [32]. The fact that serum uric acid remains in the normal range on a high purine diet appears to rule out a significant defect in tubular handling of urate.

Patients with mixed stones produce urine supersaturated with calcium oxalate and uric acid, whereas those with either calcium oxalate or uric acid stones have an imbalance in supersaturation favoring one crystal over the other [33]. The precipitation of calcium oxalate with subsequent stone formation in the hyperuricosuric patient is initiated by seed crystals of sodium hydrogen urate or uric acid through the process of heterogeneous nucleation [34]. The cause of the hyperuricosuria is also dietary overindulgence in purine-rich foods. Both calcium and oxalate excretion are usually normal in these patients [35].

Struvite Stones (Associated with Urinary Tract Infection)

Struvite stones are made of magnesium ammonium phosphate ($MgNH_4$ $PO_4 \cdot 6H_2O$) and form only in the presence of bacteria that possess urease, an enzyme capable of hydrolyzing urea to ammonia (urea-splitting organisms). The latter, in turn, hydrolyzes spontaneously to ammonium hydroxide, which increases urine pH. The alkaline milieu facilitates an increase in the concentration of deprotonated phosphate and, since magnesium is always present in the urine, the formation of struvite stones. The stones grow as bacteria multiply and are found almost exclusively in women. Their occurrence in men usually indicates the presence of additional hypercalciuria [36]. The organisms responsible for struvite stones in the elderly are the same as those reported in younger patients, with *Proteus* species being the most common [37]. Struvite stones, like uric acid stones, can become very large and are capable of filling the whole collecting system.

Hyperoxaluria

Hyperoxaluria (urinary oxalate excretion greater than 40 mg per 24 hours) occurs in the elderly with intestinal malabsorption and is secondary to increased oxalate absorption in the colon [38]. Because of the increased oxalate excretion, the urine is supersaturated with calcium oxalate, thus favoring crystallization [39]. It has been demonstrated that an increase in urinary oxalate concentration increases supersaturation even more than an equivalent increase in calcium concentration [40]. Other auxiliary factors that may be critical are low urinary output due to the presence of volume contraction in many of these patients and low urinary citrate, a reflection of citrate malabsorption and metabolic acidosis. The latter is secondary to bicarbonate losses through the gastrointestinal tract. Since urinary pH may be persistently low in such patients, uric acid stones may also form (see earlier discussion).

Hypocitruria

There is a group of elderly patients who form calcium phosphate stones in whom the only abnormality is a low urinary citrate excretion (less than 3 mmol per liter) due to the presence of mild chronic metabolic acidosis induced by carbonic anhydrase inhibitor (acetazolamide) therapy for glaucoma. Calcium phosphate stones in these patients tend to form during the first 12 months of acetazolamide therapy. Besides hypocitruria, hypermagnesiuria and perhaps an intermittent rise in urine pH due to a transient decrease in HCO_3 reabsorption (at the peak of drug action) also contribute to the calcium monohydrogen phosphate supersaturation [41, 42]. Some patients who form stones during acetazolamide administration also have an abnormality in calcium excretion when they are studied after discontinuing acetazolamide [41]. It should be noted that hypocitruria is not limited to calcium phosphate stone formers. Not infrequently, hypocitruria is the only metabolic abnormality in patients with calcium oxalate nephrolithiasis [43, 44].

CLINICAL MANIFESTATIONS
The clinical manifestations of urolithiasis in the elderly are the same as in younger patients. Flank pain radiating to the groin with gross or microscopic hematuria constitutes the most frequent presentation. Urinary infection, manifested by chills and fever and frequently associated with costophrenic angle tenderness, may be present in patients with obstructing stone disease and is also seen in patients with struvite stones. Patients with only one functioning kidney (in some of our patients a small, nonfunctioning contralateral kidney was a consequence of severe renal artery disease) may present with anuria. In a significant number of patients, particularly those with struvite stones, stones are found during an investigation for recurrent urinary tract infections or during radiologic evaluation for hematuria. On retrospective analysis, these patients often describe a dull, persistent loin discomfort of some duration.

TREATMENT AND PROGNOSIS
Since specific therapy is dependent on the specific pathogenesis, it is important to decide which patients with urolithiasis require a metabolic work-up. To answer this question, it is necessary to outline the procedure to be followed, the potential for recurrence, and the benefit(s) to be obtained from the information gained. Our initial work-up includes three 24-hour urine collections for determination of calcium, oxalate, uric acid, phosphate, citrate, pH, and volume. Blood is also taken for determination of urea, creatinine, calcium, phosphorus, total carbon dioxide, and uric acid levels. The mean values from the three collections are then determined, and, depending on the results, additional studies including the serum parathyroid hormone (PTH) level, serum vitamin D_3, urinary cyclic AMP, and others are carried out. The median time to recurrence in the elderly (i.e, the time by which 50 percent of the patients have had recurrent urolithiasis) is 11 ± 5 years, with 39 percent forming a second stone within 6.8 ± 0.6 years [2]. There appears to be no difference in the recurrence rate between patients with and without a metabolic abnormality [9]. With this background information, the de-

cision to perform an extensive evaluation must be individualized, although we will try to provide some broad guidelines.

Our approach in the elderly patient with clinical evidence of urolithiasis, as in younger patients, is to treat the acute episode with analgesics and hydration. Patients who cannot take oral fluids because of nausea or vomiting, those with fever, and those in whom there is a strong suspicion of obstruction are admitted to the hospital. Forty percent of our patients have been managed on an outpatient basis. Spontaneous stone passage in the elderly occurs in 50 percent of the cases compared to 65 percent in younger patients. In the remaining half, some form of urologic intervention is usually required [45]. The percentage of patients with residual stones on sonogram or x-ray examination (kidney-ureters-bladder [KUB] or intravenous pyelogram, which is obtained in all patients in this age group) [46] in our experience is approximately 30 percent. Twenty percent had bilateral involvement.

Once the acute episode is over, patients with organic brain syndrome, those who are frail and bedridden, and those with associated disease with a potentially poor prognosis are not studied. They are placed on a high fluid intake and followed regularly with a KUB or sonogram to assess stone recurrence or growth. Urologic evaluation for possible extracorporeal shock wave lithotripsy (ESWL) is advised (see later discussion) for patients with struvite stones less than 2 cm in size. Stones larger than 2 cm are best approached by percutaneous nephrolithotomy. This procedure also constitutes the procedure of choice for lower pole branched stones, whereas ESWL is better for stones in the upper poles. It should be noted that advanced renal insufficiency (serum creatinine > 4 mg per dl) constitutes an absolute contraindication to ESWL. Stones located in the lower ureters are usually handled through ureteroscopy. Other patients are offered the choice of either careful observation or investigation, as outlined earlier. We emphasize complete investigation for all patients with recurrences (if they have not been previously studied) [47]. Stone formers with associated osteoporosis should also be fully evaluated because the hypercalciuria in some is not accompanied by the usual compensatory intestinal hyperabsorption of calcium. This latter defect predisposes them to negative calcium balance with consequent stimulation of the parathyroids and enhanced skeletal mobilization of calcium [48].

Specific Therapy: Nonpharmacologic
Fluid intake sufficient to ensure a urine volume above 2.5 liters per day is recommended [49]. Urine dilution has been found to reduce the propensity for crystallization of calcium salts by lowering the urinary saturation of brushite (CaH_2O, which may be acting as the initial crystal nidus for certain calcium-containing renal stones) and calcium oxalate and by increasing the minimum supersaturation required to elicit spontaneous

nucleation of calcium oxalate [50]. This approach, however, when used as the sole therapeutic modality, has not been convincingly shown to prevent stone formation [51].

In patients with absorptive hyperoxaluria, beets, spinach, grapefruit, chocolate, nuts, and tea should be avoided. In addition, supplemental vitamin C should be discouraged or at least kept below 1 g per day [52]. Those with uric acid and mixed stones should moderate their intake of foods rich in animal proteins. Patients with calcium oxalate stones and hypercalciuria should consider lowering their sodium intake to below 4 g per day and moderate their protein intake, if high [53, 54]. Dietary calcium restriction does not play a role in the management of the elderly with nephrolithiasis (see Chap. 5).

Specific Therapy: Pharmacologic

In patients with recurrent calcium oxalate stones and no detectable urinary abnormality we use the regimen originally proposed by Coe [9], which consists of allopurinol, 100 mg daily, and hydrochlorothiazide, 50 mg daily, with a 2- to 4-g daily sodium diet. This regimen has, in general, been well accepted and tolerated in the elderly.

Hypercalciuria (both renal and absorptive) usually responds to thiazides and salt restriction [55], although the hypocalciuric effect of the diuretic may be attenuated in time in patients with the absorptive form of the syndrome [56]. The thiazides decrease urinary calcium excretion by acting directly on calcium reabsorption in the distal tubule [57] as well as by inducing a state of volume contraction (maintained by a low-sodium diet), which leads to enhanced proximal reabsorption of both sodium and calcium, thereby decreasing distal delivery. Finally, the thiazide-induced alkalosis may also contribute to the decrease in calcium excretion. We usually start with hydrochlorothiazide 50 mg per day. In patients in whom urinary calcium excretion is not normalized, the dose is increased to 50 mg twice a day. The majority of our elderly patients respond to this regimen. Hypokalemia develops in 10 to 15 percent of the patients; if therapy is required (see Chap. 3), we add potassium citrate 15 to 30 mEq twice a day. In the presence of persistent hypercalciuria despite a maximum dose of thiazide, amiloride 2.5 mg twice a day can be added. Since this drug increases distal tubule calcium reabsorption through a mechanism different from that of the thiazides, its hypocalciuric effect is additive [58, 59].

When attenuation or loss of the hypocalciuric response to thiazides occurs in patients with absorptive hypercalciuria, the drug may be temporarily discontinued (for 6–10 weeks). Restoration of a normal response may occur after this temporary withdrawal. Sodium cellulose phosphate, at a dosage of 10 to 15 g per day, might possibly be substituted in the interim [60].

In patients with uric acid stones, a low-purine diet is recommended along with potassium citrate, 15 to 40 mEq twice a day, the last dose given at bedtime to ensure a high overnight urine pH. The goal is to raise urine pH to 6.0. Higher levels are undesirable because they may favor secondary calcium phosphate stones [61]. Allopurinol (100–300 mg per day) is added if hyperuricosuria is present. This drug is also the agent of choice for the hyperuricosuric patient who forms calcium oxalate stones [62].

Struvite stones are usually large and are often associated with infection and parenchymal damage with progressive loss of kidney function. Antibiotic therapy alone is inadequate. Such patients should be referred for either surgery [63] or other procedures such as ESWL for small stones [64, 65]. Larger stones (2 cm) are best managed by a combination of percutaneous nephrolithotripsy and ESWL or chemical dissolution of residual infected fragments with acetohydroxamic acid, a bacterial urease inhibitor [66]. Because of potential serious side effects, we believe this drug should be handled only by people familiar with its use [67, 68].

The ideal treatment for intestinal hyperoxaluria is control of the underlying disease in addition to dietary restriction. Since this is not always feasible, other modalities have to be tried. Oral administration of large amounts of calcium, 250 to 1000 mg with meals, has been recommended [69]. This measure decreases gut absorption and urinary excretion of oxalate; however, because of a concurrent increase in urinary calcium excretion there is really no significant change in the urinary state of saturation with respect to calcium oxalate. Magnesium gluconate, a gut binder, 0.5 to 1.0 g every 8 hours, may be tried as well as cholestyramine, 8 to 16 mg per day, which can adsorb dietary oxalate, making it less available for intestinal absorption. Unfortunately, cholestyramine may interfere with the absorption of vitamin K and other drugs commonly used by the elderly (e.g., digoxin). Patients who are acidotic can be managed with potassium citrate at the usual dose outlined above. Attention should also be paid to adequate hydration [55].

In patients who form calcium phosphate stones while taking acetazolamide the drug should be discontinued if possible. If not, potassium citrate can be used to prevent stone formation [70]. Such patients should undergo metabolic evaluation to rule out abnormalities in calcium excretion.

Therapy for the hypercalcemic hypercalciuric patient who forms stones is that of the underlying cause of the hypercalcemia (see Chap. 5).

The rate of recurrence of kidney stones in the elderly undergoing therapy is not known (our short follow-up and small number of patients do not permit us to provide an answer). In one prospective study dealing with younger patients, the authors used three characteristics to identify those patients in whom relapse was most likely to occur [71]. Patients in whom there was a short interval between the time they entered the authors' program and their last episode of urolithiasis, patients who had a higher urinary calcium excretion (2.79 versus 2.39 mg per kg for the non-recurrent patients), and patients with a low urinary volume were all prone to recurrence. Other investigators [72] have used a stepwise discriminant analysis selecting plasma albumin, urinary pH, urinary calcium excretion, plasma phosphate, GFR, and nephrogenic cyclic AMP as the most important variables contributing to the difference between controls and recurrent stone formers. Patients with recurrent stones despite therapy-induced "normalization" of their urine are managed symptomatically during the acute episode. We usually continue long-term therapy since the risks associated with stone formation far exceed the risks associated with therapy [73].

OBSTRUCTIVE UROPATHY

As with younger patients, urinary obstruction in the elderly can be either unilateral or bilateral. In this section we will discuss obstruction as a cause of renal impairment in the elderly; therefore, unless the disease process involves a patient with only one functioning kidney, our focus will be mainly on bilateral obstruction.

INCIDENCE AND PREVALENCE
Obstructive uropathy is responsible for 10 to 15 percent of cases of acute renal failure in the elderly [74–77]. Since 4 to 6 percent of elderly patients in the hospital are evaluated for renal failure, the frequency of clinically significant obstructive uropathy varies between 0.4 and 0.6 percent.

ETIOLOGY
Obstruction, which may be either intrinsic or extrinsic, can occur at any level of the urinary tract in the elderly. It should be considered in any patient with renal insufficiency, whether acute or chronic. The different causes of obstructive uropathy in 116 patients are outlined in Table 8-1. Seventy-five patients (65 percent) were males, and 41 (35 percent) were females. Prostatic disease was the most common cause in males; in females, it was bladder involvement (either neurogenic or cancerous) followed by tumors of the pelvic organs (ovaries, uterus, cervix).

CLINICAL MANIFESTATIONS
A significant number of patients are asymptomatic, and the diagnosis is uncovered during investigation for renal insufficiency. This is particularly common in patients with neurogenic bladder or those with pelvic malignancy, in whom an elevated serum creatinine level may be discovered during evaluation for chemotherapy. Symptoms are variable and include anuria associated with pelvic discomfort, prostatism, dysuria if

TABLE 8-1. Etiology of obstructive uropathy in 116 elderly patients

Diagnosis		No. patients (%)
Nonmalignant causes		
Prostatic hypertrophy		41 (35)
Neurogenic bladder		18 (16)
Urolithiasis		7 (6.5)
Obstructive pyelonephritis (papillary necrosis)		7 (6.5)
Urethral stricture		4 (3)
Others (ureteropelvic junction, retroperitoneal fibrosis)		4 (3)
	Total	81 (70)
Malignant causes		
Prostatic cancer		14 (12)
Bladder cancer		9 (8)
Pelvic tumors		6 (5)
Others (colon, retroperitoneal tumors)		6 (5)
	Total	35 (30)

SOURCE: Adapted from Kumar R, Hill CM, and McGeown MG: Acute renal failure in the elderly. *Lancet* 1:90–91, 1973; and the authors' experience.

concomitant infection is present, new onset of enuresis, and gross hematuria [78]. Thirty to forty percent of our patients were clinically uremic with nausea, vomiting, changes in mentation, and asterixis. Evidence of sepsis (chills, fever, hypotension, costovertebral angle tenderness) may be present. Edema of the extremities due to venous occlusive disease or lymphatic obstruction was commonly found in patients with pelvic malignancy and lymphomas. An abdominal mass, representing an enlarged bladder, occurs in 1.7 percent of males being evaluated for prostatic hypertrophy [79]. Uterine prolapse may on occasion be responsible for obstruction [80].

The degree of renal insufficiency may vary from very mild to severe (serum creatinine up to 20 mg per dl or higher). Hyperkalemia and non-anion gap acidosis are found in 70 percent of patients, and an inappropriately elevated urine pH (> 5.5) is found in 60 percent [81]. The urine sodium may be low (< 20 mEq per liter) in early acute renal failure due to obstructive uropathy, mimicking the diagnosis of "prerenal" azotemia [82, 83]. Hematuria, either gross or microscopic, is seen in 30 percent of patients. The urine sediment is otherwise benign, with more than 2+ proteinuria present in less than 4 percent of patients.

The diagnosis of obstructive uropathy can be confirmed by the finding of dilatation of the urinary collecting system on ultrasonography or CT scan. It should be emphasized that a nondilated system does not necessarily rule out the diagnosis of obstructive uropathy [84], as seen in 3 of our 69 patients (4 percent). This figure is similar to that given in reports by others [85, 86], in which 11 of 246 patients (4.5 percent) did not have upper tract dilatation. This phenomenon is seen predominantly in the elderly. Therefore, in any patient in whom there is a high index of suspicion for obstruction (such as patients with a history of or high probability on examination of prostatic, bladder, colon, or pelvic cancer) and in those with no obvious cause of renal failure it is mandatory to perform retrograde pyelography even if imaging techniques do not point to obstruction. If retrograde pyelography is unsuccessful or impossible, percutaneous nephrostomy may be safely accomplished even in a nondilated collecting system [86]. On postmortem examination, patients with cancer and nondilated obstructive renal failure have usually had a tumor encasing both the kidneys and the ureters. Patients with retroperitoneal fibrosis may also present with nondilated obstructive uropathy [87]. It is postulated that the fibrotic process interferes with the normal peristaltic transport of urine from the renal pelvis to the bladder.

TREATMENT AND PROGNOSIS
Hyperkalemia is the most common acute life-threatening complication seen in patients with obstructive uropathy. The hyperkalemia, which is a consequence of metabolic acidosis, distal renal tubular acidosis, or hyporenin-hypoaldosteronism (see Chap. 3), should be treated promptly and aggressively with glucose-insulin and sodium bicarbonate prior to manipulation of the urinary tract. Antibiotics (see Chap. 9) should be administered for patients with clinical evidence of infection, adjusting the dose for renal failure and reassessing the choice of antibiotics depending on the results of the urine or blood cultures. We do not routinely use prophylactic antibiotics. The presence of uremic signs and symptoms does not constitute an absolute indication for dialytic intervention prior to making an attempt to relieve the obstruction. Occasionally, a patient with severe metabolic acidosis and clinical evidence of fluid overload might require dialysis with fluid removal prior to manipulation. Percutaneous nephrostomy has become the method of choice for relieving the obstruction when the upper tract is involved. Patients in whom the procedure is unsuccessful can be managed either by insertion of a ureteral catheter or stent through the bladder or by open nephrostomy. In patients with metastatic prostatic disease with associated obstructive uropathy who are not clinically uremic or hyperkalemic, intravenous administration of diphosphate stilbestrol, at a dose of 250 to 500 mg per day, may be tried [88]. Patients who respond usually do so within the first 72 hours. We rarely prolong this form of therapy beyond 4 days.

Once the obstruction has been relieved, 90 percent of patients undergo immediate diuresis. In the remaining 10 percent either superimposed volume contraction (due to poor intake, vomiting, or diarrhea) or acute tubular necrosis secondary to sepsis is responsible for the variable delay in recovery. The average time between onset of diuresis and attainment of stable kidney function varies from 10 to 14 days [89]. During the first 4 to 5 days special attention should be paid to adequate replacement of urinary losses so that volume contraction resulting from the postobstructive diuresis does not occur. The volume of losses will depend to a certain extent on the state of hydration at the time the obstruction is relieved. Tubular defects in salt and water reabsorption, involving the proximal tubule, the thick ascending limb of Henle, and the cortical collecting tubules, are also usually present and may be due to metabolic alterations sustained during obstruction [90–92]. Other factors that may contribute to the defect in salt reabsorption are atrial natriuretic peptide and medullary washout [93]. Furthermore, an inability to concentrate the urine maximally due to a tubular resistance to antidiuretic hormone (ADH), at a step beyond the intracellular generation of cyclic AMP, is frequently present [91, 94].

The degree of recovery depends primarily on the duration of the obstruction [95]. Forty percent of our patients returned to baseline kidney function that was frequently normal, particularly in those patients who acquired the obstruction while hospitalized. In the remaining 60 percent, renal insufficiency was present at the time of hospitalization and frequently was the primary reason for hospital admission. In these patients 6 percent (mainly males with prostatic disease) failed to recover at all and were placed on maintenance hemodialysis, and the remaining 54 percent recovered only partially. Half of these patients, however, may have had underlying kidney disease related to associated medical problems (diabetic nephropathy, hypertensive nephrosclerosis, analgesic nephropathy), but specific information was not available.

Once the patient's condition stabilizes, more definitive therapy is usually necessary to manage the underlying disease [96, 97]. Decisions about long-term management of the patient whose obstruction results from a malignant process depend on the extent of the disease, the tumor type, and the patient's clinical status. We usually make our decision on an individual basis after discussions with the patient, the family, the urologist, and the oncologist. Patients with tumors arising outside the pelvis have the worst prognosis. In patients with tumors arising within the pelvis the prognosis is somewhat better, with a 70 percent survival rate at 3 months and a mean survival of 7.6 months [98]. Patients with prostatic cancer have the best prognosis and should therefore be managed aggressively [99].

In patients with a benign cause of obstruction, kidney function can remain stable for long periods of time, even in those who have a creatinine clearance of between 20 and 30 ml per minute. In our experience patients have remained stable for up to 5 years as long as the obstruction was the only cause of the renal failure. Management of these patients should be the same as that for any patient with chronic renal insufficiency (see Chap. 11).

Five to ten percent of patients remain chronic salt losers, most likely because of an intrinsic inability of the distal nephron to conserve salt [100]. Clinical evidence of severe volume depletion can develop in such patients when intercurrent illnesses intervene that limit intake or increase losses through the gastrointestinal tract. The urinary sodium remains high (> 45 mEq per liter) despite volume contraction [101]. These patients are best managed chronically with either salt (NaCl tablets) supplementation or fludrocortisone 0.1 to 0.3 mg daily. Patients with persistent hyperkalemic-hyperchloremic metabolic acidosis (40 percent of our patients) can be managed as previously described (see Chap. 3).

REFERENCES

1. Johnson CM, et al: Renal stone epidemiology: a 25-year study in Rochester, Minnesota. *Kidney Int* 16:624–631, 1979.
2. Sutherland JW, Parks JH, and Coe FL: Recurrence after a single renal stone in a community practice. *Min Electrol Metab* 11:267–269, 1985.
3. Scott R: Prevalence of calcified upper urinary tract stone disease in a random population survey. Report of a combined study of general practitioners and hospital staff. *Br J Urol* 59:111–117, 1987.
4. Ljunghall S: Incidence of upper tract stones. *Min Electrol Metab* 13:220–227, 1987.
5. Nicar MJ, Hill K, and Pak CYC: Inhibition by citrate of spontaneous precipitation of calcium oxalate in vitro. *J Bone Min Res* 2:215–220, 1987.
6. Abramson PA and Smith CL: Evaluation of factors involved in calcium stone formation. *Min Electrol Metab* 13:201–208, 1987.
7. Steele TH: The pharmacology of renal lithiasis. *Ann Rev Pharmacol Toxicol* 17:11–25, 1977.
8. Bowyer RC, Brockis TS, and McCulloch RK: Glycosaminoglycans as inhibitors of calcium oxalate crystal growth and aggregation. *Clin Chem Acta* 95:23–28, 1979.
9. Coe FL: Treated and untreated recurrent calcium nephrolithiasis in patients with idiopathic hypercalciuria, hyperuricosuria and no metabolic disorders. *Ann Intern Med* 87:404–410, 1977.
10. Pak CYC, et al: Ambulatory evaluation of nephrolithiasis. Classification, clinical presentation and diagnostic criteria. *Am J Med* 69:19–30, 1980.
11. Parks JH and Coe FL: A urinary calcium-citrate index for the evaluation of nephrolithiasis. *Kidney Int* 30:85–90, 1986.
12. Baggio B, et al: Raised transmembrane oxalate flux in red blood cells in idiopathic calcium oxalate nephrolithiasis. *Lancet* 2:12–13, 1984.
13. Robertson WG and Peacock M: The cause of idiopathic calcium stone disease hypercalciuria or hyperoxaluria? *Nephron* 26:105–110, 1980.
14. Nakagawa Y, et al: Urine glycoprotein crystal growth inhibitors. Evidence

for a molecular abnormality in calcium oxalate nephrolithiasis. *J Clin Invest* 76:1455–1462, 1985.

15. Lemann J Jr, et al: Studies of the mechanism by which chronic metabolic acidosis augments urinary calcium excretion in man. *J Clin Invest* 46:1318–1328, 1967.

16. Simpson DP: Citrate excretion: A window on renal metabolism. *Am J Physiol* 244:F223–F234, 1983.

17. Stewart AF, et al: Calcium homeostasis in immobilization: An example of resorptive hypercalciuria. *N Engl J Med* 306:1136–1140, 1982.

18. Tori JA, Kewabramani LS, and Orth MS: Urolithiasis in children with spinal cord injury. *Paraplegia* 16:357–365, 1978.

19. Burr RG and Nusiebeh I: Biochemical studies in paraplegic renal stone patients. I. Plasma biochemistry and urinary calcium and saturation. *Br J Urol* 57:269–274, 1985.

20. Pak CYC, et al: The hypercalciurias. Causes, parathyroid functions and diagnostic criteria. *J Clin Invest* 54:387–400, 1974.

21. Sherwood LM: Idiopathic hypercalciuria: A mixed bag of stones. *J Lab Clin Med* 90:951–954, 1977.

22. Lau YK, et al: Proximal tubular defects in idiopathic hypercalciuria: Resistance to phosphate administration. *Min Electrol Metab* 7:237–249, 1982.

23. Evans RA, et al: The pathogenesis of idiopathic hypercalciuria: Evidence for parathyroid hyperfunction. *Q J Med* 53:41–53, 1984.

24. Kaplan RA, et al: The role of 1α,25-dihydroxyvitamin D in the mediation of intestinal hyperabsorption of calcium in primary hyperparathyroidism and absorptive hypercalciuria. *J Clin Invest* 59:756–760, 1977.

25. Shen FH, et al: Increased serum 1,25-dihydroxyvitamin D in idiopathic hypercalciuria. *J Lab Clin Med* 90:955–962, 1977.

26. Coe FL, et al: Effects of low calcium diet on urine calcium excretion, parathyroid function and serum $1,25(OH)_2D_3$ levels in patients with idiopathic hypercalciuria and in normal subjects. *Am J Med* 72:25–32, 1982.

27. Coe FL and Favus MJ: Hypercalciuric states. *Min Electrol Metab* 5:183–200, 1981.

28. Coe FL, et al: Urinary macromolecular crystal growth inhibitors in calcium nephrolithiasis. *Min Electrol Metab* 3:268–275, 1980.

29. Zerwekh JE, et al: Modulation by calcium of the inhibitor activity of naturally occurring urinary inhibitors. *Kidney Int* 33:1005–1008.

30. Millman S, et al: Pathogenesis and clinical course of mixed calcium oxalate and uric acid nephrolithiasis. *Kidney Int* 22:366–370, 1982.

31. Coe FL, et al: Uric acid saturation in calcium nephrolithiasis. *Kidney Int* 17:662–668, 1980.

32. Coe FL, Moran E, and Kavalich AG: The contribution of dietary purine overconsumption to hyperuricosuria in calcium oxalate stone formers. *J Chron Dis* 29:793–800, 1976.

33. Coe FL: Uric acid and calcium oxalate nephrolithiasis. *Kidney Int* 24:392–403, 1983.

34. Pak CYC, et al: Mechanism for calcium urolithiasis among patients with hyperuricosuria. *J Clin Invest* 59:426–431, 1977.

35. Coe FL and Kavalach KG: Hypercalciuria and hyperuricosuria in patients with calcium nephrolithiasis. *N Engl J Med* 291:1344–1350, 1974.

36. Kristensen C, et al: Reduced glomerular filtration rate and hypercalciuria in primary struvite nephrolithiasis. *Kidney Int* 32:749–753, 1987.

37. Griffith DP, Bruce RR, and Fishbein WN: Infection (Urease)-Induced Stones.

In *Contemporary Issues in Nephrology*, Vol 5. New York: Churchill Livingstone, 1980. Pp. 231–260.

38. Dobbins JW and Binder HJ: Importance of the colon in enteric hyperoxaluria. *N Engl J Med* 296:298–301, 1977.
39. Hodgkinson A and Wilkinson R: Plasma oxalate crystalluria and urine saturation in recurrent renal stone formers. *Clin Sci* 40:365–374, 1971.
41. Kass MA, et al: Acetazolamide and urolithiasis. *Ophthalmology* 88:261–265, 1981.
42. Ahlstrand C and Tiselius HG: Urine composition and stone formation during treatment with acetazolamide. *Scand J Urol Nephrol* 31:225–228, 1987.
43. Pak CYC and Fulker C: Idiopathic hypocitraturic calcium oxalate nephrolithiasis successfully treated with potassium citrate. *Ann Intern Med* 104:33–37, 1986.
44. Minisola S, et al: Studies in citrate metabolism in normal subjects and kidney stone patients. *Min Electrol Metab* 15:303–308, 1989.
45. Elliot JS: Calcium oxalate urinary calculi: Clinical and chemical aspects. *Medicine* 62:36–43, 1983.
46. Laing FC, Jeffery RB Jr, and Wing VW: Ultrasound versus excretory urography in evaluating acute flank pain. *Radiology* 154:613–616, 1985.
47. Pak CYC, et al: Is selective therapy of recurrent nephrolithiasis possible? *Am J Med* 71:615–622, 1981.
48. Sakhaee K, et al: Postmenopausal osteoporosis as a manifestation of renal hypercalciuria with secondary hyperparathyroidism. *J Clin Endocrinol Metab* 61:368–373, 1985.
49. Smith LH, Van Den Berg CJ, and Wilson DM: Current concepts in nutrition: nutrition and urolithiasis. *N Engl J Med* 298:87–89, 1978.
50. Pak CYC, et al: Evidence justifying a high fluid intake in treatment of nephrolithiasis. *Ann Intern Med* 93:36–39, 1980.
51. Ljunghall S, Fellström B, and Johansson G: Prevention of renal stones by a high fluid intake? *Eur Urol* 14:381–385, 1988.
52. Lamden MP and Chrystowskli GA: Urinary oxalate excretion by man following ascorbic acid ingestion. *Proc Soc Exp Biol Med* 85:190–195, 1954.
53. Licata AA, et al: Effects of dietary protein on urinary calcium in normal subjects and in patients with nephrolithiasis. *Metabolism* 28:895–900, 1979.
54. Pak CYC, et al: Dietary management of idiopathic calcium urolithiasis. *J Urol* 131:850–852, 1984.
55. Pak CYC: Medical management of nephrolithiasis in Dallas: Update 1987. *J Urol* 140:461–467, 1988.
56. Preminger GM and Pak CYC: Eventual attenuation of hypocalciuric response to hydrochlorothiazide in absorptive hypercalciuria. *J Urol* 137:1104–1109, 1987.
57. Costanzo LS and Windhager EE: Calcium and sodium transport by the distal convoluted tubule of the rat. *Am J Physiol* 235:F492–F496, 1978.
58. Leppla D, et al: Effect of amiloride with or without hydrochlorothiazide on urinary calcium and saturation of calcium salts. *J Clin Endocrinol Metab* 57:920–924, 1983.
59. Alon U, Costanzo LS, and Chan JCM: Additive hypocalciuric effects of amiloride on hydrochlorothiazide in patients treated with calcitriol. *Min Electrol Metab* 10:379–386, 1984.
60. Pak CYC: Kidney stones: various forms and treatment. *Nephron* 23:142–146, 1979.

61. Pak CYC, Sakhaee K, and Fuller C: Successful management of uric acid nephrolithiasis with potassium citrate. *Kidney Intern* 30:422–428, 1986.
62. Ettinger B, et al: Randomized trial of allopurinol in the prevention of calcium oxalate calculi. *N Engl J Med* 315:1386–1389, 1986.
63. Miller RA: Role of endoscopic surgery in management of renal and ureteric calculi: A review. *J R Soc Med* 78:1034–1038, 1985.
64. Riehle RA Jr, Fair WR, and Vaughn D Jr: Extracorporeal shock-wave lithotripsy for upper tract calculi: One year's experience at a single center. *JAMA* 255:2043–2048, 1986.
65. Watson GM and Wickham JEA: Initial experience with pulsed dye laser for ureteric calculi. *Lancet* 1:1357–1358, 1986.
66. Pode D, et al: Can extracorporeal shock-wave lithotripsy eradicate persistent urinary infection associated with infected stones? *J Urol* 140:257–259, 1988.
67. Williams JJ, Rodman JS, and Peterson CM: A randomized double-blind study of acetohydroxamic acid in struvite nephrolithiasis. *N Engl J Med* 311:792–794, 1984.
69. Barilla DE, et al: Renal oxalate excretion following oral oxalate loads in patients with ileal disease and with renal and absorptive hypercalciurias. Effect of calcium and magnesium. *Am J Med* 64:579–585, 1978.
70. Editorial. Citrate for calcium nephrolithiasis. *Lancet* 1:955, 1986.
71. Strauss AL, et al: Factors that predict relapse of calcium nephrolithiasis during treatment. A prospective study. *Am J Med* 72:17–24, 1982.
72. Thode J, et al: Simplified protocol for biochemical evaluation of recurrent renal calcium stone disease. *Min Electrol Metab* 14:288–296, 1988.
73. Pak CYC, Skurla C, and Harvey J: Graphic display of urinary risk factors for renal stone formation. *J Urol* 134:867–870, 1985.
74. Kumar R, Hill CM, and McGeown MG: Acute renal failure in the elderly. *Lancet* 1:90–91, 1973.
75. Oliveira DB and Winearls CG: Acute renal failure in the elderly can have a good prognosis. *Age Aging* 13:304–308, 1984.
76. McInnes EG, et al: Renal failure in the elderly. *Q J Med* 64:583–588, 1987.
77. Lameire N, et al: Acute Renal Failure in the Elderly. In Oreopoulos DG (ed): *Geriatric Nephrology: The Medical, Psychosocial, Nursing, Financial and Ethical Issues of Treating End-Stage Renal Disease in the Elderly.* Boston: Nijhoff, 1986.
78. Jones DA, O'Reilly PH, and George NJR: Reversible hypertension associated with unrecognized high pressure chronic retention of urine. *Lancet* 1:1052–1054, 1987.
79. Mukamel E, et al: Occult progressive renal damage in the elderly male due to benign prostatic hypertrophy. *J Am Geriatr Soc* 27:403–406, 1979.
80. Elkin M, Goldman SM, and Meng CH: Ureteral obstruction in patients with uterine prolapse. *Radiology* 110:289–294, 1974.
81. Battle DC, Arruda JAL, and Kurtzman NA: Hyperkalemic distal renal tubular acidosis associated with obstructive uropathy. *N Engl J Med* 304:373–380, 1981.
82. Hoffman LM and Suki W: Obstructive uropathy mimicking volume depletion. *JAMA* 236:2096–2097, 1976.
83. Miller TR, et al: Urinary diagnostic indices in acute renal failure. A prospective study. *Ann Intern Med* 89:47–50, 1978.
84. Spital A, Valvo JR, and Segal AJ: Nondilated obstructive uropathy. *Urology* 31:478–482, 1988.

85. Naidich JB, et al: Nondilated obstructive uropathy: Percutaneous nephrostomy performed to reverse renal failure. *Radiology* 160:653–657, 1986.
86. Maillet PJ, et al: Nondilated obstructive acute renal failure: Diagnostic procedures and therapeutic management. *Radiology* 160:659–662, 1986.
87. Lalli A: Retroperitoneal fibrosis and inapparent obstructive uropathy. *Radiology* 122:339–342, 1977.
88. Resnick MI: Hormonal therapy in prostatic carcinoma. *Urology* 24:518–523, 1984.
89. Nadig PW and Valk WL: Recovery from obstructive disease. *J Urol* 88:470–472, 1982.
90. Buerkert J, Head M, and Klahr S: Effects of acute bilateral ureteral obstruction on deep nephron and terminal collecting duct function in the young rat. *J Clin Invest* 59:1055–1065, 1977.
91. Hanley MJ and Davidson K: Isolated nephron segments from rabbit models of obstructive uropathy. *J Clin Invest* 69:165–174, 1982.
92. Nito H, et al: Effect of unilateral ureteral obstruction on renal cell metabolism and function. *J Lab Clin Med* 91:60–71, 1978.
93. Solez K, et al: Inner medullary plasma flow in the kidney with ureteral obstruction. *Am J Physiol* 231:1315–1321, 1976.
94. Fine LG, et al: Functional profile of the isolated uremic nephron. *J Clin Invest* 61:1519–1527, 1978.
95. Sarmina J and Resnick MI: Obstructive uropathy in patients with benign prostatic hyperplasia. *J Urol* 141:866–869, 1989.
96. Herr HW: Intermittent catheterization in neurogenic bladder disorders. *J Urol* 113:477–479, 1975.
97. Applebaum SM: Pharmacologic agents in micturitional disorders. *Urology* 16:555–568, 1980.
98. Bodner D, Kursh ED, and Resnick MI: Palliative nephrostomy for relief of ureteral obstruction secondary to malignancy. *Urology* 24:8–10, 1984.
99. Khan AV and Utz DL: Clinical management of cancer of prostate with bilateral ureteral obstruction. *J Urol* 113:816–819, 1975.
100. Bishop MC: Diuresis and renal functional recovery in chronic retention. *Br J Urol* 57:1–5, 1985.
101. Uribarri J. Oh MS, and Carroll HJ: Salt-losing nephropathy. Clinical presentation and mechanisms. *Am J Nephrol* 3:193–198, 1983.

9   URINARY INFECTIONS

INCIDENCE AND PREVALENCE

It is now well established that significant bacteriuria as defined by Kass (10^5 organisms per ml of midstream urine) [1] increases with age. This higher prevalence in the elderly occurs in both sexes, and the higher ratio of females to males seen in younger patients decreases with aging [2]. In 1,996 patients 70 years of age or older screened for bacteriuria by Nordenstam et al [3], the frequency of positive cultures ($> 10^5$ organisms per ml) was 9.0 percent among women and 2.4 percent among men. Even higher prevalence rates (10–16 percent in ambulatory men and 17–37 percent in ambulatory women) have been found by others [4–7]. For the elderly living in nursing homes or extended care facilities, the rate of infection is 17 to 33 percent in men and 23 to 31 percent in women [2, 8]. It is estimated that in elderly hospitalized patients 30 to 33 percent of the men and 32 to 50 percent of the women either have or will subsequently develop bacteriuria [2].

PATHOGENESIS

There are several reasons why the elderly are more prone to develop urinary tract infection.

COLONIZATION
In general, vaginal and periurethral colonization with the offending organism precedes the onset of cystitis in women with recurrent urinary tract infection [9]. Both increasing age and debilitation are associated with increased colonization of the skin and mucous membranes by gram-negative organisms [10].

ADHERENCE
Even though increased susceptibility to perineal and periurethral colonization with gram-negative bacteria has been found in women with recurrent urinary infections, the infection need not be with the colonizing organism [11]. Moreover, infection does not necessarily follow colonization [12], suggesting that other factors must be operative. Bacterial adherence, which represents an interaction between organisms and uroepithelial cells, appears to be important [13]. For instance, the bacte-

ria that are more likely to cause infection and are more often associated with infection have a higher adherence rate to squamous epithelium than do less virulent strains isolated from the vaginal introitus [14]. Although adherence appears to play a role it does not constitute an independent risk factor in the increased incidence of urinary tract infection in the elderly [15]. Other variables modulate the degree of adherence of a given microorganism to the uroepithelium [16] including (1) the ability of the uroepithelial cell to produce local antibody [17]; (2) the genetic susceptibility of the host [18]; (3) intravaginal pH. Only the last factor has been specifically studied in a small number of postmenopausal women. A high intravaginal pH (> 5.2) was found to be associated with increased bacterial adherence, which was reversed once the pH was brought back to normal with continuous low-dose intravaginal estrogen therapy [19].

URINE STASIS
Vesical emptying and high urine flow have been shown by Cox and associates [9, 20] to play an important role in preventing urinary tract infection. Bladder emptying is frequently impaired in the elderly by problems such as prostatic enlargement in the male and changes in bladder function and pelvic musculature in the female. Also, difficulty in micturition arising from neuromuscular disorders, dementia, and concomitant use of drugs such as anticholinergics is common in the elderly. Postvoiding residual volume is increased in both elderly men and elderly women [21, 22]. Finally, recent studies by Parsons and Mulholland [23] have provided strong evidence of the role of bladder surface glycosaminoglycans in protecting against infection. It is quite probable that with advancing age there are either quantitative or qualitative changes in this substance.

URINARY TRACT INSTRUMENTATION
It is estimated that 40 to 60 percent of hospitalized elderly or those living in nursing homes and other institutions are incontinent [24]. Despite the fact that incontinence is transient in as many as 50 percent of these patients and that two-thirds of the remainder can be cured or markedly improved, physicians often resort to catheterization. In one study, only 27.5 percent of catheterized patients had been adequately evaluated for the cause of their incontinence [25]. The presence of an indwelling catheter is guaranteed to cause an infection within a few days. The incidence is 100 percent within 4 days when an open system is used and 50 percent with a closed system. In general, catheter-associated urinary infections increase approximately 8 to 10 percent per day with a closed system [26]. The use of condom catheters is also associated with a high rate of urinary tract infection after prolonged use [27, 28].

Bacteria are usually introduced at the time of catheterization or enter the bladder either by extraluminal migration from the urethral meatus or by intraluminal migration following contamination of the drainage bag. The bacteria may originate from the patient's normal flora (e.g., *Escherichia coli*) or by cross-contamination from external sources (e.g., *Serratia marcescens*) [29]. A transient increase in the adherence of gram-negative bacteria to bladder epithelial cells has been shown to be an important early event in the development of catheter-associated bacteriuria [30].

ALTERATION IN HOST-DEFENSE MECHANISMS
There is evidence that old rats have more difficulty than younger rats in clearing bacteria introduced into the urinary tract [31]. Whether such a factor is operative in humans remains to be shown. A tenfold decrease in antigen processing, a defective primary response to mitogens, and increased intensity of delayed hypersensitivity reactions as well as diminished bactericidal activity and altered oxygen metabolism have been reported in the elderly, and these changes may increase susceptibility to infection [32–34]. Anergy and depressed cell-mediated immunity are frequently associated with a variety of disease states as well as with malnutrition, so it is possible that some of the immunologic defects observed in the elderly are related to underlying disease rather than old age per se [35].

Once the bladder has been invaded by bacteria, the patient is at risk of developing kidney infection. This process may start with bacteria adhering to the ureteral mucosa. Endotoxin produced by these bacteria alters ureteral motility, causing it to act as if mechanically obstructed and in turn causing changes in the shape of the renal papillae. Intrarenal reflux of bacteria then ensues, with subsequent adherence to the renal tubular epithelium. This sequence of events is then followed by complement activation, an inflammatory response in the kidneys, and subsequent phagocytosis of the microorganisms [36]. In a minority of patients, bacteria gain access to the kidneys by hematogenous seeding from a distant pyogenic focus.

CLINICAL MANIFESTATIONS

Asymptomatic bacteriuria is associated with leukocyturia far more commonly in the elderly (both males and females) than in their younger counterparts [8, 37]. Nonspecific urinary symptoms such as incontinence, frequency, urgency, and suprapubic pain are usually of little diagnostic importance because they are found with equal frequency in subjects with and without bacteriuria [38, 39] and should not be used as the only indications for therapy in the elderly with bacteriuria. In our experience, approximately 5 percent of patients present with significant dysuria, and 8 percent have symptomatic upper urinary tract infection (pyelonephritis).

The clinical presentation of acute pyelonephritis is similar in older and younger patients. Fever, chills, dysuria, and costovertebral angle tenderness constitute the most common presenting symptoms. Pyuria, defined as more than 10 polymorphonuclear leukocytes per high power field (a value that has been found highly predictive of significant bacteriuria in the elderly), is a universal finding [40]. Leukocytosis is present in 76 percent of cases. Blood cultures are positive in 58 percent of patients, and shock is present in 33 percent, both values being significantly higher than those found in younger patients [41]. In fact, the urinary tract is the most common source of gram-negative bacteremia in elderly hospitalized patients, particularly those with an indwelling catheter [42–45]. The presence of other medical problems (cerebrovascular disease, pulmonary disease, decubitus ulcers) may occasionally direct the clinician's attention away from the urinary tract, delaying the proper diagnosis [46].

NATURAL HISTORY AND TREATMENT

ASYMPTOMATIC BACTERIURIA

Noncatheterized Patients
As already noted, asymptomatic bacteriuria is very common in the elderly. Suntharalingham and colleagues [47], using the bladder washout method of Fairley et al [48] in 31 elderly female patients with bacteriuria, were able to locate the site of infection to the upper tract in 17 (55 percent) and to the lower tract in the remaining 14 (45 percent). Using a similar technique, Nicolle and associates [49] found a 67 percent incidence of upper tract infection in elderly institutionalized females. Unfortunately, no data were provided on the therapeutic outcome in either of these two studies. These rates of upper tract infection in the elderly are higher than the 32 percent found by Rubin et al [50] using the antibody-coated bacteria technique in younger patients. In a study of 36 elderly institutionalized men with bacteriuria, 20 were not treated and remained bacteriuric. Sixteen were treated, and although they had fewer months of bacteriuria only 1 of the 16 remained free of bacteriuria during the 2-year study period [8]. No difference was found in mortality rate nor in infectious morbidity in this study. Similar data have also been reported in elderly institutionalized women [51]. Furthermore, spontaneous reso-

lution of bacteriuria appears to be rather common in the elderly [39]. Based on these data and also on the fact that antimicrobial therapy may be associated with significant adverse effects [52], our present recommendation is not to treat the elderly patient (male or female) with asymptomatic bacteriuria [52, 53]. A reduction in survival has been found by some in bacteriuric elderly patients (symptomatic or nonsymptomatic) compared to nonbacteriuric subjects [54, 55], although others have not confirmed this finding [56]. It is possible that bacteriuria constitutes a marker for a worse outcome in some elderly people [57].

Catheterized Patients

There is a very high incidence of bacteriuria in patients catheterized for more than 4 days [58]. Recent studies have shown that bacterial counts of greater than 10^2 organisms per ml represent a more valid index of infection in the catheterized patient than the usual 10^5 organisms per ml (midstream specimen) used for the noncatheterized patient [59]. Attempts to reduce the incidence of bacteriuria through such measures as meatal care, antibiotic catheter coating, frequent bag changing, catheter irrigation, and antibiotic prophylaxis have all proved unsuccessful [60–62].

It is generally accepted that antimicrobial therapy for patients with long-term indwelling catheters should be reserved for those who develop symptoms such as fever or severe suprapubic pain or for prophylaxis if an invasive genitourinary procedure (e.g., cystoscopy) is undertaken [61, 63]. The same approach is recommended for patients requiring intermittent catheterization [64]. One exception might be the patient with asymptomatic bacteriuria who is seen after a prostatectomy [65]. In such patients the bacteriuria tends to persist (except when *Staphylococcus epidermidis* is the organism) even after the indwelling catheter has been removed. A 7- to 10-day course of therapy is indicated based on the organism isolated and the sensitivity results.

The rationale for not treating asymptomatic bacteriuric catheterized patients is that the incidence of upper tract infection is low in these patients, and the bacterial flora changes rapidly, a process that might be enhanced by antimicrobial therapy [66]. Also, the emergence of drug-resistant organisms will be promoted, making the treatment of subsequent infections more difficult [67]. As noted by some authors, in noncatheterized patients, an increase (threefold) in mortality has been found among hospitalized bacteriuric patients with indwelling bladder catheters [68]. The significance of this association has yet to be determined.

SYMPTOMATIC BACTERIURIA

The management of acute dysuria in the elderly is similar to that in younger patients [69]. There are no data available as to what constitutes

TABLE 9-1. Antibiotic therapy for the elderly with urinary tract infection

Indication	Antimicrobial agent	Administration route	Dosage per GFR (ml/min)		
			> 50	50–10	< 10
Cystitis	Trimethoprim-sulfamethoxazole, double strength	Oral	q12h	q18h	q18h
	Amoxicillin 250 mg	Oral	q6h	q8h	q12–16h
	Nitrofurantoin microcrystals 100 mg	Oral	q6h	Avoid	Avoid
	Norfloxacin 400 mg	Oral	q12h if GFR > 20 ml/min 200 mg q12h if GFR < 20 ml/min		
	Ciprofloxacin 250–750 mg	Oral	q12h if GFR > 30 ml/min q18h if GFR < 29 ml/min		
Acute bacterial pyelonephritis	Ampicillin 1–2 g	IV	q6h	q8h	q12–16h
	Cephalothin 1–2 g	IV	q6h	q6h	q12h
	Gentamicin 1 mg/kg	IM/IV	q8h	q12–72h	q72h
	Tobramycin 1 mg/kg	IM/IV	q8h	q12–72h	q72h
	Amikacin 7.5 mg/kg	IV	q12h	q24–72h	q72h
	Vancomycin 15–20 mg/kg	IV	q24–72h	q72–240h	q240h
Other infections of the urinary tract	Ethambutol 25 mg/kg	Oral	q24h	q24–36h	q48h
	Isoniazid 300 mg	Oral	q24h	q24h	q24h
	Rifampin 600 mg	Oral	q24h	q24h	q24h
	Amphotericin B 0.4–0.6 mg/kg	IV	q24h	q24h	q24–36h
	Ketoconazole 200–800 mg	Oral	q24h	q24h	q24–36h
	Flucytosine 25–37.5 mg/kg	Oral	q6h	q12–24h	q24–48h
	Methenamine hippurate 1 g	Oral	q12h	Avoid	Avoid

the optimal approach in this group. The following has been our practice. At the initial visit a complete history and physical examination are performed, paying special attention to the pelvic and urethrovaginal areas in the female and the prostate in the male. Part of a midstream urine specimen is examined microscopically, and the rest is sent to the laboratory for culture. In the presence of bacteriuria and pyuria [70], therapy is started with trimethoprim-sulfamethoxazole, one double-strength tablet twice a day. We suggest a 2-week course rather than the single-dose, 1-day treatment [71, 72]. The former regimen has been shown to be quite effective even when upper tract infection is present [73]. Other antibiotics useful in the therapy of urinary tract infection and their dosages in the elderly are listed in Table 9-1. The patient is always seen for follow-up confirmation of bacteriologic and symptomatic cure, since in the female the bacteriuria might be coincidental and the dysuria due to desiccation of the urethra or vaginal mucosa secondary to estrogen deficiency [74], various forms of vaginitis [75], or noninfectious cystitis [76]. The incidence of nonbacterial (e.g., *Chlamydia, Trachomatis*) causes of acute dysuria in the elderly is not known.

We usually do a postvoiding residual urine in every male, every diabetic female, and any patient with evidence of peripheral neuropathy who presents with symptomatic urinary tract infection. If a significant residual volume is found (> 150 ml), the patient is referred for urologic evaluation. Intravenous pyelogram and cystoscopy are recommended for males with acute dysuria not due to prostatitis and for females with recurrent infections (three or more infections in a 1-year period with the same organism) [69]. There are no studies, however, indicating the yield of these procedures in the elderly. Similar investigations should also be undertaken in both males and females with pyelonephritis.

Women with a normal genitourinary tract and recurrent symptomatic infection should be considered for a 6-month course of 40 mg trimethoprim and 200 mg sulfamethoxazole or nitrofurantoin macrocrystals, 100 mg orally at bedtime [77]. This regimen has been found to be both efficient and cost-effective [78]. In patients who cannot tolerate this regimen, methenamine hippurate, 1 g every 12 hours, can be tried [79]. It should be noted, however, that prophylaxis does not prevent recurrences after therapy has been discontinued [80]. When that occurs, a longer (5-year) course of trimethoprim-sulfamethoxazole, 40-200 mg 3 times weekly at bedtime, may be tried [81]. Also, recurrent urinary tract infection in men may require a long course of therapy (6–12 weeks) [82, 83]. Since chronic prostatitis is responsible for the bacteriuria in a great many of these patients, either a quinolone such as norfloxacin, 800 mg per day, or ciprofloxacin, 250 to 750 mg twice a day, is an effective alternative therapeutic agent [84, 85]. These antibiotics have been found to have good prostatic tissue penetration [86] (see Table 9-1).

ACUTE PYELONEPHRITIS

In all elderly patients presenting with symptoms and signs of acute pyelonephritis a urinary Gram stain should be done, and treatment with an intravenous antibiotic should be started after all the cultures (urine and blood) have been taken. In the noncatheterized patient, the microorganism is generally gram-negative with *E. coli* found in 43 percent, *Proteus mirabilis* in 25 percent, *Pseudomonas aeruginosa* in 10 percent, *Providencia* species in 7 percent, *Klebsiella pneumoniae* in 7 percent, *Streptococcus faecalis* in 4 percent, and others in 4 percent [41]. For the chronically catheterized patient, gram-negative organisms still predominate, but there is a possibility of a polymicrobial infection. In one study, polymicrobial infections were found in 77 percent of these patients [44]. Our experience with catheter-induced urosepsis in 30 elderly patients who were long-term residents of an extended care facility has been different; multiple organisms in the blood or urine were found in only 10 patients (33 percent). Increased resistance to ampicillin and first-generation cephalosporins has been the major problem. In patients with community-acquired infection we usually initiate treatment with either a cephalosporin or trimethoprim-sulfamethoxazole (see Table 9-1) administered intravenously, since *E. coli,* the most commonly isolated organism in the elderly [41], is usually sensitive to both drugs [87]. We also add a "loading dose" of aminoglycoside (gentamicin 2 mg per kg) pending culture and sensitivity results (which usually are available the next day). If the organism is sensitive to the cephalosporin or trimethoprim-sulfamethoxazole, a full 14-day course is continued; if not, the appropriate antibiotic is substituted. If it is an aminoglycoside, the maintenance dose can be calculated by determining the glomerular filtration rate (GFR) from the formula reviewed in Chap. 1. Given the marked interindividual variation and the narrow therapeutic range of aminoglycosides, it is mandatory that serum drug and creatinine levels be monitored carefully [88, 89] (see Table 9-1).

For catheterized patients, unless the urinary Gram stain shows the presence of a gram-positive organism, we start treatment with an aminoglycoside alone. Our preference is tobramycin, since *P. aeruginosa* was isolated in 47 percent of our cultures. The dose and scheduling for tobramycin are the same as those used for gentamicin [90]. If the organism is sensitive to a less toxic drug, we switch accordingly. If not, tobramycin is continued, and the dose is altered according to serum levels or the patient's GFR. The dose of amikacin, another aminoglycoside reserved for more resistant organisms, should also be adjusted in the elderly according to the measured or estimated GFR [91] (see Table 9-1). With early and adequate antibiotic administration, the outcome is generally good for the elderly with acute bacterial pyelonephritis. Most patients become afebrile within 48 to 96 hours, and death as a direct cause of sepsis is rare. Antibiotic therapy is usually administered for a total of 2 weeks.

Persistence of fever and generalized toxicity despite an adequate antibiotic regimen, or the development of acute renal failure should lead the clinician to a vigorous search for one of the following complications.

PYONEPHROSIS

Pyonephrosis is the most common complication of pyelonephritis in elderly patients when ureteral obstruction is present. A calculus is usually responsible for the obstruction, although a sloughed papilla or other obstructing lesion may occasionally be found. The diagnosis is made by either ultrasonographic examination or CT scan of the kidneys. An intravenous pyelogram (IVP) can also be used if renal function is normal or near normal and the patient is properly prepared. On confirmation of the diagnosis a urologist should be consulted to achieve early drainage.

RENAL PAPILLARY NECROSIS

Fifty-one percent of elderly patients who develop renal papillary necrosis also have acute pyelonephritis [92, 94]. Sixty-seven percent of elderly patients with pyelonephritis and renal papillary necrosis are diabetic. When the entire papillary surface is destroyed, it sloughs into the pelvis and may cause obstruction. Management consists of early drainage. In the absence of obstruction, antibiotic therapy alone may be adequate.

PERINEPHRIC ABSCESS

Perinephric abscess usually results from rupture into the perinephric space of a corticomedullary abscess, a consequence of retrograde spread of infection from the lower urinary tract. Fortunately, this complication is not common. The diagnosis is made either by IVP, ultrasound, or CT scan. CT constitutes the diagnostic technique of choice because it identifies the lesion and best defines its extent and surrounding anatomy [95, 96]. In addition to antibiotics, percutaneous drainage under sonographic guidance is usually necessary. Patients with multiple abscesses and a poorly functioning kidney often require a nephrectomy, debridement, and postoperative drainage.

EMPHYSEMATOUS PYELONEPHRITIS

This form of pyelonephritis is associated with the presence of gas in the collecting system (emphysematous pyelitis) or within the renal parenchyma (emphysematous pyelonephritis). This complication occurs primarily in diabetics, often in association with ureteral obstruction. Since the mortality is high, immediate urologic intervention is necessary when obstruction is present. In the absence of ureteral obstruction, good results have been reported in patients with pyelitis treated with antibiotics

alone [97, 98]. Forty-one percent of patients with emphysematous pyelitis and 37 percent of those with emphysematous pyelonephritis reported by Evanoff et al [98] were over the age of 60.

SPECIAL FORMS OF PYELOCYSTITIS IN THE ELDERLY

TUBERCULOSIS

In the majority of cases urinary tuberculosis represents a reactivation of
a dormant focus from earlier hematogenous spread during the primary
infection. Originally the mycobacterium lodges in the preglomerular
capillary bed. Because of acquired cellular immunity, bacterial multiplication stops, and healed granulomas form. During reactivation these
granulomas enlarge and coalesce while new foci are initiated within the
renal pyramids, followed by caseous necrosis. This process, if left untreated, will eventually destroy the kidney.

The exact incidence of renal tuberculosis in the elderly is not known,
but it is known that 10 to 16 percent of reported cases of genitourinary
tuberculosis occur in this age group [99]. Females are more commonly
affected than males.

In most patients no past history of tuberculosis can be elicited, and
dysuria is usually the most common initial presentation. In 5 (33 percent) of our 15 patients, there were no symptoms at all. The disease was
found during investigation of sterile "pyuria" or during evaluation for
unrelated problems. Systemic symptoms such as fever, weight loss, and
cachexia are rare [100]. Pyuria is a universal finding, and hematuria is
present in one-third of the patients. An old lesion can be identified on
chest x-ray in 25 percent of patients. The purified protein derivative
(PPD) is positive in over 90 percent of patients.

Renal failure due to bilateral kidney involvement is rare (one of our
patients had had previous nephrectomy for tuberculosis 10 years earlier,
and the disease was destroying the remaining kidney). The findings on
IVP vary in severity from calyceal dilatation with scarring to obstruction
and destructive dilatation of the pyelocaliceal system. Occasionally, the
appearance is that of a space-occupying lesion secondary to a large cortical abscess. Calcification is common.

The diagnosis of renal tuberculosis is based on the isolation of the organism in the urine. It is recommended that first morning specimens be
obtained and cultured 3 times. On occasion, the diagnosis may be established by biopsy material obtained at the time of cystoscopy.

The initial therapy is usually medical, consisting of isoniazid (INH),
300 mg orally once a day, together with 50 mg daily of pyridoxine supplementation to prevent neuropathy. Kinetic data concerning the disposition

of INH in a large group of elderly are lacking [101]. It is recommended that serum transaminases be monitored monthly during treatment, and if any value exceeds 3 times normal the drug should be temporarily discontinued. The sensation of hyperexcitability occasionally reported by the elderly taking this drug can be avoided by using a divided dose regimen of 100 mg every 8 hours [102]. In all instances a second drug should be given; either ethambutol, 25 mg per kg per day for the first 2 months followed by 15 mg per kg per day thereafter, or rifampin, 600 mg daily (see Table 9-1). Ophthalmologic evaluation is routinely necessary in the elderly prior to treatment with ethambutol. Side effects of rifampin are mainly hepatic, and no dosage alteration is necessary in the elderly [103]. Some authors recommend adding streptomycin for the first 6 months in advanced cases [100]. Our practice is to perform a yearly sonogram (or IVP) to detect the presence of obstructive uropathy, which is usually secondary to the development of a ureteral stricture. The prognosis for cure with a 24-month course of double antibiotic therapy is generally good. Although this is the approach recommended by the authors, good results have also been reported with a course of daily rifampin and INH for 2 months, switching to a regimen of either twice a week for 7 additional months or 3 times a week for 2 additional months [104]. Five of our patients died from cardiovascular causes, and autopsy was performed in three with no residual active disease found.

In some patients surgery may be necessary. The indications include intractable pain, persistent bleeding, suspicion of malignancy in a nonfunctioning kidney [105], and refractory hypertension associated with a poorly functioning kidney. For the latter, nephrectomy is the treatment of choice after demonstrating that the offending kidney is renin-producing [106].

XANTHOGRANULOMATOUS PYELONEPHRITIS
Xanthogranulomatous pyelonephritis is a severe chronic form of renal parenchymal infection characterized by the accumulation of large numbers of lipid-laden macrophages in the inflamed areas. These foamy macrophages may be mistaken for the clear cells of renal carcinoma when closely packed. This progressive granulomatous reaction generally results from prolonged, low-grade suppuration in a kidney in which urine flow is retarded by either a calculus or other abnormality affecting the ureteropelvic junction [107]. The disease is usually unilateral and reaches a peak incidence in the sixth and seventh decades; 45 percent of reported patients were older than 60 years, mainly females [108, 109]. Fever, flank pain, and chills are the most common presenting manifestations. Malaise, weight loss, and lower urinary tract complaints have also been reported [110]. Physical examination usually reveals abdominal distention and a palpable mass on the involved side. The sedimentation

rate is usually elevated, leukocytosis is common, and the urine culture is positive in 70 percent of cases, *E. coli* and *P. mirabilis* being the predominant organisms. On x-ray examination of the abdomen, an upper tract calculus (plain or staghorn) is found in 71 percent of patients. The IVP reveals either a nonfunctioning kidney (76 percent) or a poorly functioning one. The abdominal CT scan is the most useful diagnostic test because the extent of perirenal involvement and the details of the intrarenal lesions (calculi, necrosis, hydronephrosis, abscesses) can be seen in the greatest detail. Cure is possible only with surgical treatment (usually complete nephrectomy) [111].

FUNGAL INFECTIONS

Urinary fungal infections in the elderly present either as primary infections or as manifestations of systemic infection. In nonhospitalized patients the incidence of fungal urinary tract infection (defined as $> 10^3$ organisms per ml) is not known, but it is rather unusual in our experience and occurs most often in diabetics. The asymptomatic patient may be monitored carefully with periodic reassessment [112]. In the presence of diabetes mellitus, good glycemic control should be attempted first. In the symptomatic patient (with urgency or hematuria), oral flucytosine, 100 to 150 mg per kg daily in divided doses, is recommended [113, 114]. The duration of treatment is not well established. Relapses have been noted after 2 weeks of therapy; however, in one study the initial response rate with this regimen was 94 percent [115]. This drug should probably not be used in the elderly with renal insufficiency. Ketoconazole, 200 to 800 mg orally, has also been found effective in a small number of patients [116] (see Table 9-1).

In hospitalized patients, fungiuria (most commonly due to *Candida albicans*) is not uncommon in elderly patients who have been on systemic antibiotic therapy, particularly if they have intravenous or bladder catheters inserted. In the absence of any evidence of systemic fungal infection (such as a rising serum *Candida* antibody titer or retinal lesions), all catheters should be removed and, if possible, antibiotics discontinued. The fungus generally disappears from the urine within 4 to 5 days with this approach. If the organism persists, the bladder may be irrigated continuously with a solution of 200 to 300 ml of sterile water containing 1 mg per dl of amphotericin B. The double-lumen catheter used for this purpose should be cross-clamped for 60 to 90 minutes at regular intervals [117]. This regimen should be continued for 5 to 7 days, and cultures then repeated. The persistence of a positive culture constitutes an indication for systemic antifungal therapy (see Table 9-1).

Urinary infection through the hematogenous route (fungemia) can occur with any of the fungi known to produce clinically important disease in humans. In some instances (e.g., histoplasmosis) the patient may first seek medical attention because of urinary complaints [118]. Therapy consists of parenteral administration of amphotericin B. It is recommended that 0.3 mg per kg per day be used as an initial dose, gradually increasing to 0.4 to 0.6 mg per kg per day, while monitoring kidney function closely [119] (see Table 9-1). Duration of therapy depends on the clinical response, the fungus involved, and the site of involvement [118].

ANTIBIOTIC PROPHYLAXIS FOR UROLOGIC SURGERY

A detailed analysis of prophylactic use of antibiotics for urologic surgery in the elderly is beyond the scope of this discussion. The reader is referred to a recently published review [120]. In general, antibiotic prophylaxis is considered beneficial for (1) transrectal biopsy; (2) cystoscopy in patients with chronic indwelling catheters; (3) transurethral prostatectomy, particularly in patients with pre-existing bacteriuria and indwelling catheters, with some controversy over the benefits of prophylaxis in other patients [121, 122]; and (4) ureteral and renal stone surgery. The choice of antibiotic should be based on the results of urine culture in patients with chronic catheters. For other patients, any antibiotic with broad gram-negative coverage should be used. The drug should be given 1 or 2 hours prior to surgery and continued for 24 hours postoperatively, noting that the renal clearance of many of the commonly used antibiotics is reduced in the elderly [123].

REFERENCES

1. Kass EH: Bacteriuria and the diagnosis of infection in the urinary tract. *Arch Intern Med* 100:709–713, 1957.
2. Kaye D: Urinary tract infections in the elderly. *Bull NY Acad Med* 56:209–220, 1980.
3. Nordenstam GR, et al: Bacteriuria and mortality in an elderly population. *N Engl J Med* 314:1152–1156, 1986.
4. Dean NC, Yamamura R, and Yoshikawa TT: Pyuria: Its predictive value of asymptomatic bacteriuria in ambulatory elderly men. *J Urol* 135:520–522, 1986.
5. Wolfson SA, et al: Epidemiology of bacteriuria in a predominantly geriatric male population. *Am J Med* 250:168–173, 1965.
6. Dontas AS, et al: Bacteriuria and survival in old age. *N Engl J Med* 304:939–943, 1981.
7. Norman DC and Yoshikawa TT: Frequency of asymptomatic bacteriuria in ambulatory elderly males. *Clin Res* 36:96A, 1988.
8. Nicolle LE, et al: Bacteriuria in elderly institutionalized men. *N Engl J Med* 309:1420–1425, 1983.

9. Cox CE, Lacy SS, and Hinman F Jr: The urethra and its relationship to urinary infection II. The urethral flora in the female with recurrent urinary infection. *J Urol* 99:632–634, 1968.

10. Johnson WG, Pierce AK, and Sanford JP: Changing pharyngeal bacterial flora of hospitalized patients. *N Engl J Med* 281:1137–1140, 1969.

11. Brumfitt W, Gargan RA, and Hamilton-Miller JMT: Periurethral enterobacterial carriage preceding urinary infection. *Lancet* 1:824–826, 1987.

12. Kunin CM, Polyach F, and Posted F: Periurethral bacterial flora in women. Prolonged intermittent colonization with E. coli. *JAMA* 243:143, 1980.

13. Fowler JE and Stamey TA: Studies on introital colonization in women with recurrent urinary infections. VIII: The role of bacterial adherence. *J Urol* 117:472–476, 1977.

14. Schaeffer AJ, et al: Variable adherence of uropathogenic E. coli to epithelial cells from women with recurrent urinary tract infection. *J Urol* 128:1227–1230, 1982.

15. Sobel JD and Muller G: Pathogenesis of bacteriuria in elderly women: The role of E. coli adherence to vaginal epithelial cells. *J Gerontol* 39:682–685, 1984.

16. O'Hanley P, et al: Gal-Gal binding and hemolysin phenotypes and genotypes associated with uropathogenic E. coli. *N Engl J Med* 313:414–420, 1985.

17. Stamey TA, et al: The immunologic basis of recurrent bacteriuria. *Medicine* 57:47–56, 1978.

18. Schaeffer AJ, Jones JM, and Dunn JK: Association of in-vitro E. coli adherence to vaginal and buccal epithelial cells with susceptibility of women to recurrent urinary tract infections. *N Engl J Med* 304:1062–1066, 1981.

19. Parsons CL and Schmidt JD: Control of recurrent lower urinary tract infection in the post-menopausal woman. *J Urol* 128:1224–1226, 1982.

20. Cox CE: The urethra and its relationship to urinary tract infection: The flora of the normal female urethra. *South Med J* 59:621–623, 1966.

21. Andersen JT, et al: Bladder function in healthy elderly males. *Scand J Urol Nephrol* 12:123–127, 1978.

22. Brocklehurst JC and Dillane JB: Studies of the female bladder in old age. I: Cystometrograms in non-incontinent women. *Gerontol Clin* (Basel) 8:285–305, 1966.

23. Parsons CL and Mulholland SG: Bladder surface mucin: Its antibacterial effect against various bacterial species. *Am J Pathol* 93:423–432, 1978.

24. Resnick NM and Yalla SV: Management of urinary incontinence in the elderly. *N Engl J Med* 313:800–805, 1985.

25. Ribeiro BJ and Smith SR: Evaluation of urinary catheterization and urinary incontinence in a general nursing home population. *J Am Geriatr Soc* 33:479–482, 1985.

26. Garibaldi RA, et al: Factors predisposing to bacteriuria during indwelling urethral catheterization. *N Engl J Med* 291:215–218, 1974.

27. Johnson ET: The condom catheter: Urinary tract infection and other complications. *South Med J* 76:579–582, 1983.

28. Ouslander JG, Greengold B, and Chen S: External catheter use and urinary tract infections among incontinent male nursing home patients. *J Am Geriatr Soc* 35:1063–1070, 1987.

29. Maki DG, Henekens GG, and Phillips CW: Nosocomial urinary tract infection with S. marcescens: An epidemiologic study. *J Infect Dis* 128:579–587, 1973.

30. Daifukee R and Stamm WE: Bacterial adherence to bladder uroepithelial

cells in catheter-associated urinary tract infection. *N Engl J Med* 314:1208–1213, 1986.

31. Freedman LR: Experimental pyelonephritis. XV: Increased susceptibility to *E. coli* infection in old rats. *Yale J Biol Med* 42:30–38, 1969.
32. Gross JS: Infections in the elderly. *Med Times* 113:93–104, 1985.
33. Kaack MB, et al: Immunology of pyelonephritis. VIII: *E. coli* causes granulocytic aggregation and renal ischemia. *J Urol* 136:1117–1122, 1986.
34. Saltzman RL and Peterson PK: Immunodeficiency in the elderly. *Rev Infect Dis* 9:1127–1139, 1987.
35. Kniker WI, et al: Multitest MCI for the standardized measurement of delayed cutaneous hypersensitivity and cell-mediated immunity. *Ann Allergy* 52:75–82, 1984.
36. Roberts JA: Pathogenesis of pyelonephritis. *J Urol* 129:1102–1106, 1983.
37. Boscia JA, et al: Pyuria and asymptomatic bacteriuria in elderly ambulatory women. *Ann Intern Med* 110:404–405, 1989.
38. Brocklehurst JC, et al: Dysuria in old age. *J Am Geriatr Soc* 19:582–592, 1971.
39. Boscia JA, et al: Lack of association between bacteriuria and symptoms in the elderly. *Am J Med* 81:979–982, 1986.
40. Norman DC, Yamamura R, and Yoshikawa TT: Pyuria: Its predictive value of asymptomatic bacteriuria in ambulatory elderly men. *J Urol* 135:520–522, 1986.
41. Gleckman R, et al: Community-acquired bacteremic urosepsis in elderly patients: A prospective study of 34 consecutive episodes. *J Urol* 128:79–81, 1982.
42. Stamm WE, Martin SM, and Bennett JV: Epidemiology of nosocomial infections due to gram-negative bacilli: Aspects relevant to development and use of vaccines. *J Infect Dis* 136:S151–S160, 1977.
43. Esposito AL, et al: Community-acquired bacteremia in the elderly: Analysis of one hundred consecutive episodes. *J Am Geriatr Soc* 28:315–319, 1980.
44. Gleckman R, et al: Catheter-related urosepsis in the elderly: A prospective study of community-derived infections. *J Am Geriatr Soc* 30:255–257, 1982.
45. Rudman D, et al: Clinical correlates of bacteremia in a Veterans Administration extended care facility. *J Am Geriatr Soc* 36:726–732, 1988.
46. Milnes JP and Swain DG: Severe renal sepsis in the very elderly. *Postgrad Med* 62:643–645, 1986.
47. Suntharalingham M, Seth V, and Moore-Smith B: Site of urinary tract infection in elderly women admitted to an acute geriatric assessment unit. *Age Aging* 12:317–322, 1983.
48. Fairley KF, et al: Simple test to determine the site of urinary tract infection. *Lancet* 2:427–428, 1967.
49. Nicolle LE, et al: Localization of urinary tract infection in elderly institutionalized women with asymptomatic bacteriuria. *J Infect Dis* 157:65–70, 1988.
50. Rubin RH, et al: Single-dose amoxicillin therapy for urinary tract infection. *JAMA* 244:561–564, 1980.
51. Nicolle LE, Mayhew WJ, and Bryan L: Prospective randomized comparison of therapy and no therapy for asymptomatic bacteriuria in institutionalized elderly women. *Am J Med* 83:27–33, 1987.
52. Boscia JA, et al: Therapy versus no therapy for bacteriuria in elderly ambulatory non-hospitalized women. *JAMA* 257:1067–1071, 1987.
53. Abruytyn E, Boscia JA, and Kaye D: The treatment of asymptomatic bacteriuria in the elderly. *J Am Geriatr Soc* 36:473–475, 1988.
54. Sourander LB and Kasanen A: A 5-year follow-up of bacteriuria in the aged. *Gerontol Clin* 14:274–281, 1972.

55. Dontas AS, et al: Bacteriuria and survival in old age. *N Engl J Med* 304:939–943, 1981.
56. Nicolle LE, et al: The association of bacteriuria with resident characteristics and survival in elderly institutionalized men. *Ann Intern Med* 106:682–686, 1987.
57. Nordenstam GR, et al: Bacteriuria and mortality in an elderly population. *N Engl J Med* 314:1152–1156, 1986.
58. Gleckman RA: The chronically catheterized elderly patient. A selective review. *J Am Geriatr Soc* 33:489–491, 1985.
59. Stark RP and Maki DG: Bacteriuria in the catheterized patient. What quantitative level of bacteriuria is relevant? *N Engl J Med* 311:560–564, 1984.
60. Reid RI, et al: Comparison of urine bag-changing regimens in elderly catheterized patients. *Lancet* 2:754–756, 1982.
61. Warren JW, et al: Sequelae and management of urinary infection in the patient requiring chronic catheterization. *J Urol* 125:1–8, 1981.
62. McFarlane DE: Prevention and treatment of catheter-associated urinary tract infection. *J Infect* 10:96–106, 1985.
63. Siler WO and Stahclin HB: Practical management of catheter-associated urinary tract infections. *Geriatrics* 43:43–50, 1988.
64. Mohler JL, Cowen DL, and Flanigan RC: Suppression and treatment of urinary tract infection in patients with an intermittently catheterized neurogenic bladder. *J Urol* 138:336–340, 1987.
65. Gordon DL, et al: Diagnostic criteria and natural history of catheter-associated urinary tract infections after prostatectomy. *Lancet* 2:1269–1271, 1983.
66. Stovall CW, Mihaldzic N, and Lloyd FA: Incidence of renal bacteriuria in the presence of long standing bladder infections. In *Proceedings of the 16th VA Spinal Cord Injury Conference, 1967.* Pp. 172–176.
67. Breitenbucher RB: Bacterial changes in the urine samples of patients with long-term indwelling catheters. *Arch Intern Med* 144:1585–1589, 1984.
68. Platt R, et al: Mortality associated with nosocomial urinary tract infection. *N Engl J Med* 307:637–642, 1982.
69. Komaroff AL: Acute dysuria in women. *N Engl J Med* 310:368–375, 1984.
70. Stamm WE, et al: Diagnosis of coliform infection in acutely dysuric women. *N Engl J Med* 307:463–468, 1982.
71. Schultz HJ, et al: Acute cystitis: A prospective study of laboratory tests and duration of therapy. *Mayo Clin Proc* 59:391–397, 1984.
72. Lerner SA and Fekete T: Single-dose therapy for cystitis. *JAMA* 247:1865–1866, 1982.
73. Stamm WE, McKevitt M, and Counts GW: Acute renal infection in women. Treatment with trimethoprim-sulfamethoxazole or ampicillin for two or six weeks. *Ann Intern Med* 106:341–345, 1987.
74. Fihn S and Stamm WE: Management of Women with Acute Dysuria. In Rund DA (ed), *Emergency Medicine Annual 1983*, Norwalk, CT: Appleton-Century-Crofts, 1983. Pp. 225–246.
75. Komaroff AL, et al: Management strategies for urinary and vaginal infections. *Arch Intern Med* 138:1069–1073, 1978.
76. Tauscher JW and Shaw DC: Eosinophilic cystitis. *Clin Pediatr* 20:741–743, 1981.
77. Stamm WE, et al: Antimicrobial prophylaxis of recurrent urinary tract infections. A double-blind, placebo-controlled trial. *Ann Intern Med* 92:770–775, 1980.
78. Stamm WE, et al: Is antimicrobial prophylaxis of urinary tract infections cost effective? *Ann Intern Med* 94:251–255, 1981.

79. Cronberg S, et al: Prevention of recurrent acute cystitis by methenamine hippurate: Double-blind controlled cross-over long-term study. *Br Med J* 294:1507–1508, 1987.

80. Kunin CM: Duration of treatment of urinary tract infections. *Am J Med* 71: 849–854, 1981.

81. Nicolle LE, et al: Efficacy of five years of continuous, low dose trimethoprim-sulfamethoxazole prophylaxis for urinary tract infection. *J Infect Dis* 157: 1239–1242, 1988.

82. Smith JW, et al: Recurrent urinary tract infections in men. Characteristics and response to therapy. *Ann Intern Med* 91:544–548, 1979.

83. Lipsky BA: Urinary tract infections in men. Epidemiology, pathophysiology, diagnosis and treatment. *Ann Intern Med* 110:138–150, 1989.

84. Childs SJ and Goldstein EJC: Ciprofloxacin as treatment for genitourinary tract infection. *J Urol* 141:1–5, 1989.

85. Sant GR and Weinstein BS: Therapy of urinary tract infections in the elderly: Role of fluoroquinolones. *Urology* [Suppl] 35:19–21, 1990.

86. Hamus PM and Danziger LH: Treatment of chronic bacterial prostatitis. *Clin Pharmacol* 3:49–55, 1984.

87. Johnson JR and Stamm WE: Urinary tract infections in women. Diagnosis and treatment. *Ann Intern Med* 111:906–917, 1989.

88. Bauer LA and Blovin RA: Gentamicin pharmacokinetics: Effects of aging in patients with normal renal function. *J Am Geriatr Soc* 30:309–311, 1982.

89. Zaske DE, et al: Wide interpatient variations in gentamicin dose requirements for geriatric patients. *JAMA* 248:3122–3126, 1982.

90. Bauer LA and Blouin RA: Influence of age on tobramycin pharmacokinetics in patients with normal renal function. *Antimicrob Agents Chemother* 20: 587–589, 1981.

91. Bauer LA and Blouin RA: Influence of age on amikacin pharmacokinetics in patients without renal disease. *Eur J Clin Pharmacol* 24:639–642, 1983.

92. Eknoyan G, et al: Renal papillary necrosis: An update. *Medicine* 61:55–73, 1982.

93. Harvald B: Renal papillary necrosis. A clinical survey of sixty-six cases. *Am J Med* 35:481–486, 1963.

94. Faubert PF and Porush JG: Unpublished observations, 1987.

95. Sheinfeld J, et al: Perinephric abscess. Current concepts. *J Urol* 137:191–194, 1987.

96. Edelstein H and McCabe RE: Perinephric abscess: Modern diagnosis and treatment in 47 cases. *Medicine* 67:118–131, 1988.

97. Ahlering TE, et al: Emphysematous pyelonephritis: A 5-year experience with 13 patients. *J Urol* 134:1086–1088, 1985.

98. Evanoff GV, et al: Spectrum of gas within the kidney. *Am J Med* 83:149–154, 1987.

99. Alvarez S and McCabe WR: Extrapulmonary tuberculosis revisited. A review of experience at Boston City and other hospitals. *Medicine* 63:25–55, 1984.

100. Simon HB, et al: Genitourinary tuberculosis. Clinical features in a general hospital population. *Am J Med* 63:410–420, 1977.

101. Advemeier C, et al: Pharmocokinetics of isoniazid in the elderly [letter]. *Br J Clin Pharmacol* 10:167–169, 1980.

102. Yoshikawa TT and Nagami PH: Adverse drug reactions in tuberculous therapy. Risks and recommendations. *Geriatrics* 37:61–66, 1982.

103. Advemier C, et al: Pharmacokinetic studies of rifampicin in the elderly. *Ther Drug Monit* 5:61–65, 1983.

104. Weinberg AC and Boyd SD: Short-course chemotherapy and role of surgery in adult and pediatric genitourinary tuberculosis. *Urology* 31:95–102, 1988.
105. Lattimer JK and Wechsler MW: Editorial comment. *J Urol* 124:191, 1980.
106. Flechner SM and Gow JC: Role of nephrectomy in the treatment of non-functioning or very poorly functioning unilateral tuberculous kidney. *J Urol* 123:822–825, 1980.
107. McDonald GSA: Xanthogranulomatous pyelonephritis. *J Pathol* 133:203–213, 1981.
108. Tolia BM, et al: Xanthogranulomatous pyelonephritis: Detailed analysis of 29 cases and a brief discussion of atypical presentations. *J Urol* 126:437–442, 1981.
109. Petronic V, Buturovic J, and Isvaneski M: Xanthogranulomatous pyelonephritis. *Br J Urol* 64:336–338, 1989.
110. Grainger RG, Longstaff AJ, and Parsons MA: Xanthogranulomatous pyelonephritis: A reappraisal. *Lancet* 1:1398–1401, 1982.
111. Malek RS and Elder JS: Xanthogranulomatous pyelonephritis. A critical analysis of 26 cases and of the literature. *J Urol* 119:589–593, 1978.
112. Schonebeck J: Studies on *Candida* infection of the urinary tract and on the antimycotic drug 5-fluorocytosine. *Scand J Urol Nephrol* [Suppl] 11:7–48, 1972.
113. Fisher J, et al: Fungus balls of the urinary tract. *South Med J* 72:1281–1284, 1979.
114. Rohner TJ Jr and Tuliszewski RM: Fungal cystitis: Awareness, diagnosis and treatment. *J Urol* 124:142–143, 1980.
115. Wise GJ, Kozinn PJ, and Goldberg P: Fluocytosine in the management of genitourinary candidiasis: 5 years of experience. *J Urol* 124:70–72, 1980.
116. Gaybill JR, et al: Ketoconazole therapy for fungal urinary tract infections. *J Urol* 129:68–70, 1983.
117. Fisher JF, et al: Urinary tract infections due to *Candida albicans*. *Rev Infect Dis* 4:1107–1118, 1982.
118. Frangos DN and Nyberg LM Jr: Genitourinary fungal infections. *South Med J* 79:455–459, 1986.
119. Bennett JE: Chemotherapy of systemic mycosis. *N Engl J Med* 290:30–31, 1974.
120. Larsen EH, Gasser TC, and Madsen PO: Antimicrobial prophylaxis in urologic surgery. *Urol Clin North Am* 13:591–604, 1986.
121. Coptcoat MJ, et al: Is antibiotic prophylaxis necessary for routine urodynamic investigations? A controlled study in 100 patients. *Br J Urol* 61:302–303, 1988.
122. Grabe M: Antimicrobial agents in transurethral prostatic resection. *J Urol* 138:245–252, 1987.
123. Ljungberg B and Nilsson-Ehle I: Pharmacokinetics of antimicrobial agents in the elderly. *Rev Infect Dis* 9:250–264, 1987.

10 ACUTE RENAL FAILURE

Acute renal failure (ARF), defined as an increase in the BUN or serum creatinine, can be due to prerenal, renal, or postrenal causes. Postrenal (or obstructive) uropathy is discussed in Chap. 8. In this chapter the discussion involves mainly acute prerenal and renal failure, complications that occur in approximately 8 percent of admissions of patients over 60 years of age at our hospital. Among this group, prerenal failure occurred in 52 percent of the cases, similar to the 47 percent reported by Pascual et al [1] and the 55 percent reported by McInnes et al [2]. The remaining 48 percent had intrinsic renal failure (acute tubular necrosis). The incidence of the latter form of ARF in the elderly has significantly increased during the past decade [3]. For instance, in a series of ARF (intrinsic renal disease) in adult patients reported prior to 1980, 24 to 46 percent of the patients were elderly [4–6], compared to 60 to 76 percent in more recent studies [6–9]. Our experience is similar, a phenomenon that cannot be solely explained by a higher percentage of elderly patients occupying hospital beds. The population of our hospitalized elderly patients has increased by only 30 percent during this same period.

PRERENAL FAILURE (PRERENAL AZOTEMIA)

ETIOLOGY
The etiology of prerenal azotemia in our hospitalized elderly patients, in order of decreasing frequency, includes volume contraction, uncontrolled congestive heart failure, and drugs such as nonsteroidal anti-inflammatory drugs (NSAIDs), converting enzyme inhibitors, diuretics, and antibiotics.

PATHOGENESIS AND CLINICAL MANIFESTATIONS
As noted, volume contraction is the most common cause of prerenal azotemia in the elderly [1]. The typical patient is admitted for congestive heart failure, given a diuretic, and put on a low-sodium diet. Frequently, aggressive diuresis is continued after the patient has improved significantly, leading to volume contraction with an increase in BUN and serum creatinine (the latter often disproportionately less). In elderly patients with congestive heart failure, the diuresis may be so aggressive that acute prerenal azotemia ensues even though the patient is still wet. This phenomenon is seen more frequently in patients receiving a loop diuretic in combination with a thiazide [10]. Other groups at risk include

elderly patients with mild pre-existing renal insufficiency who are hospitalized for either elective surgery or an acute illness and placed on a salt-restricted diet or a diuretic for hypertension. Symptoms vary from non-specific complaints such as generalized weakness to those related to a decrease in circulating plasma volume such as increased thirst and postural lightheadedness or vertigo. On physical examination, poor skin turgor and an orthostatic drop in blood pressure may be noted.

The sensitivity of the physical examination in concert with the history and record review in the diagnosis of volume contraction in the elderly is not very high. Indeed, in one prospective study involving adult patients of various ages the sensitivity was found to be only 49 percent and specificity was 51 percent [11]. Besides the disproportionate rise in the BUN compared to the serum creatinine, hyponatremia is present in 30 percent of the patients. Hypernatremia may be seen in confused, bedridden elderly patients without access to water. Unless there is concomitant pre-existing renal disease, the urine sediment may be benign. In our last 30 elderly patients with prerenal azotemia, urinary indices revealed a urine-plasma creatinine of 31 ± 8 (which is generally compatible with prerenal azotemia). The urine sodium (Na) concentration, which is expected to be low in prerenal azotemia (< 10 mEq per liter), when assessed by the renal failure index (RFI) (UNa $\div$ Ucreatinine/Pcreatinine) or fractional excretion of Na (FE_{Na}) (UNa/PNa $\div$ Ucreatinine/Pcreatinine), was 1.5 ± 0.8. In prerenal azotemia the RFI or FE_{Na} is usually less than 1.0 percent. In general, the presence of prerenal azotemia accompanying diuretic use is associated with a high urinary sodium concentration and thus is not helpful. When prerenal azotemia occurs in the setting of metabolic alkalosis with bicarbonaturia, the urinary Na concentration may be relatively high (> 40 mEq per liter), and the urinary chloride is more diagnostic (< 10 mEq per liter) [12]. Both proximal and distal nephron segments participate in the enhanced salt reabsorption seen with volume contraction, the stimulus including renal factors such as a decreased glomerular filtration rate (GFR), peritubular physical factors related to an elevated filtration fraction and a decrease in papillary plasma flow [13], and humoral factors including catecholamines, angiotensin, aldosterone, and vasopressin [14]. In addition to hemodynamic factors, the decrease in kidney function seen in such patients may also be related to a decrease in the glomerular ultrafiltration coefficient [15].

In patients with worsening kidney function due to uncontrolled congestive heart failure, the diagnosis is not difficult because dyspnea, distended neck veins, S_3 gallop, or hepatic congestion is usually present. The RFI and FE_{Na} are low (below 1.0 percent), occasionally even in patients receiving diuretic therapy. A combined decrease in the transcapillary hydraulic pressure and glomerular ultrafiltration coefficient appears to be responsible for the decline in kidney function seen in these patients [16]. In general, the reduction in GFR tends to be more severe in the elderly, possibly reflecting an age-associated hemodynamic pattern governing GFR in this age group [17].

The ARF secondary to NSAIDs is usually of the prerenal variety and is a complication encountered almost exclusively in the elderly, since more than 80 percent of reported patients have been over the age of 60 [18, 19]. Males are affected as frequently as females. The most commonly responsible agents are indomethacin, ibuprofen, zomepirac, sulindac, naproxen, and salicylates. The acute worsening in kidney function tends to occur early after initiation of the drug, usually during the first 3 to 5 days, and does not depend on dose (see section on drug-induced hyperkalemia in Chap. 3). It develops in patients with an "ineffective" circulatory volume (congestive heart failure, liver cirrhosis, sepsis, dehydration) and chronic renal insufficiency. The degree of renal failure varies in severity, with some patients developing symptoms and signs of uremia [20]. Most patients (71 percent) with NSAID-induced ARF are nonoliguric. Hyperchloremic metabolic acidosis and a rise in serum potassium (K) occur in virtually every patient. The severity of the hyperkalemia depends on the pre-existing K level and the rate of urine formation. Findings suggestive of interstitial nephritis (another complication of NSAIDs; see later discussion) such as skin rash, eosinophilia and eosinophiluria, and proteinuria are usually absent. The urinary sediment is benign, and the RFI or FE_{Na} is less than 1 percent in more than 80 percent of patients. Histologic examination of the kidney in two of our patients who died (one from a cardiac arrhythmia and the other from a massive pulmonary embolism) failed to show any significant abnormalities. Both prostaglandin E_2 (PGE_2) and 6-keto-$PGF_{1\alpha}$ (a stable breakdown product of prostacyclin or PGI_2) have been found to be significantly decreased in such patients. Renal function appears to decline in parallel with the decrease in 6-keto-$PGF_{1\alpha}$ rather than PGE_2 [21, 22]. Glomerular and vascular prostaglandins, mainly PGE_2 and PGI_1, play an important homeostatic role in modulating or antagonizing the vasoconstriction induced by angiotensin II and activation of the renal autonomic nervous system. Thus, the administration of NSAIDs to patients with the risk factors noted earlier induces renal failure by removing the negative feedback or modulatory role of vasodilatory prostaglandins (mainly prostacyclin), thereby accentuating renal vasoconstriction [23].

ARF secondary to the angiotensin-converting enzyme inhibitors (ACEi) occurs in 27 percent of patients taking captopril and in 17 percent of those taking enalapril with bilateral renal artery stenosis or renal artery stenosis in a solitary kidney [24, 25]. The rise in serum creatinine can be attributed to the fall in blood pressure and efferent glomerular arteriolar tone, which decreases transglomerular hydraulic pressure and thereby GFR. The fact that 25 percent of patients on captopril and 23 percent of those on enalapril with unilateral renal artery stenosis and a normally functioning contralateral kidney also develop ARF suggests that factors other than angiotensin II blockade might be responsible for the effects of these agents on kidney function [24]. The urinary sediment in such patients is usually benign, and the RFI and FE_{Na} suggest prerenal azotemia. Serum creatinine may also rise in patients with advanced congestive heart failure and pre-existing chronic mild to moderate renal insufficiency (serum creatinine 1.5–2.0 mg per dl) following the administration of captopril or enalapril [26]. Renal failure in such circumstances may be the result of excessively rapid diuresis, since lowering the dose of the diuretic without changing that of the ACEi may return kidney function to baseline. The long-acting ACEi enalapril, however, may be detrimental to renal function in some patients regardless of their extracellular volume status. In these instances the relative hypotension induced may be responsible for the decrease in kidney function [27].

ARF has been reported in elderly patients with pre-existing renal insufficiency who are receiving potassium-sparing diuretics [28]. In this study, involving 19 elderly patients, the drug most commonly used was amiloride in combination with hydrochlorothiazide (10 patients), followed by triamterene with hydrochlorothiazide (8 patients) and amiloride alone (1). Six patients were taking other diuretics, and 5 were using an NSAID. Hypovolemia might have been a contributing factor in some of these patients. The renal insufficiency was reversible on discontinuing the involved drugs in 17 patients, suggesting that a functional rather than a structural abnormality was responsible for the renal failure. Of the remaining 2 patients, 1 did not improve, and 1 died with renal failure. It is clear that renal function must be regularly monitored in these patients.

Finally, the use of tetracycline for correction of hyponatremia (mainly in patients with pre-existing liver disease) may be associated with prerenal azotemia due to increased urinary salt losses (see Chap. 2).

TREATMENT AND PROGNOSIS

The prognosis is usually good in the elderly with prerenal azotemia due to volume contraction. Unless sepsis develops, exposure to nephrotoxic agents occurs, or other problems arise to alter the course of the prerenal azotemia by producing acute tubular necrosis (a complication seen in 2–3 percent of our patients), recovery is the rule. Patients who are symptomatic with orthostatic hypotension and those with uremic symptoms should receive fluid parenterally, the rate of infusion being adjusted according to the quantity and electrolyte content of the fluid lost. In the others, a more gradual approach can be used, changing the diet to a regular salt diet and liberalizing oral fluid intake. Diuretics should be discontinued. Weight and kidney function should be monitored frequently. The dosage of all drugs excreted by the kidneys (e.g., digoxin) should be reassessed regularly as GFR improves.

Most patients with declining kidney function secondary to congestive heart failure per se will improve on a low-salt diet, bed rest, judicious use of inotropic agents, vasodilators, and diuretic administration. Furosemide and bumetanide are the most widely used diuretics in these patients; the intravenous method of administration is preferred because pharmacodynamics in these patients are altered [29]. In the elderly, 30 to 50 percent less furosemide reaches the renal tubules compared to younger subjects with normal renal function [30]. In general, doses of 160 to 200 mg of furosemide or 3 to 5 mg of bumetanide are sufficient to produce a maximum diuretic response [31]. If necessary, hydrochlorothiazide, 50 to 100 mg per day, or metolazone, 5 to 10 mg per day orally, can be added to the loop diuretic [10, 32]. If all else fails, dialysis or continuous arteriovenous hemofiltration (CAVH) may be necessary [33]. The mortality is high in patients who fail to respond to diuretics and vasodilator therapy; however, the chances of recovering baseline kidney function in patients in whom the heart failure is controlled are good except in diabetics, in whom the incidence of irreversible losses of function of varying degree is well above 30 percent in our experience.

In approximately 85 percent of patients with ARF secondary to NSAID use, kidney function returns to baseline within 5 to 6 days of discontinuing the drug. Dialysis may be required in the remaining 15 percent, but eventually these patients recover sufficient kidney function to be able to stop dialysis. In these latter patients, FE_{Na} was greater than 1 percent, suggesting that they may have developed acute tubular necrosis. The reason for this more severe form of ARF is not clear.

The renal insufficiency precipitated by use of ACEi also reverts on discontinuing therapy. In patients in whom impairment in kidney function is mild (a rise in serum creatinine of 1–1.5 mg per dl), creatinine clearance stabilizes over time and may even increase despite continuing the drug [24].

ACUTE TUBULAR NECROSIS

ETIOLOGY
The etiology of acute renal failure due to the syndrome called acute tubular necrosis (ATN) in 250 elderly patients is outlined in Table 10-1, showing that hypovolemic and septic shock and nephrotoxic agents are responsible for 69 percent of the cases. Multiple etiologic factors are

TABLE 10-1. Etiology of acute tubular necrosis in 250 elderly patients

		No. patients	Percentage
Medical			
Hypovolemic shock		96	38.4
Septic shock		41	16.4
Nephrotoxic agents		35	14.0
Cardiovascular catastrophes		19	7.6˙
Hepatobiliary diseases		8	3.2
Pigments (myoglobin, hemoglobin)		5	2.0
	Total	204	81.6
Surgical		46	18.4

found in more than 44 percent of elderly patients with ATN [1]. ARF secondary to atheroembolic disease is dealt with in Chap. 13.

CLINICAL MANIFESTATIONS

In the elderly, as in younger patients, ATN is manifested by a rise in BUN of 10 to 20 mg per dl per day and a rise in creatinine of 1 to 2 mg per dl per day. Prior to the 1980s, the reported incidence of oliguria, defined as a daily urine output of less than 500 ml, was in the range of 60 to 75 percent of patients with ATN [5]. In more recent reports, however, oliguria has been reported in only 30 to 45 percent [36]. Our experience has been about the same, both in the general population and in the elderly. Anuria, defined as a urinary output less than 100 ml per day, occurs in 8 to 12 percent. Hyperkalemia is seen almost exclusively in the oliguric group, more so in patients with increased muscle and other tissue breakdown. Acidosis is generally mild, with a serum bicarbonate concentration of 18 to 20 mEq per liter in 80 percent of the patients. RFI and FE_{Na} are usually greater than 3 percent, similar to that reported in younger patients [35, 37]. Defects in inner medullary collecting duct sodium reabsorption appear to play an important role in the increased FE_{Na} seen in ATN [38]. Five to ten percent of elderly patients, however, have a low FE_{Na} in the presence of ATN. This phenomenon is most often seen in the early stages of radiocontrast nephropathy [39] and myoglobinuric renal failure, in which spasm of the glomerular capillaries may be playing a role. The urinary sodium in ATN may also be misleadingly low in patients in shock and those who have congestive heart failure or the hepatorenal syndrome. The measurement of urinary osmolality is usually of limited value in differentiating prerenal azotemia from ATN in the elderly, given the diminished ability to concentrate the urine generally present in the aged [40]. Microscopic examination of the urine may reveal large numbers of tubular cells, tubular cell casts, and coarsely granular pigmented casts. Such a characteristic urinary sediment was present in approximately 60 percent of our patients with ATN.

SPECIFIC FORMS OF ACUTE TUBULAR NECROSIS
Ischemic
Ischemic ARF due to inadequate renal perfusion such as occurs with hypovolemia, sepsis, or cardiogenic shock accounts for 62.4 percent of all cases of ATN in the elderly, a somewhat higher rate than the 50 percent reported in the general population [41]. In the initiation phase of this form of ARF, adenosine triphosphate (ATP) is depleted following the ischemic episode, resulting in inactivity of the Na-K-ATPase pump with subsequent water uptake by the cell and cell swelling, erythrocyte aggregation, congestion, and stasis [42]. In general, the metabolic and functional severity is related to the degree of loss of residual nucleotides during the ischemic episode [43]. The decrease in cortical blood flow resulting from vascular congestion could induce medullary ischemia [44], which is responsible for intraluminal tubular obstruction and a decrease in the glomerular ultrafiltration coefficient [45, 46]. These factors, together with tubular backleak of glomerular ultrafiltrate and activation of the tubuloglomerular feedback loop, contribute to the maintenance phase of ATN [47–49]. The predominance of one mechanism over the other may vary significantly among individual patients and may help to explain why some patients are oliguric and others are not and why some have a protracted course and others a shorter one.

The biochemical changes responsible for cell injury during the maintenance phase of ATN are still unsettled. Several pathways are involved including the accumulation of free radicals and free fatty acids, a decrease in phospholipids, and an increase in membrane permeability with subsequent increased intracellular calcium [50], the end point being mitochondrial and plasma membrane damage [51]. In patients with sepsis it is not unusual for the drop in urinary output to precede by hours the temperature spike and hypotension. This phenomenon most likely represents endotoxin-induced renal ischemia due to renal nerve activation [52] and increased release of platelet-activating factor [53], thromboxane A_2, and leukotrienes [54]. It is, therefore, prudent for a clinician facing a sudden, otherwise unexplained drop in urinary output in an elderly patient at risk (those with respiratory failure or an indwelling catheter) to start adequate antibiotic coverage after all the appropriate cultures have been taken.

Nephrotoxin-Induced
Nephrotoxin-induced ATN accounts for 14 percent of cases seen in the elderly (Table 10-1). The agents responsible for this disorder are outlined in Table 10-2.

TABLE 10-2. Agents responsible for nephrotoxin-induced ATN

Agent	Frequency (%)
Antibiotics	40
Nonsteroidal anti-inflammatory drugs	22
Contrast media	18
Cancer chemotherapy	9
Other drugs or a combination of nephrotoxic drugs	11
	100

ANTIBIOTICS. Aminoglycoside-induced nephrotoxicity occurs in 8 to 20 percent of patients receiving any one of the three commonly used drugs: gentamicin, tobramycin, and amikacin [55–58]. The incidence is particularly high in the elderly because these drugs are handled mainly through glomerular filtration, which tends to decrease with age. The usually recommended dose not infrequently is associated in the elderly with higher peak and trough levels as well as with abnormal proximal tubular cell accumulation of the antibiotic [59]. Therefore, when using aminoglycosides in the elderly the best approach is to measure serum concentrations and calculate each patient's dosage requirement individually early during treatment. By so doing the incidence of nephrotoxicity can be lowered significantly [60]. Data similar to those existing for the general population comparing the relative nephrotoxicity of one aminoglycoside with another are not available for the elderly [61, 62]. Besides age, other factors associated with an increased risk of nephrotoxicity include pre-existing renal insufficiency, liver disease, concomitant administration of drugs such as furosemide or a cephalosporin, volume depletion, hypokalemia, and duration of therapy [63–65]. As in younger patients, the elderly with aminoglycoside-induced nephrotoxicity have a progressive increase in BUN and creatinine starting around the second week of therapy. Nonoliguria is the rule. Since a vasopressin-resistant concentrating defect and an increase in FE_{Na} generally precede the rise in BUN and creatinine [66], 70 to 80 percent of our patients also showed evidence of volume contraction at the time of diagnosis. The defect in Na reabsorption appears to involve both the proximal and distal tubules. Renal tubular epithelial casts are frequently found on examination of the urine sediment. Enzymuria and proteinuria (usually less than 1 g per 24 hours) are frequently observed. The exact mechanisms responsible for the ARF seen with aminoglycoside-induced nephrotoxicity are not clear. The final common pathway, as in ischemic ATN, is renal tubular cell injury, including binding by the drug to cell membrane phospholipids, provoking changes in renal phospholipid content and in plasma membrane permeability and transport, as well as direct effects on cell mitochondrial and lysosomal functions [63].

Besides the aminoglycosides, the cephalosporins can also induce renal injury, particularly when the two agents are used in combination [67, 68]. ATN due to either cephalothin or cephalexin use has been reported in the elderly [69–71]. The clinical picture is identical to that characteristic of aminoglycoside toxicity. Renal failure is more common with high doses, occurs anytime between the third and fourteenth day of therapy, and can be severe enough to require dialysis. Changes compatible with ATN are seen on examination of kidney tissue [72]. The mechanisms by which these antibiotics induce renal tubular cell necrosis are not clear. It should be noted that cefoxitin can interfere with the creatinine assay, thereby causing a false elevation in serum creatinine levels, more so in patients with pre-existing chronic renal insufficiency [73].

An increase in BUN and serum creatinine occurs in virtually every elderly patient receiving the antifungal agent amphotericin B. No correlation seems to exist between the degree of renal failure and the total dose of drug administered. Although renal function improves when the drug is discontinued, a certain percentage of elderly patients (more so than younger patients) are left with a persistent reduction in creatinine clearance compared to pretreatment values [74]. The usual recommendation is to withhold therapy when the serum creatinine exceeds 3 mg per dl [75]. The renal failure is generally nonoliguric. Proteinuria is minimal, and tubular casts are frequently found in the urine sediment. Histologically, necrosis of proximal and distal tubule epithelial cells with intracellular and intratubular calcium deposits is seen, the severity correlating with the degree of renal insufficiency [76, 77]. Besides ARF, patients receiving amphotericin B may also develop various forms of tubular dysfunction manifested by hypokalemia, nephrogenic diabetes insipidus, and renal tubular acidosis. These complications most likely result from direct tubular epithelial cell damage produced by the drug [78].

ATN, not always reversible, has been reported in the elderly with pre-existing renal insufficiency who have received a tetracycline other than doxycycline. The exact mechanism responsible for the worsening in kidney function is unclear. It is, therefore, recommended that other antibiotics be used in such patients whenever feasible [79].

NSAIDs. Histologically proven ATN has been reported in the elderly taking NSAIDs [80]. The overall clinical picture is no different from that found in patients who develop prerenal azotemia, except that renal indices are compatible with ATN and the course is more prolonged after the offending agent has been withdrawn. Some patients, as discussed earlier, may even require dialysis, and recovery of 100 percent of baseline kidney function may not take place.

TABLE 10-3. Risk factors associated with dye-induced ATN

Pre-existing renal insufficiency (mainly due to nephrosclerosis)
Diabetic nephropathy
"Ischemic" kidney due to either volume contraction or
   congestive heart failure
Multiple myeloma
Prior contrast-induced ATN

CONTRAST MEDIA. Eighteen percent of cases of nephrotoxin-induced ATN in the elderly are due to contrast agent administration (see Table 10-2) and occur almost exclusively in patients with underlying kidney disease. This form of ATN may develop after any intravascular injection of contrast media, whether it is for angiography, intravenous pyelography, computed tomography (CT), or intravenous cholangiography. The incidence of ATN, however, appears to be highest among patients undergoing arteriography. The nonionic, low-osmolality contrast agents, although better tolerated by patients, have neither prevented the development nor lowered the incidence of ATN [81–85]. Of 151 patients reported with contrast-induced ATN, 115 (76 percent) were over the age of 60. One or several of the proposed risk factors (Table 10-3) were present in 94 percent of the older patients and 89 percent of the younger ones [86–96]. Therefore, it seems unlikely that old age per se, in the absence of any risk factor, increases the likelihood of development of ARF following contrast dye administration.

The BUN and serum creatinine start to rise within 24 to 48 hours after injection of the radiocontrast agent, reaching a peak by the third to fourth day [94]. Most of the patients are nonoliguric, with oliguria present in only 16 to 20 percent [86–96]. In our experience renal tubular epithelial cell or muddy-brown casts in the urinary sediment are unusual. In general, FE_{Na} is greater than 1 percent, but values of less than 1 percent have been reported [93, 97]. The pathogenesis of radiocontrast-induced ATN is probably multifactoral, with direct tubular toxicity and renal ischemia due to dye-induced vasoconstriction playing roles. The latter may lead to disruption of the medullary oxygen balance, possibly contributing to the initiating insult [98, 99]. Tubular obstruction caused by Tamm-Horsfall protein precipitation with contrast media and perhaps a decrease in the glomerular ultrafiltration coefficient have been implicated in the maintenance phase [100–102]. As a rule, if dye has to be given to a patient with underlying renal insufficiency, it is prudent to make sure the patient is neither volume contracted nor in congestive heart failure. We routinely administer furosemide (dose in mg = 4,000 per creatinine clearance, either measured or calculated) or 250 ml of 20 percent mannitol at the time of dye infusion. This regimen has been associated with a

75 percent decrease in the incidence of dye-induced ATN at our institution [103]. It has also been suggested that administering an amount of dye estimated by the following formula (5 ml of contrast × body weight [kg] ÷ serum creatinine [mg per dl], up to a maximum of 300 ml) could significantly lower the risk of developing ATN with radiocontrast media use [104].

CHEMOTHERAPY. As in younger patients, drugs such as methotrexate, streptozocin, mitomycin (see section on hemolytic uremic syndrome in Chap. 7), and cisplatin can induce ATN in the elderly [105]. With methotrexate, intratubular precipitation of the drug occurs in concentrated and acid urines, resulting in obstruction. This complication is now seen with less frequency because hydration and alkalinization are routinely carried out prior to therapy [106]. The nephrotoxicity of streptozotocin is dose related, occurring most frequently at doses exceeding 1.5 g per m^2 per week. The renal failure, which is oliguric, is usually preceded by clinical evidence of tubular damage, manifested by proteinuria, Fanconi's syndrome, or nephrogenic diabetes insipidus [107]. Cisplatin is the anticancer drug most frequently associated with renal failure in the elderly. Age per se, despite the decrease in GFR, does not constitute a risk factor as long as the dose is kept at or below 60 mg per m^2 per month [108]. The nephrotoxicity, which is dose related, results in direct damage to the S_3 segments of the proximal tubule. A reduction in renal blood flow and transglomerular hydrostatic pressure, accounting for the decrease in GFR, has been demonstrated in animals [109]. Hypomagnesemia and nephrogenic diabetes insipidus may develop. Acute uric acid nephropathy, a consequence of intratubular urate deposition, which was originally described in patients with lymphoproliferative disorders undergoing chemotherapy, has become a rarity nowadays because preventive measures such as volume expansion and allopurinol adminstration are routine [110].

Anesthetic agents such as methoxyfluorane may be associated with nonoliguric ATN. The pathogenesis is not clear. ATN may be seen in patients taking paracetamol at either excessive or therapeutic doses [111, 112]. Clinical evidence of hepatotoxicity may not be present. Finally, several other drugs have been associated with ATN [113]; however, in many of these reports it is not clear whether one is dealing with ATN or acute interstitial nephritis, since histologic examination of kidney tissue was not included in the report.

Hepatobiliary Disease

Hepatobiliary diseases are responsible for 8 percent of cases of ATN in the elderly (Table 10-1). The renal failure associated with acute cholecystitis, acute cholangitis, and acute hepatitis is oliguric in 57 percent of patients and tends to occur early, although in patients with acute chol-angitis or cholecystitis it may become manifest during the postoperative period. The FE_{Na} is usually greater than 1 percent. A lower value should suggest the possibility of hepatorenal syndrome. Several mechanisms acting singly or in concert contribute to the high incidence of ATN seen with hepatobiliary diseases; these include sepsis, hypotension related to the cardiodepressor or natriuretic effect of cholemia, circulating endo-toxin, and changes in vascular reactivity [114–119]. Bailey [120] has re-ported a high correlation between the presence of circulating endotoxin and decreased creatinine clearance seen in patients with obstructive jaun-dice. These high levels of endotoxin may be derived from increased gut absorption due to the absence of bile salts in the intestinal lumen. Bile salts apparently exert an inhibitory effect on endotoxin absorption. ATN complicates acute pancreatitis in 1.4 percent of elderly patients [121]. In our experience, oliguria is present in approximately 65 percent of the pa-tients. Blood pressure is usually in the normotensive range, although it is lower compared to that seen following recovery (by 10–20 mm Hg in every patient). The incidence of hypocalcemia is no different from that observed in other forms of ATN. The studies of Levy et al [122] suggest that hypovolemia induced by the release of specific enzymes from the inflamed pancreas, with subsequent loss of protein-rich plasma from the vascular space, appears to be responsible for the renal damage.

Pigment-Induced
This form of ATN occurs less frequently in the elderly compared to younger patients [35]. The nontraumatic form of rhabdomyolysis sec-ondary to influenza-like illness, seizures, alcoholism, and muscle necro-sis associated with gangrene due to vascular occlusion [123] are more prevalent in the elderly compared to the post-traumatic variety. Also, ARF associated with hemolysis is far less common than that associated with rhabdomyolysis in our experience. As in younger patients with these complications, volume contraction is almost universally present. Oliguria is present in 40 percent of patients and hypocalcemia in 65 per-cent [124]. The exact mechanisms by which myoglobin or hemoglobin induce renal failure are not clear. Since both substances contain iron, it is quite possible that intracellular formation of toxic oxygen radicals and the generation of potentially cytotoxic fatty acids are involved [125]. Since volume contraction plays a significant role in pigment-induced nephropathy, it is suggested that an alkaline solute diuresis be imme-diately instituted in such patients [126].

Acute Tubular Necrosis in Surgical Patients
ATN complicates the course in 18.4 percent of elderly surgical patients (see Table 10-1). Except in abdominal aortic aneurysmectomy and inter-

vention in the jaundiced patient (see previous section on hepatobiliary disease), in our experience the rate of ATN does not depend on the type of procedure being performed. Hypotension, particularly in patients who are volume contracted (owing to continuation of diuretics and a low-salt diet during the preoperative period in a patient with pre-existing chronic renal insufficiency), and sepsis secondary to abscess formation or a perforated viscus are responsible for most of the cases occurring during the perioperative period. At various times during the recovery period, cardiovascular catastrophes or sepsis due to wound, lung, or genitourinary infections become the predominant factors. Multiple factors were present in 78 percent of our patients.

The overall incidence of ATN in the elderly undergoing abdominal aortic surgery varies between 14 and 24 percent [127, 128]. In this group, the majority of patients (68 percent in one study) [129] had undergone emergency surgery for a ruptured aneurysm. Hypotension, prolonged ischemic time in patients requiring suprarenal aortic clamping, and atheroembolic disease (see Chap. 13) are primarily responsible for the renal failure [130, 131], which is nonoliguric in the majority of patients, reflecting the current practice of rapid fluid replacement and intraoperative use of mannitol. Since the presence of ARF unfavorably alters the outcome, Swan-Ganz catheterization and volume loading should be undertaken whenever feasible before, during, and after surgery. In one study, in which fluid balance was carefully monitored and the pulmonary artery wedge pressure was kept at 10 mm H_2O, the occurrence of ARF was decreased by one-third [128].

TREATMENT

Therapy for ATN is supportive. Attention should be paid to fluid homeostasis, particularly in the oliguric patient. In our experience, volume overload in an elderly patient with pre-existing cardiac disease constitutes the most common indication for initiating dialytic therapy (60 percent). Uncontrolled hyperkalemia and acidosis necessitate dialysis in 15 percent. The remaining 25 percent of patients requiring dialysis is made up in large part of patients with multiple organ failure in addition to ATN. It has been our approach to start dialysis early, although no firm data are available to suggest that this approach necessarily improves the mortality rate.

Since oliguria in itself constitutes a risk factor for increasing mortality, large doses of furosemide (200–500 mg) with or without dopamine (1–3 μg per kg per minute) should be administered [5, 140–144]. Using this approach, 40 percent of patients can be converted from an oliguric to a nonoliguric form of ATN. The transition from oliguria to nonoliguria, however, does not hasten recovery. We usually start with 200 mg of furosemide administered intravenously and increase the dose every 2 to

3 hours if there is no response up to a maximum single dose of 500 mg. About a third of our patients who responded to this regimen reverted to oliguria within a short period of time, often following a second renal insult. Mortality in this group approaches 100 percent.

Dialysis
All three dialytic interventions presently available, including peritoneal dialysis, hemodialysis, and continuous arteriovenous hemofiltration with dialysis (CAVHD, a combination of dialysis with hemofiltration), have been used successfully in the elderly [145–147]. In general, these modalities are as well tolerated in the elderly as in younger patients. The choice of one over another is dictated by the treating physician's experience. We use peritoneal dialysis as our first choice for most patients. For elderly patients with severe hyperkalemia (serum K > 6.5 mEq per liter) accompanied by acidosis and marked catabolism, hemodialysis is preferred. Patients requiring the removal of large amounts of fluid, those with recent or old abdominal surgical scars, and those requiring large amounts of fluid for nutritional purposes can be treated by CAVHD [148]. In our experience, the specific mode of renal replacement therapy does not directly influence the mortality rate, although the morbidity associated with hemodialysis or CAVHD (bleeding related to the administration of heparin and hypotension) is somewhat higher than that seen with peritoneal dialysis (hyperglycemia, peritonitis, and bloody dialysate returns). Twenty to sixty percent of elderly patients with ATN require dialysis [1, 34].

Nutrition
In the critically ill elderly patient, attention should be paid to providing adequate nutrition. The gastrointestinal tract remains the optimal route for the delivery of nutrients and should be used first unless there are clear contraindications. In patients who are unable to ingest food normally, a nasogastric tube may be necessary. If this situation is prolonged, a feeding gastrostomy or jejunostomy may be necessary [149, 150]. Once the method of delivery has been chosen, a continuous infusion of any of the available feeding mixtures can be used. We generally start with a half-strength concentration at a rate of 50 ml per hour and gradually increase the strength as well as the infusion rate, depending on the patient's tolerance, until the desired volume and caloric requirements are achieved. Formulas for calculating caloric requirements in the basal as well as in the stressed state are available [151–153]. For patients in whom enteral feeding, is not possible, peripheral vein total parenteral nutrition or central venous hyperalimentation should be used. We prefer the latter approach in the postoperative patient. The composition of the infusate is similar to that outlined by Abel et al [154]. Although the use of specific

nutritional support does provide a marginal improvement in nitrogen balance and reduces catabolism, in our experience this intervention has not changed the course or the outcome of ATN in the elderly.

PROGNOSIS

A higher mortality has been found in older patients with ATN compared with younger patients in most series published prior to 1980 [132, 133]. Since 1980, age as a risk factor for increased mortality in patients with ATN has been found in only a few studies [3, 7, 8, 134]. Based on our personal experience and that of many others [1, 5, 6, 9, 34, 35, 129, 135–137], we doubt that age per se has any bearing on the prognosis of the patient with ATN except in those who develop renal failure following aortic aneurysmectomy. In this group, patients over 70 years of age definitely have a statistically higher mortality than younger patients [128, 130]. Most studies suggest (as does our personal experience) that the concomitant presence of pulmonary complications such as respiratory failure, jaundice, cardiovascular complications, sepsis, and oliguria are associated with a poor outcome in the elderly with ATN [1, 3, 35, 138]. The overall mortality for ATN in the elderly is 36 to 58 percent [1, 8, 9, 34, 133, 139].

Seventy-five to eighty percent of the elderly with ischemic ATN die during the maintenance phase of renal failure. The average recovery time for those who survive varies between 16 and 20 days and follows a pattern similar to the B pattern described by Myers and Moran [155]. A small number of patients with congestive heart failure, diabetes mellitus, or renovascular disease who develop ischemic ATN superimposed on chronic renal insufficiency do survive but rarely recover premorbid kidney function and often require maintenance hemodialysis. The long-term outcome in such patients has been generally poor.

Mortality in our population of elderly patients with nephrotoxic ATN is less than 10 percent. The overall incidence in the adult population is approximately 13 percent [3, 156]. Dialytic intervention is required in 20 percent of patients, with permanent renal damage ensuing in 8 percent, mainly diabetics. In general, the recovery period tends to be significantly longer in the elderly.

As noted, the serum creatinine in patients with ATN secondary to contrast nephropathy usually peaks on the third or fourth day, and recovery is usually complete by 10 to 14 days, with the great majority of patients returning to the pretreatment level of kidney function [94]. Dialysis is rarely necessary, except in diabetics who occasionally are left with a persistently lower level of kidney function that only rarely requires maintenance dialysis.

Mortality in the elderly with ARF associated with liver disease is high, approaching 100 percent in those with the hepatorenal syndrome. The recovery rate in patients with biliary tract disease and renal failure varies between 44 and 76 percent [114, 115, 118]. With acute pancreatitis, no specific data are available, but all of our elderly patients recovered kidney function.

Most elderly patients with pigment-induced ATN do well, particularly those with nontrauma-related rhabdomyolysis.

Mortality for patients with ARF following aortic aneurysm repair is between 63 and 77 percent and is worse in patients over 70 years of age. Mortality is only 12 percent in patients who do not develop renal failure [128, 130]. A significant number of patients who survive have residual chronic renal insufficiency, which may be severe enough to require maintenance dialysis. This complication is particularly common in patients with pre-existing renovascular disease and is usually a result of cholesterol embolization [130].

DIFFERENTIAL DIAGNOSIS

The diagnosis of ATN is usually made on the basis of the history, physical examination, and routine laboratory data. Once the diagnosis has been established, patients follow a fairly predictable course. In 5 to 15 percent of elderly with ARF in whom the findings are confusing, particularly when no precipitating event is evident, or in whom the clinical course is atypical, other diagnostic steps such as a percutaneous kidney biopsy or a renal angiogram are needed [1, 3, 157]. In this group of patients ATN is found in 15 percent, acute interstitial nephritis in 30 percent, acute atheroembolic disease in 30 percent, acute glomerulonephritis in 19 percent, and other diseases in 6 percent [35, 157–159].

ACUTE INTERSTITIAL NEPHRITIS

Acute interstitial nephritis (AIN) is a disorder characterized on biopsy by diffuse infiltration of the renal interstitium by mononuclear inflammatory cells and eosinophils, tubulitis, and, on occasion, scattered noncaseating granulomas with multinucleated giant cells [160]. A cell-mediated immune mechanism involving activated T cells that release lymphokines and eosinophil chemotactic factors appears to be primarily responsible for the renal findings [161, 162]. Eosinophil activation and degranulation with release of the eosinophil basic protein, a known epithelial toxin, are also of pathogenetic importance (Fig. 10-1) [163, 164].

AIN may be idiopathic or related to an infection or a drug [165]. The idiopathic and infectious varieties occur infrequently in the elderly in our experience. Drug-induced AIN is the most common form of this disease seen in the elderly. Its true incidence in this age group is not known,

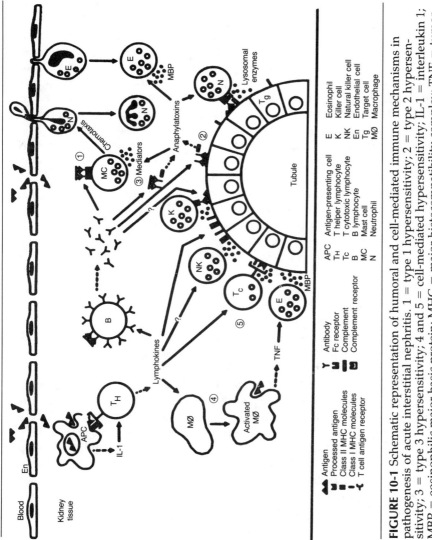

FIGURE 10-1 Schematic representation of humoral and cell-mediated immune mechanisms in pathogenesis of acute interstitial nephritis. 1 = type 1 hypersensitivity; 2 = type 2 hypersensitivity; 3 = type 3 hypersensitivity; 4 and 5 = cell-mediated hypersensitivity; IL-1 = interleukin 1; MBP = eosinophilic major basic protein; MHC = major histocompatibility complex; TNF = tumor necrosis factor. (From Ten RM, et al: Acute interstitial nephritis: Immunologic and clinical aspects. *Mayo Clin Proc* 63:921–930, 1988.)

but it was present in 15 to 30 percent of the patients in whom biopsies were done and 6.7 percent of all cases of ARF reported by Lameire and associates [35, 166, 167]. Eight percent of elderly patients with acute intrinsic renal failure evaluated by us in 1989 had findings and a clinical course compatable with AIN.

The list of drugs implicated in the etiology of AIN is quite extensive [165], but in the elderly the major offenders are NSAIDs (fenoprofen and meclofenamate more so than the others), antibiotics (penicillins, cephalosporins, sulfonamides, rifampin), diuretics (furosemide, potassium-sparing agents), and others (allopurinol, cimetidine, captopril). Acute deterioration of renal function is the most common manifestation of AIN, which can occur anytime from hours to months after the offending drug has been started [155, 168]. Skin rash, fever, and eosinophiluria were found in less than one-third of our patients. The urine indices (U_{Na}, RFI, and FE_{Na}) are similar to those characteristic of patients with ATN and therefore are not specifically helpful diagnostically [169]. Eosinophiluria, defined as eosinophils constituting more than 1 percent of urinary leukocytes, is a very helpful sign when detected (this may require Hansel's stain) but is present in only a minority of patients and may also be seen in patients with rapidly progressive glomerulonephritis, a relatively common cause of ARF in the elderly [170]. Hematuria is uncommon. Proteinuria is common, usually less than 1 g of protein per 24 hours, but may reach nephrotic range when AIN is due to an NSAID (see Chap. 7). The value of the gallium scan of the kidneys has been limited in our experience [171]. The urinary level of eosinophilic major basic protein as measured by radioimmunoassay has been found to be elevated in patients with AIN compared to those with other forms of kidney disease [164]. Further experience with this test is necessary before its value in the diagnosis of AIN can be assessed.

Since the definitive diagnosis of AIN can be made only on kidney biopsy, which may not be immediately feasible in all patients in whom the disease is suspected, it is prudent to discontinue the suspected drug if the diagnosis is entertained. In patients taking multiple drugs, we usually start with the one with the highest probability of inducing AIN. Withdrawal of the offending drug usually leads to resolution of symptoms over a variable period of time (days to weeks). Glucocorticoids (prednisone 60 mg per day given orally, with rapid tapering once kidney function stabilizes or returns to baseline) can be used. The beneficial effect of this therapy is supported by several retrospective studies [165]. The prognosis of AIN is good in the elderly, the majority of patients recovering baseline kidney function. In some patients (less than 5 percent in our experience) permanent loss of kidney function may occur, particularly in diabetics.

OTHER FORMS OF ARF

Renal artery occlusion and cholesterol embolization may produce ARF (see Chap. 13). Acute glomerulonephritis is responsible for 19 percent of cases of ARF in the elderly. Extracapillary glomerulonephritis, either idiopathic or associated with a systemic disease, is responsible for 69 percent of these cases [159]. Among the remaining 31 percent, various other forms of glomerular diseases have been found on histologic examination, IgA nephritis being the most common. Hematuria, red cell casts, and proteinuria are usually present in these patients.

Other disorders such as multiple myeloma, amyloidosis, scleroderma, and hemolytic uremic syndrome can induce ARF and are discussed elsewhere (see Chap. 7).

REFERENCES

1. Pascual J, et al: Incidence and prognosis of acute renal failure in older patients. *J Am Geriatr Soc* 38:25–30, 1990.
2. McInnes EG, et al: Renal failure in the elderly. *Q J Med* 243:583–588, 1987.
3. Turney JH, et al: The evolution of acute renal failure, 1956–1988. *Q J Med* 273:83–104, 1990.
4. Scott RB, et al: Why the persistently high mortality in acute renal failure? *Lancet* 2:75–79, 1972.
5. Minuth AN, Terrell JB Jr, and Suki WN: Acute renal failure: a study of the course and prognosis of 104 patients and of the role of furosemide. *Am J Med Sci* 271:317–324, 1976.
6. Abreo K, Moarthy A, and Osborne M: Changing patterns and outcome of acute renal failure requiring hemodialysis. *Arch Intern Med* 146:1338–1341, 1986.
7. Lien J and Chan V: Risk factors influencing survival in acute renal failure treated by hemodialysis. *Arch Intern Med* 145:2067–2069, 1985.
8. Bullock ML, et al: The assessment of risk factors in 462 patients with acute renal failure. *Am J Kidney Dis* 2:97–103, 1985.
9. Rosenfeld JB, et al: Acute renal failure: a disease of the elderly? *Adv Nephrol* 16:159–168, 1987.
10. Wollam GL, et al: Diuretic potency of combined hydrochlorothiazide and furosemide therapy in patients with azotemia. *Am J Med* 72:929–938, 1982.
11. Chung HM, et al: Clinical assessment of extracellular fluid volume in hyponatremia. *Am J Med* 83:905–908, 1987.
12. Anderson RJ, Gabow PA, and Gross PA: Urinary chloride concentration in acute renal failure. *Min Electrol Metab* 10:92–97, 1984.
13. Chou, SY, et al: Inner medullary hemodynamics in chronic salt-depleted dogs. *Am J Physiol* 246:F146–F154, 1984.
14. Shapiro JI and Anderson RJ: Sodium Depletion States. In *Contemporary Issues in Nephrology*, Vol. 16. New York: Churchill Livingstone, 1987. Pp. 246–276.
15. Steiner RW, Tucker BJ, and Blantz RC: Glomerular hemodynamics in rats with chronic sodium depletion. *J Clin Invest* 64:503–512, 1979.
16. Myers BD, et al: Dynamics of glomerular ultrafiltration following open-heart surgery. *Kidney Int* 20:366–374, 1981.

17. Cody RJ, et al: Relation of glomerular filtration rate in chronic congestive heart failure patients. *Kidney Int* 34:361–367, 1988.
18. Blackshear JL, Davidman M, and Stillman T: Identification of risk for renal insufficiency from nonsteroidal anti-inflammatory drugs. *Arch Intern Med* 143:1130–1134, 1983.
19. Corwin HL and Bonventre JV: Renal insufficiency associated with non-steroidal anti-inflammatory agents. *Am J Kidney Dis* 4:147–152, 1984.
20. McCarthy JT, et al: Acute intrinsic renal failure induced by indomethacin. Role of prostaglandin synthetase inhibition. *Mayo Clin Proc* 57:289–296, 1982.
21. Cinotti GA, et al: Effects of sulindac and ibuprofen in patients with chronic glomerular disease. Evidence of the dependence of renal function on prostacyclin. *N Engl J Med* 310:279–283, 1984.
22. Abraham PA and Stillman TM: Salsalate exacerbation of chronic renal insufficiency. Relation to inhibition of prostaglandin synthesis. *Arch Intern Med* 147:1674–1676, 1987.
23. Horton R, Zipser R, and Fichman M: Prostaglandins, renal function and vascular regulation. *Med Clin North Am* 64:891–914, 1981.
24. Franklin SS and Smith RD: Comparison of effects of enalapril plus hydrochlorothiazide versus standard triple therapy on renal function in renovascular hypertension. *Am J Med* (Suppl 3C) 79:14–23, 1985.
25. Hollenberg NK: The treatment of renovascular hypertension: surgery, angioplasty and medical therapy converting-enzyme inhibitors. *Am J Kidney Dis* (Suppl 1) 10:52–60, 1987.
26. Packer M, et al: Functional renal insufficiency during long term therapy with captopril and enalapril in severe chronic heart failure. *Ann Intern Med* 106:346–354, 1987.
27. Packer M, et al: Comparison of captopril and enalapril in patients with severe chronic heart failure. *N Engl J Med* 315:847–853, 1986.
28. Lynn KL, Bailey RR, and Swainson CP: Renal failure with potassium-sparing diuretics. *NZ Med J* 98:629–633, 1985.
29. Brater DC, et al: Bumetanide and furosemide in heart failure. *Kidney Int* 26:183–189, 1984.
30. Kerremans ALM, et al: Furosemide kinetics and dynamics in aged patients. *Clin Pharmacol Ther* 34:181–189, 1983.
31. Voelker JR, et al: Comparison of loop diuretics in patients with chronic renal insufficiency. *Kidney Int* 32:572–578, 1987.
32. Oster JR, Epstein M, and Smoller S: Combined therapy with thiazide-type and loop-type diuretic agents for resistant sodium retention. *Ann Intern Med* 99:405–406, 1983.
33. Bartlett RH, et al: Continuous arteriovenous hemofiltration for acute renal failure. *Trans Am Soc Artif Intern Organs* 34:67–77, 1988.
34. Kumar R, Hill CM, and McGeown MG: Acute renal failure in the elderly. *Lancet* 1:90–91, 1973.
35. Lameire N, et al: Acute Renal Failure in the Elderly. In Oreopoulos DG (ed), *Geriatric Nephrology*. Boston: Martinus Nijhoff, 1986. Pp. 103–116.
36. Anderson RJ, et al: Non-oliguric acute renal failure. *N Engl J Med* 296:1134–1138, 1977.
37. Oken DE: On the differential diagnosis of acute renal failure. *Am J Med* 71:916–920, 1981.
38. Wilson DR and Honrath U: Inner medullary collecting duct function in ischemic acute renal failure. *Clin Invest Med* 11:157–166, 1988.
39. Fang LS, et al: Low fractional excretion of sodium with contrast media-induced acute renal failure. *Arch Intern Med* 140:531–533, 1980.

40. Sporm NI, Lancestremere RG, and Papper S: Differential diagnosis of oliguria in aged patients. *N Engl J Med* 267:130–132, 1962.
41. Dixon BS and Anderson RJ: Non-oliguric acute renal failure. *Am J Kidney Dis* 6:71–80, 1985.
42. Mason J: The pathophysiology of ischemic acute renal failure. A new hypothesis about the initiation phase. *Renal Physiol* 9:129–147, 1986.
43. Stromski ME, et al: Metabolic and functional consequences of inhibiting adenosine deaminase during renal ischemia in rats. *J Clin Invest* 82:1694–1699, 1988.
44. Brezis M, et al: Renal ischemia: A new perspective. *Kidney Int* 26:375–383, 1984.
45. Moran SM and Myers BD: Pathophysiology of protracted acute renal failure in man. *J Clin Invest* 76:1440–1448, 1985.
46. Oken DE: Hemodynamic basis for human acute renal failure (vasomotor nephropathy). *Am J Med* 76:702–710, 1984.
47. Myers BD, et al: Pathophysiology of hemodynamically mediated acute renal failure in man. *Kidney Int* 18:495–504, 1980.
48. Meyers BD, et al: Glomerular and tubular function in non-oliguric acute renal failure. *Am J Med* 72:642–649, 1982.
49. Thurau K and Boylan JW: Acute renal success: The unexpected logic of oliguria in acute renal failure. *Am J Med* 61:308–315, 1976.
50. McCoy CE, et al: Adenosine triphosphate depletion induces a rise in cytosolic free calcium in canine renal epithelial cells. *J Clin Invest* 82:1326–1332, 1988.
51. Epstein FH and Brown RS: Acute renal failure: A collection of paradoxes. *Hosp Pract* 1:171–194, 1988.
52. Henrich WL, et al: Dissociation of systemic and renal effects of endotoxemia. Prostaglandin inhibition uncovers an important role of renal nerves. *J Clin Invest* 69:691–699, 1982.
53. Wang J and Dunn MJ: Platelet-activating factor mediates endotoxin-induced acute renal insufficiency in rats. *Am J Physiol* 253:F1283–F1289, 1987.
54. Badr KF, et al: Roles for thromboxane A_2 and leukotrienes in endotoxin induced acute renal failure. *Kidney Int* 30:474–480, 1986.
55. Law WK, et al: Comparative efficacy and toxicity of amikacin/carbenicillin versus gentamicin/carbenicillin in leukopenic patients. *Am J Med* 62:959–966, 1977.
56. Smith CR, et al: Controlled comparison of amikacin and gentamicin. *N Engl J Med* 296:349–353, 1977.
57. Smith CR, et al: Double-blind comparison of the nephrotoxicity and auditory toxicity of gentamicin and tobramycin. *N Engl J Med* 30:1106–1109, 1980.
58. Lane AZ, Wright GE, and Blair DC: Ototoxicity and nephrotoxicity of amikacin: An overview of phase II and phase III in the United States. *Am J Med* 62:911–918, 1977.
59. Schentag JJ, et al: Gentamicin tissue accumulation and nephrotoxic reactions. *JAMA* 240:2067–2069, 1978.
60. Zaske DE, et al: Wide interpatient variations in gentamicin dose requirements for geriatric patients. *JAMA* 248:3122–3126, 1982.
61. Kumin GD: Clinical nephrotoxicity of tobramycin and gentamicin. A prospective study. *JAMA* 244:1808–1810, 1980.
62. Whelton A and Solez K: Aminoglycoside nephrotoxicity. A tale of 2 transports. *J Lab Clin Med* 99:148–155, 1982.
63. Humes HD, Weinberg JM, and Knauss TC: Clinical and pathophysiologic aspect of aminoglycoside nephrotoxicity. *Am J Kidney Dis* 2:5–29, 1982.
64. Moore RD, Smith CR, and Lietman PS: Increased risk of renal dysfuncion

due to interaction of liver disease and aminoglycosides. *Am J Med* 80:1092–1097, 1986.

65. Smith CR, Moore RD, and Lietman PS: Studies of risk factors for aminoglycoside nephrotoxicity. *Am J Kidney Dis* 8:308–313, 1986.

66. Hsu CH, et al: Renal tubular sodium and water excretion in antibiotic-induced nephrotoxicity. Renal function in antibiotic nephrotoxicity. *Nephron* 20:227–234, 1978.

67. Player JE: Association of renal injury combined with cephalothin-gentamicin therapy among patients severely ill with malignant disease. *Cancer* 37:1937–1941, 1976.

68. Foord D: Cephaloridine, cephalothin and the kidney. *J Antimicrob Chemother* (Suppl 1) 1:119–133, 1975.

69. Burton JR, et al: Acute renal failure during cephalothin therapy. *JAMA* 229:679–682, 1974.

70. Carling PC, et al: Nephrotoxicity associated with cephalothin administration. *Arch Intern Med* 135:797–801, 1975.

71. Fung-Herrera CG and Mulvaney WP: Cephalexin nephrotoxicity. Reversible nonoliguric acute renal failure and hepatotoxicity associated with cephalexin therapy. *JAMA* 229:318–319, 1974.

72. Barientos A, Bello I, and Gutierrez-Millet V: Renal failure and cephalothin. *Ann Intern Med* 84:612, 1976.

73. Saah AJ, Koch TR, and Drusano GL: Cefoxitin falsely elevates creatinine levels. *JAMA* 247:205–206, 1982.

74. Miller RP and Bates JH: Amphotericin B toxicity. A follow-up report of 53 patients. *Ann Intern Med* 71:1089–1095, 1969.

75. Terrell CL and Hermans PE: Antifungal agents used for deep-seated mycotic infections. *Mayo Clin Proc* 62:1116–1128, 1987.

76. Iovine G, et al: Nephrotoxicity of amphotericin B. *Arch Intern Med* 112:853–862, 1963.

77. Wertlake PT, et al: Nephrotoxic tubular damage and calcium deposition following amphotericin B therapy. *Am J Pathol* 43:449–457, 1963.

78. Androli TE: On the anatomy of amphotericin B-cholesterol pores in lipid bilayer membranes. *Kidney Int* 4:337–345, 1973.

79. Phillips ME, et al: Tetracycline poisoning in renal failure. *Br Med J* 2:149–151, 1974.

80. Adams DH, et al: Non-steroidal antiinflammatory drugs and renal failure. *Lancet* 1:57–60, 1986.

81. Smith HJ, et al: High dose urography in patients with renal failure: A double-blind investigation of iohexol and metrizoate. *Acta Radiol Diagn* 26:213–220, 1985.

82. Adgard S, et al: Acute renal insufficiency after administration of low-osmolar contrast media. *Lancet* 2:1281, 1986.

83. Cavaliere G, et al: Tubular nephrotoxicity after intravenous urography with ionic high-osmolal and non-ionic low-osmolal contrast media in patients with chronic renal insufficiency. *Nephron* 46:128–133, 1987.

84. Jerrikar AM, et al: Nephrotoxicity of high- and low-osmolality contrast media. *Nephron* 48:300–305, 1988.

85. Schwab SJ, et al: Contrast nephrotoxicity: A randomized controlled trial of a nonionic and an ionic radiographic contrast agent. *N Engl J Med* 320:149–153, 1989.

86. Swartz RD, et al: Renal failure following major angiography. *Am J Med* 65:31–37, 1978.

87. Carvallo A, et al: Acute renal failure following drip infusion pyelography. *Am J Med* 65:38–45, 1978.

88. Van Zee B, et al: Renal injury associated with intravenous pyelography in non-diabetic and diabetic patients. *Ann Intern Med* 89:51–54, 1978.
89. Byrd L and Sherman RL: Radiocontrast-induced acute renal failure: a clinical and pathophysiologic review. *Medicine* 58:268–279, 1979.
90. Ansari Z and Baldwin DS: Acute renal failure due to radio-contrast agents. *Nephron* 17:28–40, 1976.
91. Krumlovsky FA, et al: Acute renal failure: Association with administration of radiographic contrast material. *JAMA* 239:125–127, 1978.
92. Alexander RD, Berkes SL, and Abuelo JG: Contrast media-induced oliguric renal failure. *Arch Intern Med* 138:381–384, 1978.
93. Fang LST, et al: Low fractional excretion of sodium with contrast media-induced acute renal failure. *Arch Intern Med* 140:531–533, 1980.
94. Shafi T, et al: Infusion intravenous pyelography and renal function: Effects in patients with chronic renal insufficiency. *Arch Intern Med* 138:1218–1221, 1978.
95. Arkonen S and Kjellstrand CM: Intravenous pyelography in nonuremic diabetic patients. *Nephron* 24:268–270, 1979.
96. Anto HR, et al: Infusion intravenous pyelography and renal function: Effects of hypertonic mannitol in patients with chronic renal insufficiency. *Arch Intern Med* 141:1652–1656, 1981.
97. D'Elia JA, et al: Inadequacy of fractional excretion of sodium test. *Arch Intern Med* 141:818, 1981.
98. Norby LH and DiBona GF: The renal vascular effects of meglumine diatrizoate. *J Pharmacol Exp Ther* 193:932–940, 1975.
99. Brazis M and Epstein FH: A closer look at radiocontrast-induced nephropathy. *N Engl J Med* 320:179–181, 1989.
100. McKenzie JK, Patel R, and McQueen EG: The excretion rate of Tamm-Horsfall urinary mucoprotein in normals and in patients with renal disease. *Aust NZ J Med* 13:32–39, 1964.
101. Vari RC, et al: Induction, prevention and mechanisms of contrast media-induced acute renal failure. *Kidney Int* 33:699–707, 1988.
102. Berns AS: Nephrotoxicity of contrast media. *Kidney Int* 36:730–740, 1989.
103. Porush JG, et al: Infusion intravenous pyelography and renal function: Effects of hypertonic mannitol and furosemide in patients with chronic renal insufficiency. In Eliahou HE (ed), *Acute Renal Failure*. London: John Libbey, 1982. Pp. 161–167.
104. Cigarroa RG, et al: Dosing of contrast material to prevent contrast nephropathy in patients with renal disease. *Am J Med* 86:649–652, 1989.
105. Schilsky RL: Renal and metabolic toxicities of cancer chemotherapy. *Semin Oncol* 9:75–83, 1982.
106. Ries F and Klastersky J: Nephrotoxicity induced by cancer chemotherapy with special emphasis on cisplatin toxicity. *Am J Kidney Dis* 8:368–379, 1986.
107. Sadoff I: Nephrotoxicity of streptozotocin (NSC-85998). *Cancer Chemother Rep* 54:457–459, 1979.
108. Hrushesky WJM, Shimp W, and Kennedy BJ: Lack of age-dependent cisplatin nephrotoxicity. *Am J Med* 76:579–584, 1984.
109. Safirstein R, et al: Cisplatin nephrotoxicity. *Am J Kidney Dis* 8:356–367, 1986.
110. Klinenberg JR, et al: Urate deposition disease: How is it regulated and how can it be modified. *Ann Intern Med* 78:99–111, 1973.
111. Kleinman JG, Breitenfield RV, and Roth DA: Acute renal failure associated with acetaminophen ingestion: Report of a case and review of the literature. *Clin Nephrol* 14:201–205, 1980.
112. Gabriel R, et al: Acute Renal Failure Following Therapeutic Dose of Parace-

tamol (Acetaminophen). In Eliahou HE (ed), *Acute Renal Failure.* London: John Libbey, 1982. Pp. 125–128.

113. Roxe DM: Toxic nephropathy from diagnostic and therapeutic agents: Review and commentary. *Am J Med* 69:759–774, 1980.

114. Anderson JB, Sorensen FH, and Skjoldborg H: Acute renal failure in association with choledocholithiasis. *Acta Clin Scand* 137:81–86, 1971.

115. Bismuth H, Kuntziger H, and Corlette MB: Cholangitis with acute renal failure. Priorities in therapeutics. *Ann Surg* 181:881–887, 1975.

116. Green J, et al: The "jaundiced heart": A possible explanation for postoperative shock in obstructive jaundice. *Surgery* 100:14–20, 1986.

117. Better OS: Renal and cardiovascular dysfunction in liver disease. *Kidney Int* 29:598–607, 1986.

118. Wait RB and Kahng K: Renal failure complicating obstructive jaundice. *Am J Surg* 157:256–263, 1989.

119. Coratelli P and Passovanti G: Pathophysiology of renal failure in obstructive jaundice. *Min Electrol Metab* 16:61–65, 1990.

120. Bailey ME: Endotoxin, bile salts and renal function in obstructive jaundice. *Br J Surg* 63:774–778, 1976.

121. Park J, Fromkes J, and Cooperman M: Acute pancreatitis in elderly patients. Pathogenesis and outcome. *Am J Surg* 152:638–642, 1986.

122. Levy M, Guller R, and Hymovitch S: Renal failure in dogs with experimental acute pancreatitis: Role of hypovolemia. *Am J Physiol* 251:F969–F977, 1986.

123. Haimovici H: Muscular, renal and metabolic complications of acute arterial occlusions: Myonephropathic-metabolic syndrome. *Surgery* 85:461–468, 1979.

124. Gabow PA, Kaehny WD, and Kelleher SP: The spectrum of rhabdomyolysis. *Medicine* 61:141–152, 1982.

125. Peller MS: Hemoglobin- and myoglobin-induced acute renal failure in rats: Role of iron in nephrotoxicity. *Am J Physiol* 255:F539–F544, 1988.

126. Ron D, et al: Prevention of acute renal failure in traumatic rhabdomyolysis. *Arch Intern Med* 144:277–280, 1984.

127. McComb's PR and Brooke R: Acute renal failure following resection of abdominal aortic aneurysm. *Surg Gynecol Obstet* 148:175–178, 1979.

128. Hesdorffer CS, et al: The value of Swan Ganz catheterization and volume loading in preventing renal failure in patients undergoing abdominal aneurysmectomy. *Clin Nephrol* 28:272–276, 1987.

129. Beaman M, et al: Changing pattern of acute renal failure. *Q J Med* 237:15–23, 1987.

130. Gornick CC and Kjellstrand CM: Acute renal failure complicating aortic aneurysm surgery. *Nephron* 35:145–157, 1983.

131. Myers BD, et al: Nature of renal injury following total renal ischemia in man. *J Clin Invest* 73:329–341, 1984.

132. Balslov JT and Jorgenson HE: A survey of 499 patients with acute anuric renal insufficiency. Causes, treatment, complications and mortality. *Am J Med* 34:753–764, 1963.

133. Scott RB, et al: Why the persistently high mortality in acute renal failure? *Lancet* 2:75–79, 1972.

134. Wheeler DC, Feehally J, and Walls J: High risk acute renal failure. *Q J Med* 234:977–984, 1986.

135. Rasmussen HH, et al: Prediction of outcome in acute renal failure by discriminant analysis of clinical variables. *Arch Intern Med* 145:2015–2018, 1985.

136. Corwin HL, et al: Prediction of outcome in acute renal failure. *Am J Nephrol* 7:8–12, 1987.
137. Menashe PI, Ross SA, and Gottlieb JE: Acquired renal insufficiency in critically ill patients. *Crit Care Med* 16:1106–1109, 1988.
138. Amerio A, et al: Prognosis in acute renal failure accompanied by jaundice. *Nephron* 27:152–154, 1981.
139. Oliveira DBG and Winearls CG: Acute renal failure in the elderly can have a good prognosis. *Age Aging* 13:304–308, 1984.
140. Kleinknecht D, et al: Furosemide in acute oliguric renal failure. A controlled trial. *Nephron* 17:51–58, 1976.
141. Brown CB, Ogg CS, and Cameron JS: High dose furosemide in acute renal failure. A controlled trial. *Clin Nephrol* 15:90–96, 1981.
142. Lindner A, et al: Dopamine and Furosemide in Acute Renal Failure. In Eliahou HE (ed), *Acute Renal Failure*. London: John Libbey, 1982. Pp. 174–175.
143. Parker S, et al: Dopamine administration in oliguria and oliguric renal failure. *Crit Care Med* 9:630–632, 1981.
144. Henderson IS, Beattie TJ, and Kennedy AC: Dopamine hydrochloride in oliguric states. *Lancet* 2:827–828, 1980.
145. Sonnenblick M, et al: Acute renal failure in the elderly treated by one-time peritoneal dialysis. *J Am Geriatr Soc* 36:1039–1044, 1988.
146. Gibney NRT, et al: Continuous arteriovenous hemodialysis: an alternative therapy for acute renal failure with critical illness. *Can Med Assoc J* 139:861–866, 1988.
147. Peachey TD, et al: Pump control of continuous arteriovenous haemodialysis. *Lancet* 2:878, 1988.
148. Mault JR, et al: Continuous arteriovenous filtration: An effective treatment for surgical acute renal failure. *Surgery* 101:478–484, 1987.
149. Delaney HM, et al: Postoperative nutritional support using needle catheter feeding jejunostomy. *Ann Surg* 186:165–170, 1977.
150. Ponsky JL: Percutaneous endoscopic gastrostomy: A closer look. *Endoscopy Rev* 24–29, 1984.
151. Anderson CF, Loosbrook LM, and Moxness KE: Nutrient intake in critically ill patients: Too many or too few calories? *Mayo Clin Proc* 61:853–858, 1986.
152. Staats BA, Gastineau CF, and Offord KP: Predictive equations for basal caloric requirement derived from the data of Boothby, Berkson and Dunn. *Mayo Clin Proc* 63:409–410, 1988.
153. Miller LS, et al: Enteral and parenteral nutrition in the critically ill patient. *Hosp Formul* 21:672–682, 1986.
154. Abel RM, et al: Improved survival from acute renal failure after treatment with intravenous essential L-aminoacids and glucose. Results of a prospective double-blind study. *N Engl J Med* 288:695–699, 1973.
155. Myers BD and Moran SM: Hemodynamically mediated acute renal failure. *N Engl J Med* 314:97–105, 1986.
156. Kleinknecht D, Landais P, and Goldfarb B: Drug-associated acute renal failure. A prospective multicenter report. *Kidney Int* 28:226A, 1985.
157. Faubert PF and Porush JGP: Unpublished observations, 1988.
158. DeMarco S, et al: Acute renal failure in the elderly: A retrospective clinicopathological analysis of 17 cases. *Min Electrol Metab* 12:259A, 1986.
159. Tanter Y, et al: Acute renal failure secondary to glomerular disease in patients over 65 years. *Min Electrol Metab* 12:273A, 1986.
160. Mignon F, Méry JP, and Morel-Maroger L: Granulomatous tubulointerstitial nephritis. *Adv Nephrol* 13:219–245, 1984.

161. Husby G, Tung KSK, and Williams RC Jr: Characterization of renal tissue lymphocytes in patients with interstitial nephritis. *Am J Med* 70:31–38, 1981.
162. Finkelstein A, et al: Fenoprofen nephropathy: Lipoid nephrosis and interstitial nephritis. A possible T-lymphocyte disorder. *Am J Med* 72:81–87, 1982.
163. Ten RM, et al: Localization of eosinophil major basic protein (MBP) in kidney disease. *Kidney Int* 31:339A, 1987.
164. Ten RM, et al: Acute interstitial nephritis: Immunologic and clinical aspects. *Mayo Clin Proc* 63:921–930, 1988.
165. Cameron JS: Allergic interstitial nephritis: Clinical features and pathogenesis. *Q J Med* 250:97–115, 1988.
166. Preston RA, et al: Renal biopsy in patients 65 years of age or older: An analysis of the results of 334 biopsies. *J Am Geriatr Soc* 38:669–674, 1990.
167. Modesto-Segondo A, et al: Renal biopsy in the elderly. *Kidney Int* 38:1237A, 1990.
168. Linton AL, et al: Acute interstitial nephritis due to drugs. Review of the literature with a report of nine cases. *Ann Intern Med* 93:735–741, 1980.
169. Lins RL, et al: Urinary indices in acute interstitial nephritis. *Clin Nephrol* 26:131–133, 1986.
170. Nolan CR III, Auger MS, and Kelleher SP: Eosinophiluria. A new method of detection and definition of the clinical spectrum. *N Engl J Med* 315:1516–1519, 1986.
171. Linton AL, et al: Gallium[67] scintigraphy in the diagnosis of acute renal disease. *Clin Nephrol* 24:84–87, 1985.

11 CHRONIC RENAL FAILURE

In general, renal failure is defined as an elevation of the BUN or serum creatinine, the latter being a more reliable parameter. In younger patients a significant loss of kidney function (up to 50 percent or more) may be present without producing an abnormal BUN or serum creatinine. In the elderly, detection of renal failure is even more of a problem because they frequently eat less protein or have a decreased muscle mass, either of which can significantly lower the BUN and/or serum creatinine. As noted in Chap. 1, there is a formula (Cockcroft and Gault) that can be used to derive the creatinine clearance from the serum creatinine level and the weight and age of the patient. In patients with abnormal results of urinalysis or other suggestions of kidney disease, a creatinine clearance (or other more accurate measurement of glomerular filtration rate [GFR]) should be obtained because the formula for deriving the creatinine clearance is only an approximation. For the purpose of this discussion an elevated BUN or serum creatinine (particularly the latter) is used as the definition of renal insufficiency; however, when contemplating the use of a nephrotoxic drug in an elderly patient, a creatinine clearance should be obtained or derived from the Cockcroft and Gault formula to make appropriate dose adjustments, if necessary.

INCIDENCE AND PREVALENCE

Chronic renal failure (CRF) is a relatively common problem in the elderly. Among elderly patients admitted to three geriatric units, 4.5 to 8.3 percent had an elevated BUN or serum creatinine, with intrinsic renal disease present in 30 to 40 percent [1]. Renal failure was the final diagnosis in 201 (15.3 percent) of 1,310 hospitalized elderly patients reported by Llera and Gregorio [2]. One-third of the patients evaluated by us during a 5-year period (1978–1982) for CRF were 60 years or older. Because the BUN and serum creatinine are rather insensitive parameters for detecting a decrease in renal function (particularly in the elderly), it is clear that the actual incidence of renal insufficiency in this group of patients must be significantly higher than the literature suggests. At the present time the highest rate of new patients entering the end-stage renal disease (ESRD) program in the United States occurs in the age group 65 years or older (Table 11-1).

TABLE 11-1. Annual percentage increase in patients
entering the end-stage renal disease program in the United States

Year	All age groups	65–74 yr old	75+ yr old
1980–1981	4.9	5.2	5.1
1981–1982	12.9	16.1	28.2
1982–1983	14.6	30.8	52.7
1983–1984	5.2	1.4	6.6
1984–1985	10.1	12.5	17.2
5-year average	9.5	13.2	22.0

SOURCE: Health Care Financing Administration, Bureau of Data Management and Strategy: Data from the program management and medical information system, August 1987.

ETIOLOGY

We evaluated 274 elderly patients with an elevated serum creatinine (> 1.5 mg per dl) between 1978 and 1982. As noted by others [3], nephrosclerosis and diabetic nephropathy constituted the two most common causes of CRF in these patients (Table 11-2). These two entities are also responsible for CRF in more than 40 percent of patients 65 years or older entering the U.S. ESRD program [4]. Sixty percent of these 274 patients (163) were male, and 39 percent (106) were black. Blacks constitute approximately 40 percent of our renal patient population.

In general, it is possible to classify patients with CRF into broad diagnostic categories on the basis of a urinalysis and 24-hour urinary protein excretion rate.

1. Glomerular disease (either primary or secondary): proteinuria of greater than 3 g per 24 hours
2. Tubulointerstitial disease: proteinuria of between 1 and 2 g per 24 hours
3. Vascular (either major arterial or arteriolar) disease: proteinuria of less than 1 g per 24 hours

It is important to note that this classification is not inclusive and that overlaps do exist. Obstructive uropathy should be ruled out either by sonography or by computed tomography (CT) in every patient with renal insufficiency. An intravenous pyelogram should be avoided in patients with CRF. Small kidneys reflect chronic advanced disease with minimal chance of reversibility. Obviously, it may be necessary to do a kidney biopsy in order to make a definitive diagnosis, particularly in patients with one of the glomerulopathies.

TABLE 11-2. Etiology of CRF in 274 elderly patients seen at the Brookdale Hospital Medical Center (1978–1982)

Diagnosis	No. patients (%)
Nephrosclerosis	113 (41.0)
Diabetic nephropathy	61 (22.0)
Tubulointerstitial disorders	37 (13.5)
Obstructive uropathy	30 (10.9)
Glomerular diseases	29 (10.6)
Hereditary: Polycystic kidney disease	4 (2.0)
Total	274 (100.0)

PATHOGENESIS AND CLINICAL MANIFESTATIONS

Unless the GFR is very low (usually less than 10 ml per minute), symptoms attributable to chronic renal disease per se are either nonspecific (such as nocturia) or completely absent. Therefore, it is not surprising that most cases of CRF are discovered during evaluation of a systemic disease known to be associated with kidney involvement or during a visit to a physician's office or hospitalization for a completely unrelated problem.

SPECIFIC DISEASE ENTITIES
Nephrosclerosis, diabetic nephropathy, obstructive uropathy, and glomerular disease have been reviewed in other chapters, as have myeloma kidney and staghorn calculi, which are the two most common forms of tubulointerstitial disease in the elderly. In this section, we will specifically address other chronic tubulointerstitial disorders and hereditary nephropathies.

Tubulointerstitial Disorders
Chronic tubulointerstitial diseases may be due to (1) drugs (analgesics, lithium), (2) metabolic disturbances (urate and oxalate nephropathy), (3) heavy metals (lead), (4) physical factors (radiation nephritis), or (5) others (sarcoidosis, chronic idiopathic interstitial nephritis).

DRUGS. The risk of developing CRF increases in daily users of phenacetin and acetaminophen, acetylsalicylic acid–acetaminophen combined (especially when taken with caffeine), and perhaps other nonsteroidal anti-inflammatory drugs as well [5, 6]. The true incidence of chronic tubulointerstitial disease in the elderly is not known but probably varies widely according to geographic area [7, 8]. We systematically take a history of analgesic use in our elderly patients and have on only very few occasions been able to attribute renal disease to analgesic abuse. Females are more commonly affected than males. Renal insufficiency of varying degree, proteinuria of less than 2,000 mg per day, sterile pyuria, and inability to concentrate urine are present in most patients. Severe volume contraction and papillary necrosis are not uncommon complications [9]. Morphologically, the early lesions consist of patchy areas of necrosis of interstitial cells, loops of Henle, and capillaries (a consequence of drug accumulation in the renal medulla), which interfere with medullary blood flow and result in medullary tissue ischemia [10]. Late findings consist of glomerular sclerosis, tubular atrophy, and interstitial as well as periglomerular fibrosis. Discontinuing the analgesic may result in stabilization or even improvement in kidney function in some patients [11, 12]. The risk of developing renal pelvic cancer appears to be higher in patients with phenacetin-induced nephropathy [13].

Tubular atrophy, interstitial fibrosis, and sclerotic glomeruli have been reported in patients on chronic therapeutic doses of lithium carbonate [14]. In a recent critical evaluation of the available evidence it was concluded that the danger of chronic renal damage from lithium per se is quite small in patients on well-controlled therapy [15]. Rather, it seems that the incidence of tubulointerstitial damage is higher in psychiatric patients taking drugs other than lithium [16]. It is recommended that a creatinine clearance be performed in every patient taking lithium prior to starting the drug and at yearly intervals thereafter. Decreasing kidney function constitutes an indication for discontinuing the drug. Lithium has also been associated with polyuria by interfering with the effect of antidiuretic hormone (ADH) on the cortical collecting tubule. Patients with this form of nephrogenic diabetes insipidus can be managed with amiloride, 5 to 10 mg administered twice a day [17]. Also, hydrochlorothiazide, 25 mg twice a day, may have an additive effect.

METABOLIC DISTURBANCES AND LEAD NEPHROPATHY. The interstitial disease caused by urates is characterized by the presence of uric acid crystals within the tubule and interstitium of the renal pyramids, accompanied by mononuclear and giant cell infiltration and fibrosis. Tophi are occasionally found in the interstitium. This form of kidney disease is rare now that allopurinol is frequently prescribed for gouty or hyperuricemic patients. Moreover, because most patients with gout are also hypertensive, it is not clear to what extent the latter contributes to the renal insufficiency. Recently, some authors have proposed that the kidney damage apparent in gouty patients might represent lead rather than uric acid toxicity [18, 19]. Histologically, the so-called gouty and lead nephropathies share the same characteristics—tubulointerstitial scarring and nephrosclerosis—making it difficult to differentiate between them. When in doubt, lead excretion should be measured 24 to 72 hours after parenteral administration of 1 to 2 g of EDTA. More than 600 mg per 24 hours of urinary lead constitutes a positive test result [20]. We have used allopurinol in hyperuricemic patients with gout and renal insufficiency and a negative EDTA test; however, in our limited experience, this approach has not prevented further progression of the kidney disease. Experience with the chronic use of EDTA as a chelating agent to treat lead nephropathy is limited [21] but should probably be tried. Other therapeutic modalities such as BAL, D-penicillamine, 2,3-dimercaptosuccinic acid have also been tried with some success [22].

Oxalate nephropathy should be suspected in any elderly patient with a history of chronic inflammatory bowel disease or following intestinal bypass surgery for massive obesity [23]. Hyperoxaluria (> 40 mg per 24 hours) is present in virtually every patient. Renal biopsy findings are nonspecific (unless oxalate crystal deposition is seen) and consist of periglomerular and interstitial fibrosis as well as tubular atrophy and hyalinization of glomeruli. The presence of granular deposits of immunoglobulins and C3 in the glomeruli of some patients suggests a possible immune pathogenesis. The possible beneficial effect of control of the hyperoxaluria or the underlying bowel disease (including the dismantling of the bypass) on the natural history of the nephropathy has not been demonstrated but in our opinion should be tried.

RADIATION NEPHRITIS. Chronic radiation nephritis is characterized clinically by proteinuria, hypertension, and renal insufficiency. The time elapsing between exposure (usually following an excess of 2,500 rads to both kidneys) and development of renal disease is 1 to 14 years [24]. With the newer techniques of radiation administration, this form of kidney disease is seen less frequently. Our own experience is limited to only one elderly patient who developed progressive renal insufficiency following treatment for lymphoma compressing the spinal cord. Treatment is supportive and is directed mainly at controlling the hypertension.

SARCOIDOSIS. Granulomas are commonly found on autopsy in the renal interstitium of patients with sarcoidosis. Clinical renal involvement, however, manifested by renal insufficiency, proteinuria in the range of 700 to 1,500 mg per 24 hours, and tubular dysfunction, occurs less frequently. Most cases reported have occurred in patients less than 60 years old, so this entity appears to be rare in the elderly [25–27]. On histologic evaluation, noncaseating granulomas with giant cells are present in the interstitium. Tubular atrophy and interstitial fibrosis are seen with more advanced disease. Apart from the presence of mild mesangial expansion, the glomeruli are unremarkable. Dramatic improvement in kidney function may be seen following steroid administration (40 to 60 mg daily).

IDIOPATHIC INTERSTITIAL NEPHRITIS. Occasionally, interstitial nephritis is found in elderly patients on kidney biopsy during evaluation for renal insufficiency and proteinuria for which no cause can be found. In the absence of advanced interstitial fibrosis and focal glomerular obsolescence, a short course (4 to 6 weeks) of prednisone (40 to 60 mg daily) is worth trying as long as no contraindications to its use exist. We have seen an occasional dramatic response, suggesting that the patient had a prolonged active interstitial nephritis of unknown origin.

Hereditary Nephropathies

ADULT POLYCYSTIC KIDNEY DISEASE. Adult polycystic kidney disease (APKD) is an autosomal dominant disorder in which the causative gene is linked to the short arm of chromosome 16 ($APKD_1$) [28]. There is a small fraction of individuals in whom a second locus may be responsible for the disease ($APKD_2$) [29]. Only 3 to 4 percent of patients with APKD are 60 years or older at the time of initial diagnosis [30, 31]. In 13 elderly patients seen during the past 12 years, the diagnosis of APKD was established by sonographic examination during investigation for hypertension and renal insufficiency, which are seen at presentation more often in the elderly than in younger patients with this disease. The incidence of other symptoms such as back pain, renal colic, hematuria, and urinary tract infection is similar to that in younger patients [32, 33]. The renal insufficiency in APKD is progressive. The rate of progression, however, varies from patient to patient and, as recently shown, depends on (1) the patient's genetic makeup—those with $APKD_2$ tend to progress slower than those with $APKD_1$ [34]; (2) blood pressure—extensive arterio- and arteriolar nephroscleroses are common histologic findings in APKD patients with advanced renal failure [33]; (3) left ventricular mass [35]; (4) gender—males do worse than females [35]; and (5) renal volume [35]. APKD patients also have a higher incidence of intracranial saccular aneurysms, various cardiac valvular abnormalities (mitral valve prolapse or aortic or tricuspid insufficiency), and inguinal hernia [36]. The prevalence of these associated abnormalities in the elderly with APKD is not known.

The cause and mechanism of cyst formation in patients with APKD is not clear. Renal tubular epithelial cells taken from patients with APKD synthesize an abnormal basement membrane in tissue culture [37], lending support to the hypothesis that the cysts result from collapse or atrophy of tubules with a primary defect in the basement membrane [38]. Also, epithelial cells within the cyst wall with an altered basement membrane could dedifferentiate and exhibit increased proliferation. Cysts with either proximal or distal tubular characteristics have been found in APKD patients [39]. The solute content of proximal cyst fluid is similar to that of serum taken from the patient, whereas distal cysts contain fluid that has a lower sodium (Na) and chloride (Cl) and a higher potassium (K), creatinine, and urea concentration than the serum.

The management of hypertension, nephrolithiasis, and urinary tract infection in the elderly with APKD is similar to that described for these conditions in other elderly patients. Infection, however, may be present in the absence of pyuria or bacteriuria when it is confined to the cyst cavity (pyocyst). Clues to the diagnosis include the development of a new discrete area of palpable tenderness in the involved kidney, particularly if blood cultures are positive [40, 41]. Also, thickening and irregularity of the cyst wall or an increase in the attenuation value of the cyst content on CT scan, although not pathognomonic for infection, is suggestive [42]. Follow-up scans should be repeated in these patients because the findings are similar in the presence of renal cell carcinoma, which occurs with higher frequency in APKD patients [43]. Trimethoprim, norfloxacin, ciprofloxin, or clindamycin, at the usual doses, can be used. Patients who have abdominal pain or gross hematuria are best managed with bed rest, liberal fluid intake, and analgesics. Symptoms usually resolve within 48 to 72 hours. We have never needed to resort to surgical reduction of a cyst for pain control in our elderly APKD patients [44].

NATURAL HISTORY OF CRF

In the elderly, as in younger patients, CRF tends to progress to ESRD long after the initial injurious event has subsided. Several factors appear to play a role in this phenomenon:

1. The host. The decline in renal function in patients with presumed hypertensive nephrosclerosis is greater in men and blacks [45, 46].
2. The disease. Some disease entities are associated with more rapid decline than others [47].
3. The degree of proteinuria. A strong positive correlation has been found by some investigators between the 24-hour urine protein excretion and the progression of CRF regardless of the cause of the renal disease [48, 49]. The postulate is that excessive glomerular protein filtration may be injurious and may lead to glomerulosclerosis because of the constant stimulation of mesangial cells.
4. Hypertension (discussed in the following section).

5. Ca deposition in the kidney. As will be discussed later, abnormalities in Ca/P metabolism are universally found in patients with advanced CRF. Because the calcium content of kidney tissue from patients with renal disease of varying severity correlates significantly with the serum creatinine and phosphorus [50, 51], it has been postulated that renal calcium deposition may play a secondary pathogenetic role in accelerating the progression of the renal failure. Dietary phosphate restriction has been shown to preserve kidney function in renal disease in experimental rats [52]. Unfortunately, similar data are unavailable in humans [53].

6. Hyperlipidemia. There is some experimental evidence to suggest that abnormal lipid metabolism, a relatively common finding in patients with CRF [54], may be an independent risk factor in the pathogenesis or progression of renal disease [55, 56]. Presumably, changes in glomerular permeability increase the filtration of lipoproteins. Their accumulation in the mesangial cells could stimulate them to proliferate and produce excess basement membrane material [57, 58]. Hyperlipidemia may also increase platelet aggregation with subsequent release of platelet growth factor. The latter could bind to receptors on the mesangial cells and induce cellular proliferation [57].

7. Finally, several intraglomerular adaptive changes, such as glomerular hyperfiltration and hypertension or glomerular hypertrophy, follow experimental renal injury or a reduction in renal mass. Control of these adaptive changes by blood pressure reduction or protein restriction appears to slow the progression of the renal disease in these animals [59–61]. Whether similar results can be obtained in humans remains to be demonstrated.

In recent years the rate of decline in kidney function in patients with CRF has been mapped by plotting the reciprocal of the serum creatinine (1/serum creatinine) against time, which usually is represented by a straight line, unique for each patient [62]. This approach is clinically useful in that changes in the slope of the line can be used to assess the result of a therapeutic intervention or to determine the effects of a new acute process on kidney function. The use of the latter is particularly helpful in situations that are potentially reversible such as volume contraction, congestive heart failure, or urinary tract obstruction. There are certain drawbacks to this method, however. Spontaneous changes, not readily attributable to a complication or therapy, can occur [63]. Also, it has been recently shown that there is a poor overall correlation between the decline in GFR and the 1/creatinine slope [64, 65], although the correlation is better when the serum creatinine is greater than 2.5 mg per dl. Despite these shortcomings, this method of gauging the progression of CRF is still used and is still found to be helpful.

PROBLEMS RELATED TO CRF
AND THEIR MANAGEMENT

HYPERTENSION

Hypertension per se not only is the primary cause of renal insufficiency in a large number of our elderly patients (particularly blacks) but also is frequently present in all forms of CRF; the incidence varies with the type of disease and is most common in patients with glomerular and polycystic kidney disease. Ninety-five percent of elderly patients entering our ESRD program either have or have had a history of hypertension. The incidence of hypertension in patients with CRF before starting dialysis is approximately 85 percent in all age groups [66].

In general, the patient with underlying renal disease is salt-sensitive, so salt and water retention appears to be an important initiating event in the pathogenesis of the hypertension [67]. Once initiated, hypertension may be maintained because the vasculature is unable to accommodate the increased volume owing to an inadequate balance between the circulating vasoconstrictors and vasodilators normally produced by the kidneys [68]. Since there is evidence to suggest that there is a significant positive correlation between mean arterial pressure (MAP) and the rate of decline in kidney function, hypertension in the presence of kidney disease should be managed aggressively [69, 70]. The ideal target level for blood pressure control has not been determined; however, we recommend achieving a MAP of approximately 100 mm Hg (140/80) in elderly hypertensives with associated renal disease. Patients should be monitored closely in anticipation of side effects related to decreased organ perfusion, particularly those with coronary artery disease [71]. In our experience, the elderly are able to tolerate this level of pressure as long as it is achieved slowly and precipitous drops in blood pressure are avoided. Control of hypertension has been shown to slow the progression of the renal disease, particularly in patients with arteriolar nephrosclerosis, diabetic nephropathy, and polycystic kidney disease [72–77]. Based on a variety of experimental evidence, it has been postulated that hypertension contributes to glomerular damage because it enhances transmission of the systemic pressure to the adapted glomerulus in the presence of a reduced renal mass [78]. The converting enzyme inhibitors or calcium channel blockers, by reversing these effects on the glomerulus, have been shown in animals to offer superior renal protection compared to other agents. Similar benefits in humans remain to be convincingly demonstrated [79–82].

Since the hypertension of CRF is associated with expansion of the plasma volume, patients should be placed on a low-sodium diet (2–3 g per day). In those who do not adhere to the salt restriction, a diuretic

TABLE 11-3. Antihypertensive drugs requiring dose modification in renal failure

Drug	GFR		
	> 50 ml per min (mg per day)	25–50 ml per min	< 25 ml per min
Atenolol	25–150	Lower by 50%	Lower by 75%
Nadolol	50–320	Lower by 50%	Lower by 75%
Methyldopa	125–2,000	No change	Lower by 50%
Clonidine HCl	0.1–1.2	No change	Lower by 50%
Captopril	25–150	Lower by 50%	Lower by 75%
Enalapril	2.5–30	Lower by 50%	Lower by 75%
Lisinopril	5–40	Lower by 50%	Lower by 75%

(furosemide or bumetanide) should be used as the initial drug, either daily or intermittently depending on the degree of weight loss. Kidney function should be monitored carefully during the first 2 to 3 weeks of therapy, since there is a risk of superimposed acute renal failure secondary to volume contraction. The dose of furosemide is 40 to 320 mg per day and of bumetanide 0.5 to 5 mg per day.

If blood pressure is not controlled with salt restriction and a diuretic, any of the available antihypertensive drugs can be added, the choice of specific agent being tailored to the individual patient. The dosage schedule of these drugs in the elderly with renal disease is identical to that outlined in Table 12-3 (see Chap. 12). Drugs that require maintenance dose modification are reviewed in Table 11-3 [83, 84]. With the availability of potent antihypertensive drugs, it is possible to control the blood pressure in patients with CRF without using a diuretic, although some degree of salt restriction is usually necessary.

PHOSPHATE RETENTION

Despite the changes in serum phosphate, parathyroid hormone (PTH), and $1,25(OH)_2D_3$ that occur with age (see Chap. 5), neither hyperphosphatemia nor renal osteodystrophy differs in severity in older compared to younger patients with CRF. No correlation was found between plasma $1,25(OH)_2D_3$ and age in patients with CRF [85]. Mean PTH and mean plasma phosphate levels in a group of 20 patients aged 55 years or younger were similar to those of 25 elderly patients evaluated by us who had a creatinine clearance of less than 10 ml per minute. None were on phosphate binders when studied. The degree of hypocalcemia was also similar in the two groups. The hyperphosphatemia of CRF results mainly from a decrease in renal phosphate excretion because of a lower GFR. Serum levels of $1,25(OH)_2D_3$ decrease because of decreased synthesis by the damaged proximal renal tubular cells [86]. In addition to hypocalcemia, hyperphosphatemia and a low $1,25(OH)_2D_3$ independently stimulate the parathyroid gland, resulting in hyperparathyroidism [87]. The hypocalcemia is a consequence of decreased intestinal calcium absorption as well as skeletal resistance to the calcemic action of PTH and an altered feedback relationship between ionized calcium and PTH secretion [88–90].

The first step in controlling hyperphosphatemia is dietary (see later section on dietary management of renal failure). This approach, unfortunately, is rarely successful by itself, necessitating the addition of phosphate binders. In recent years we have reserved the use of aluminum hydroxide for the occasional patient who has a very high serum phosphorus level (> 10 mg per dl). Once the serum phosphorus has decreased to less than 6 mg per dl, we switch to calcium carbonate administered with meals [91, 92]. If the serum phosphorus concentration is less than 6 mg per dl to start, we avoid aluminum hydroxide altogether and initiate therapy with calcium carbonate. The average daily dose required in our elderly population has been approximately 2,000 mg of elemental calcium. Patients who have difficulty with the tablets can be switched to calcium glubionate syrup (neocalglucon). Each tablespoonful (15 ml) contains 345 mg of calcium. Sixty-five percent of our patients, despite achieving normophosphatemia, remain hypocalcemic (serum Ca < 8.5 mg per dl). In these patients, we add $1,25(OH)_2D_3$ (calcitriol), starting at a dose of 0.125 μg per day and gradually increasing the dose until the serum calcium reaches 10.5 to 11.5 mg per dl. Serum PTH levels gradually decrease within a few months after this therapy is initiated. We have not routinely performed a bone biopsy prior to and after therapy in our patients, but in studies in which patients older than 65 years have been included, a significant improvement in hyperparathyroid bone disease has been observed when this approach has been used [93, 94]. The average patient will require between 0.25 and 0.50 μg per day of calcitriol. Like others [95], we have not seen any deleterious effect of this drug on kidney function, and calcitriol does not increase the risk of aluminum bone disease.

METABOLIC ACIDOSIS

Despite lower plasma aldosterone levels and a lower urinary ammonium excretion in the elderly compared to younger patients when subjected to an acid load, the acidosis seen in elderly patients with a given level of renal insufficiency is no more severe than that seen in younger patients. The urine pH is usually 5.5 or less except when the renal disease is associated with a "voltage-dependent" renal tubular acidosis (see Chap. 3), in which case the acidosis is pronounced.

Initially, the metabolic acidosis is of the hyperchloremic type (nonanion gap). As the GFR falls below 20 ml per minute, organic anions such as sulfate, phosphate, and others, which are not completely oxidized, are retained, thus giving way to an anion gap acidosis [96]. The inability of the surviving nephrons to produce sufficient amounts of ammonia to meet the requirement for excretion of the daily metabolic acid production constitutes a major factor in the pathogenesis of the acidosis associated with renal insufficiency. Also, some derangement in the intrarenal handling of filtered bicarbonate probably plays a role [97]. In 30 percent of our elderly patients the acidosis was severe enough (serum bicarbonate < 15 mEq per liter) to require therapy. We use sodium bicarbonate, starting with 0.5 mEq per kg per day in divided doses, with slow upward titration to maintain the serum pH above 7.35 or HCO_3 above 19 mEq per liter. Patients who cannot tolerate sodium bicarbonate can be given sodium citrate (bicitra). Each milliliter of bicitra is equivalent to 1 mEq of bicarbonate. Potassium citrate (polycitra K, 2 mEq K and the equivalent of 2 mEq bicarbonate per milliliter) is available for patients who cannot handle the amount of sodium required with sodium bicarbonate or citrate. Since citrate increases intestinal aluminum absorption, these two compounds should never be used together [98].

ANEMIA

Anemia is present in most elderly patients with CRF. In general, the lower the GFR, the more severe the anemia. Significant variations do occur among individual patients [99], however, so it is necessary to rule out other causes such as gastrointestinal blood loss or other chronic diseases such as rheumatoid arthritis or a malignancy before attributing the anemia to the renal disease. The most common malignancy found in our elderly population with anemia and renal failure is multiple myeloma. Since the erythrocyte sedimentation rate is frequently elevated in the elderly with CRF, reaching values over 100, particularly in those with diabetic nephropathy [100, 101], the possibility of multiple myeloma is frequently an issue.

The anemia associated with CRF is, for the most part, secondary to a decrease in erythropoietin production by the peritubular interstitial cells (endothelial?) [102, 103]. However, factors related to the uremic milieu per se are also of pathogenetic importance because the endogenous amount of erythropoietin required to maintain the same level of erythropoiesis following renal transplantation is far less than the relatively large doses of exogenous erythropoietin needed in patients with uremia [104].

The anemia is relatively well tolerated in most patients; however, in a small number the presence of concomitant conditions such as recurring angina pectoris, congestive heart failure, marked fatigue, or malignancy makes it necessary to either resort to periodic transfusions or administer erythropoietin. Erythropoietin requires thrice weekly administration either intravenously or subcutaneously [105]. We usually start our elderly patients with a dose of 50 units per kg. Hematocrit, serum ferritin, iron and total iron-binding capacity, blood pressure, and serum creatinine are monitored weekly for the first month and twice monthly thereafter until the therapeutic goal (generally a hematocrit of 35 percent) is achieved. A maintenance dose can then be used, which in our limited experience involving a small number of elderly patients averages 50 to 100 units per kg per week. The drug is well tolerated and is associated with an increase in exercise tolerance as well as an overall sense of well being. Hypertensive patients may require additional antihypertensive therapy. For those who develop iron deficiency, supplemental iron at the usual dosage is needed. Like others [106], we have not seen any acute worsening in kidney function with the use of erythropoietin. At the present time this drug is quite expensive, a factor that limits its use to those who can afford the expense or have drug insurance coverage. A reasonable substitute, although of lesser efficacy, is an androgen such as nandrolone decanoate, 1 to 1.5 mg per kg per week. Careful examination of the prostate should be performed in the male prior to initiating therapy with this drug.

DIETARY MANAGEMENT OF THE ELDERLY WITH CRF

Several studies have been carried out to evaluate whether lowering dietary protein can slow the progression of kidney failure through its effect on glomerular hyperfiltration, urinary concentrating ability, ammoniagenesis, and possibly other actions as well [107, 108]. Although patients over the age of 60 have been included in these studies, not enough information is available in the elderly (or for that matter in all age groups) to make a strong specific dietary recommendation. It is hoped that the large multicenter study being conducted in the United States, to be completed in 1992, will help settle the matter in all patients with renal disease, old as well as young.

The estimated rate of body protein synthesis in the elderly is approximately 3 g per kg per day, and the dietary protein requirement is 0.60 to 0.75 g per kg per day [109]. Presently, a prudent approach is to reduce protein intake to approximately 0.6 g per kg per day in patients who are ingesting more than this amount, as determined from a 24-hour urine collection using the following formulas: Protein intake (g per day) = urea nitrogen intake (g per day) × 6.25. Urea nitrogen intake (g per day) = urine urea nitrogen (g per day) + 0.031 g per kg body weight per day [110]. Since the average protein intake in our elderly population with CRF is 1.04 ± 0.40 g per kg, it is evident that most people require some form of restriction. Compliance is, however, difficult to achieve. We strongly suggest that the patient be followed carefully by a dietitian, since a reduction in dietary caloric intake is often associated with protein restriction, leading to malnutrition [111], particularly in patients with a very low GFR [112].

CONCURRENT MEDICAL PROBLEMS
AND THEIR MANAGEMENT

The majority of elderly patients with CRF have other co-morbid problems such as heart disease and heart failure, peripheral vascular disease, and organic brain syndrome that predispose them to frequent hospitalizations and put them at increased risk of further deterioration of renal function. Acute renal failure superimposed on CRF is the most common complication encountered in the hospitalized elderly. Volume contraction due to vigorous diuresis during the management of heart failure and continuance of a diuretic and a low-sodium diet in the hospitalized hypertensive elderly patient with poor oral intake are the most common causes of acute worsening of kidney function in these patients. The usual evidence of volume contraction, such as poor skin turgor or an orthostatic drop in blood pressure, may not be present. Weight loss, a low urine sodium concentration (< 20 mEq per liter, not always present when prerenal azotemia is superimposed on CRF), and an unchanged urinary sediment are helpful signs. Management is straightforward, but the patient must be monitored carefully to prevent fluid overload. Prognosis for recovery is excellent.

The use of nephrotoxic antibiotics and nonsteroidal anti-inflammatory drugs (NSAIDs), contrast media administration, and acute tubular necrosis due to sepsis or cardiogenic shock are the other major causes of worsening of kidney function in the elderly. In these patients the history and physical findings are quite useful, and the presence of a urinary sodium of greater than 40 mEq per liter helps to distinguish these forms of acute renal failure from the prerenal azotemia described above. These complications add significantly to the morbidity and mortality in this group. Although the acute renal failure may be reversible, in some patients dialysis may be necessary. Furthermore, particularly in patients with diabetes, kidney function may not return to premorbid levels, and the patient may require maintenance dialysis.

Obstruction, mainly in males and especially in those receiving sedatives, must be ruled out. In addition, acute interstitial nephritis (AIN) secondary to drugs (or infection) should be kept in mind. AIN, particularly when secondary to NSAID use, may occur in the absence of the usual clinical picture of fever, rash, eosinophilia, or eosinophiluria. Renal artery occlusion, particularly in patients with an abdominal aortic aneurysm or direct evidence of renal vascular disease (abdominal bruit, discrepancy in kidney size) or vascular disease elsewhere, will cause acute worsening of renal function that can be detected by a renal scan or angiogram. Finally, although rare, the possibility of acute glomerulonephritis should always be kept in mind and adequately ruled out by careful examination of the urinary sediment (red cell casts, proteinuria).

SURGERY IN THE ELDERLY WITH CRF

Preoperative, perioperative, and postoperative management of the elderly with CRF is similar to that in patients with normal kidney function. Even patients with advanced disease (serum creatinine of 3.5 mg per dl or greater or a creatinine clearance of 15 to 20 ml per minute or less) do not necessarily require prophylactic dialysis; however, attention should be paid to fluid balance, blood pressure control, acid-base status, and the serum potassium during the preoperative period. Patients with anemia should be transfused to achieve a hematocrit of 30 percent. When potentially nephrotoxic drugs are needed, the dose should be adjusted and blood levels monitored carefully. For patients with a diastolic blood pressure of greater than 110 mm Hg who cannot take oral medication, blood pressure control should be achieved with any of the parenteral drugs discussed in Chap. 12. Despite careful monitoring of all these factors, the incidence of worsening kidney function is increased in these patients, particularly those who have advanced disease prior to surgery.

THE ELDERLY WITH END-STAGE RENAL DISEASE

As already mentioned, the number of elderly patients entering the ESRD program has been increasing in the United States. Similar trends are also reported from Europe [113, 114]. Since it is not possible to identify which elderly will adapt to dialysis, it should be offered to all patients (except those in whom death is imminent from other problems) [115, 116], even though age per se constitutes an independent risk factor for increased mortality [117–121].

INDICATIONS FOR INITIATING DIALYSIS IN THE ELDERLY

The indications for starting maintenance dialysis in the elderly are identical to those in younger patients. Uremic encephalopathy, pericarditis, gastritis, colitis, and neuropathy constitute absolute indications for immediate dialysis. These complications have been seen less frequently in recent years because most elderly patients with CRF are diagnosed prior to reaching end stage. Most patients are now started on dialysis when the complications of uremia are less severe. Table 11-4 summarizes the symptoms and signs present at the time of the first dialysis in 118 elderly patients seen by us.

TABLE 11-4. Symptoms and signs present in
118 elderly patients prior to starting maintenance dialysis

	No. patients (%)
Nonspecific	
Generalized weakness	68 (58)
Anorexia, weight loss	72 (61)
Nervous system	
Encephalopathy (dementia)	58 (49)
Peripheral neuropathy (symptomatic)	8 (7)
Gastrointestinal	
Nausea, vomiting	48 (41)
Bleeding	12 (10)
Cardiovascular	
Difficulty with volume homeostasis	
(fluid overload)	19 (16)
Pleuropericarditis	2 (2)
Other	
Markedly elevated serum creatinine	
(> 15 mg per dl)	19 (16)

HEMODIALYSIS VERSUS CHRONIC PERITONEAL DIALYSIS

The choice of hemodialysis (HD) as opposed to peritoneal dialysis, usually in the form of chronic ambulatory peritoneal dialysis (CAPD), depends on the patient's overall condition, the physician's expertise, and the available resources, since neither method offers any advantage as far as survival rate is concerned when patients with similar risk factors are compared [122–124]. Both HD and CAPD appear to be associated with better survival than intermittent peritoneal dialysis (IPD). Elderly patients on home hemodialysis have a better survival rate than those receiving in-center HD or CAPD [125].

Hemodialysis in the Elderly

Hemodialysis is generally as well tolerated in the elderly as in younger patients [126, 127]. An attempt should always be made to place a Brescia-Cimino fistula to be used as a route for angioaccess, since the overall complication rate is lower in patients with a fistula than with a graft. This technique, unfortunately, has been possible in only 30 percent of our elderly patients owing mainly to venous disease. In the remaining 70 percent, a graft was required. Our 1-year patency rate for fistulas is 40 percent, considerably better than that reported by others [128]. Our 1-year graft patency rate is approximately 70 percent, similar to the 69 percent found by the same investigators [128].

The most common problem associated with angioaccess in the elderly is clotting, which is usually amenable to thrombectomy. Clotting may be recurrent in patients with intradialytic hypotension from whatever cause and in those with systemic infection. Also, it is imperative to do an angiogram in these patients to rule out stenosis of the graft venous anastomotic site, which usually can be surgically corrected. Steal syndrome is seen more frequently in diabetic patients and in those with severe peripheral vascular disease. Patients with access infection (usually a graft) should be hospitalized and started on antibiotics such as vancomycin or a penicillinase-resistant penicillin, since *Staphylococcus* is almost always the offending agent (99 percent of our cases). In the remaining 1 percent, *Enterococcus* or *Pseudomonas* was isolated. We have not had any success with medical therapy alone, and in every instance the graft required removal. The new access is usually placed 8 to 10 days later, after all signs of infection have subsided. In the interim, HD is continued through either femoral or subclavian vein catheterization.

Adequacy of HD in the elderly is assessed in the same way as in younger patients, using the sense of well-being, nerve conduction velocity, and monthly estimation of the urea index (urea index = Kt/V, where K = urea clearance through the dialyzer, t = treatment time, and V = the volume of distribution of urea). The clinician should aim for a urea index of 1.0 to 1.5 [129]. Other methods of estimating Kt/V have been described [130]. The incidence of intradialytic hypotension and transfusion requirements are similar in older and younger patients [131, 132].

Symptomatic aluminum toxicity is quite rare in our experience. Routinely measured serum aluminum levels in our elderly patients have been low. Aluminum toxicity is manifested primarily by CNS involvement including speech disturbances, dementia, convulsions, and extrapyramidal signs [133]. Patients with osteomalacia may complain of generalized bone pain or proximal muscle weakness. These patients have a tendency to develop hypercalcemia when given calcitriol and usually have an elevated serum alkaline phosphatase [134]. The serum aluminum level is often elevated but not necessarily so. A more than 20 percent rise in the serum aluminum level 5 hours after infusion of deferoxamine (28.5 mg per kg) has been found to correlate better with the presence of stainable bone aluminum [135]. The infusion is administered during dialysis, the rate not exceeding 15 mg per kg per hour. Definitive diagnosis of aluminum bone disease is made histologically [136], however. Deferoxamine, 20 to 80 mg per kg per week in single or divided doses administered either intravenously, intramuscularly, or intraperitoneally, constitutes the agent of choice for the management of these patients [137]. A high incidence of mucormycosis has been reported in patients treated with this drug [138].

The most important differential diagnosis of aluminum bone disease is hyperparathyroid bone disease (osteitis fibrosa cystica), which can be distinguished histologically from the former. In the past, patients with this form of bone disease were usually routinely referred for parathyroidectomy [139]. Since $1,25(OH)_2D_3$ administered intravenously can directly inhibit PTH secretion [140] and ameliorate the biochemical and histologic picture of osteitis fibrosa cystica in patients on maintenance hemodialysis [141], it is now the treatment of choice, with surgery reserved only for refractory cases. Our limited experience, involving a small number of elderly patients with this form of therapy, has been quite encouraging. The recommended starting dose is 1.0 μg administered into the venous line during the last few minutes of each dialysis treatment (3 times weekly), with monthly or bimonthly increments of 0.5 μg up to a maximum of 2.5 μg as long as the serum calcium remains less than 11.5 mg per dl. Hypercalcemia is the major side effect.

Pruritus is more common in the elderly than in the younger uremic patient. This may be related in part to the skin changes that take place with aging. Pruritus, which can be either localized or generalized, tends to be worse during dialysis. The pathogenesis of uremic pruritus is probably multifactorial, including increased divalent ion skin content [142], lower skin water content, increased sensitivity to pruritogens, ischemic neuropathy, and an abnormal pattern of cutaneous innervation [143]. Therapy is generally unsatisfactory. We usually start treatment with maneuvers that contribute to keeping the skin moist such as use of an oatmeal soap and baby oil applications. These simple maneuvers may provide some relief in a significant number of patients. Lidocaine infusion during dialysis, oral charcoal, and antihistamines have been used unsuccessfully. Ultraviolet irradiation within the sunburn spectrum, either through a real effect on skin or through a placebo effect, has been found helpful [144, 145].

Elderly patients on hemodialysis spend an average of 15 to 30 days a year in the hospital [122, 146–148]. Approximately 30 percent of hospital time is for fluid overload or complications directly related to dialysis, such as angioaccess clotting and infection. The remaining causes of hospitalization include cardiovascular complications such as ischemic heart disease (3 times as common in the elderly as in younger patients), congestive heart failure, or vascular insufficiency, which account for over 30 percent of the time spent in the hospital. Gastrointestinal bleeding accounts for another 10 percent. The remainder is for a variety of other problems, including cancer.

Bleeding gastritis in elderly patients on dialysis is due mainly to uremia or the use of NSAIDs. Blood loss is usually minimal, since the bleeding tends to stop within 24 hours when dialysis time is increased or therapy is given with any of the H_2-blockers or misoprostol (for those on NSAIDs), 200 μg with meals and at bedtime. More severe bleeding occurs in patients with angiodysplasia, which is the second most common cause of gastrointestinal bleeding in the elderly with ESRD in our experience. The lesions can occur anywhere along the gastrointestinal tract and are usually multiple [149]. The outcome is variable. In some patients bleeding stops spontaneously. In others a single bleeding site may be located by endoscopy and managed with laser photocoagulation or electrocautery [150]. In still others, surgery may be necessary, particularly if the site of bleeding is localized (which is not always possible). The indications for surgery in these patients should be the same as those used for other patients with gastrointestinal bleeding. We usually continue with HD under tight heparinization (or no heparin) as long as blood pressure is well maintained. Otherwise, we switch to peritoneal dialysis. Patients with a prolonged bleeding time can be given dDAVP, 0.3 mg per kg intravenously in one dose, or 0.6 mg per kg of conjugated estrogen 4 to 5 times at 24-hour intervals [151, 152]. Patients with recurrent bleeding may be managed with long-term norethynodrel-mestranol therapy in dose ratios varying from 2.5 to 5 μg of norethynodrel per 0.075 to 0.1 mg of mestranol [153]. Patients should be watched carefully for side effects related to the use of estrogens. We tend to discontinue the drug in patients who continue to bleed after 2 to 3 months of therapy and in those who have not bled for the same length of time. This latter approach is used by us and is not based on any controlled study.

Patients on maintenance HD can tolerate major surgery quite well. Dialysis is scheduled the day before for the patient undergoing elective surgery. Postsurgery HD can be safely performed as long as the amount of heparin used is kept to a minimum [154]. Elderly males who require prostatectomy are given dDAVP or estrogens prophylactically, as described previously, since they tend to bleed profusely after the procedure.

The great majority of elderly patients at the time of initiation of HD have at least one and usually multiple medical problems [155]. Despite this, most of them adapt well to HD [147, 156]. Thirty to forty-five percent of elderly patients on HD die from cardiovascular disease, and infections account for an additional 10 to 30 percent of deaths [120, 122, 131, 146]. It has been estimated that one of every six patients over the age of 60 on dialysis dies from stopping the treatment [157]. In our experience the incidence of voluntary discontinuation of HD is extremely low in all age groups, including the elderly.

CAPD in the Elderly
CAPD is generally well accepted by the elderly, with 67 percent remaining on CAPD at 1 year, 37 percent at 2 years, and 29 percent at 2.5 years [124, 158]. The number of elderly patients switching to HD because of infectious complications (50 percent), personal preference (18 percent), inadequate clearance (7 percent), or other reasons (25 percent) is similar to the numbers and reasons for change seen in the overall CAPD population. Hospitalization in the elderly on CAPD varies among centers be-

tween 19 and 58 days per patient per year, with infections (peritonitis, exit-site, or tunnel infection) and cardiovascular problems accounting for the great majority of cases [122, 124, 158]. As noted earlier, mortality in the elderly on CAPD is similar to that seen with HD. Cardiovascular and infectious causes account for 49 to 54 percent and 12 to 22 percent of the deaths, respectively [122, 124, 158, 159]. A higher incidence of inguinal hernia, fluid leaks, and vascular ischemia of the lower extremities has been found in older patients on CAPD compared with younger patients [158]. Clinical manifestations, bacteriologic findings, and management of peritonitis in the elderly are similar to those seen in the general CAPD population. Abdominal pain associated with a cloudy effluent containing more than 100 white blood cells per ml was present in all our patients. *Staphylococcus epidermidis, Staphylococcus aureus,* and *Pseudomonas aeruginosa* are the most commonly encountered organisms. Antibiotic treatment is initiated intraperitoneally and is continued for 3 to 5 days following either a negative peritoneal fluid culture or an effluent WBC count of less than 100 cells per ml [160]. In patients who fail to respond after 96 hours of an appropriate antibiotic regimen and in those with fungal or tunnel infections, the catheter should be removed [161, 162]. Serious intra-abdominal or gynecologic pathology should also be ruled out in these patients. Persistent exit-site infections despite 2 to 3 weeks of antibiotic therapy are another indication for removing the catheter. A list of the currently used antibiotics for treating peritonitis and their dosages is given in Table 11-5.

The optimal time period between catheter removal for peritonitis and insertion of a new one is usually given as 2 to 3 weeks. In our own limited experience and that of others [163], however, the two procedures may be successfully carried out at the same sitting, but additional data are needed before recommending this approach for the elderly on CAPD.

TABLE 11-5. Dosage of antibiotics currently used in the treatment of peritonitis in CAPD patients

Drug	Initial dose (mg per 2-liter bag)	Maintenance dose (mg per 2-liter bag)
Vancomycin	1,000	30
Cefazolin	500–1,000	250–500
Cefuroxime	1,500	500
Cephalothin	2,000	500
Azlocillin	500	500
Tobramycin, gentamicin	120	8–12
Amikacin	350	12–15
Amphotericin B	1.0	4–8

In the diabetic patient the extra glucose load associated with CAPD may necessitate an increase in insulin dose. The insulin can be administered either subcutaneously or intraperitoneally. The latter route has been found to be associated with a higher incidence of peritonitis in one recent study [164], however.

RENAL TRANSPLANTATION IN THE ELDERLY

Age per se should not be considered a contraindication to renal transplantation [165–168], even though only 6 percent of dialysis patients 56 years of age or older receive a kidney transplant compared to 27 percent of the total population on dialysis [169]. The higher incidence of complications and poor outcome reported in the elderly in earlier years were most likely related to aggressive conventional immunosuppression [170]. With the current use of cyclosporine and lower maintenance doses of steroids the outcome in the elderly recipient of a cadaver kidney is presently similar to that in younger patients. The 18-month allograft survival is 67 percent for recipients 60 to 65 years old and 75 percent for those over 65 years of age in the United States [171]. In Canada, the 1-, 2-, and 3-year graft survival in patients younger than 60 years is 73 percent, 64 percent, and 60 percent, respectively, and 72 percent, 61 percent, and 55 percent for those 60 years and older [172].

Cyclosporine-associated nephrotoxicity during the first year following transplantation occurs more commonly in the elderly than does graft rejection [173, 174]. The 1-year survival in elderly with renal transplants is approximately 87 percent [175]. Cardiovascular complications and sepsis constitute the most common causes of death.

Age per se does not constitute a contraindication for donation of a kidney; however, the 1-year graft survival rate for a kidney harvested from an elderly donor is lower than that for a kidney originating from a younger doner (52 versus 70 percent) [176].

REFERENCES

1. McInnes EG, et al: Renal failure in the elderly. *Q J Med* 243:583–588, 1987.
2. Llera FG and Gregorio PG: Incidence of Renal Diseases in a Geriatric Unit. In Macia Nuñez JF and Cameron JS (eds), *Renal Function and Disease in the Elderly*. London: Butterworths, 1987. Pp. 208–236.
3. Burkart J, et al: Major causes of ESRD in geriatric patients in northwest North Carolina. Paper presented at 22nd annual meeting of the American Society of Nephrologists (Abstract 48), Washington, D.C., December 1989.
4. Blagg CR: Chronic Renal Failure in the Elderly. In Oreopoulos DG (ed), *Geriatric Nephrology*. Boston: Martinus Nijhoff, 1986. Pp. 117–126.
5. Sandler DP, et al: Analgesic use and chronic renal disease. *N Engl J Med* 320:1238–1243, 1989.

6. Adams DH, et al: Non-steroidal antiinflammatory drugs and renal failure. *Lancet* 1:57–59, 1986.
7. Murray TG, et al: Epidemiologic study of regular analgesic use and end-stage renal disease. *Arch Intern Med* 143:1687–1693, 1983.
8. Buckalew VM Jr and Schey HM: Renal disease from habitual antipyretic analgesic consumption: An assessment of the epidemiologic evidence. *Medicine* 11:291–303, 1986.
9. Sabatini S: Analgesic-induced papillary necrosis. *Semin Nephrol* 8:41–54, 1988.
10. Bennett WM and DeBroe ME: Analgesic nephropathy. A preventable renal disease. *N Engl J Med* 320:1269–1271, 1989.
11. Linton AL: Renal disease due to analgesics. *Can Med Assoc J* 107:749–751, 1972.
12. Henrich WL: Analgesic nephropathy. *Am J Med Sci* 295:561–568, 1988.
13. McCredie M, et al: Phenacetin and papillary necrosis: Independent risk factor for renal pelvic cancer. *Kidney Int* 30:81–84, 1985.
14. Hestbech J, et al: Chronic renal lesions following long-term treatment with lithium. *Kidney Int* 12:205–213, 1977.
15. Boton R, Gaviria M, and Battle DC: Prevalence, pathogenesis and treatment of renal dysfunction associated with chronic lithium therapy. *Am J Kidney Dis* 10:329–345, 1987.
16. Walker RG, Davies BM, and Holwill BJ: A chronic pathological study of lithium nephrotoxicity. *J Chron Dis* 35:685–695, 1982.
17. Battle DC, et al: Amelioration of polyuria by amiloride in patients receiving long term lithium therapy. *N Engl J Med* 312:409–414, 1985.
18. Batuman V, et al: The role of lead in gouty nephropathy. *N Engl J Med* 304:520–523, 1981.
19. Colleoni N and D'Amato G: Chronic lead accumulation as a possible cause of renal failure in gouty patients. *Nephron* 44:32–35, 1986.
20. Wedeen RP: Use of CaNa$_2$EDTA Pb-mobilization test to detect occult lead nephropathy. *Uremia Inv* 9:127–130, 1985.
21. Wedeen RP, Mallich DK, and Batuman V: Detection and treatment of occupational lead nephropathy. *Arch Intern Med* 139:53–57, 1979.
22. Bennett WM: Lead nephropathy. *Kidney Int* 28:212–220, 1985.
23. Drenick EJ, et al: Renal damage with intestinal bypass. *Ann Intern Med* 89:594–599, 1978.
24. Luxton RW: Radiation nephritis. A long term study of 54 patients. *Lancet* 2:1221–1224, 1961.
25. Bolton WK, et al: Reversible renal failure from isolated granulomatous renal sarcoidosis. *Clin Nephrol* 5:88–92, 1976.
26. Muther RS, McCarron DA, and Bennett WM: Granulomatous sarcoid nephritis: A cause of multiple renal tubular abnormalities. *Clin Nephrol* 14:190–197, 1980.
27. Farge D, et al: Granulomatous nephritis and chronic renal failure in sarcoidosis. *Am J Nephrol* 6:21–27, 1986.
28. Reeders ST and Grimino GG: The molecular genetics of autosomal dominant polycystic kidney disease. *Semin Nephrol* 9:122–134, 1989.
29. Romeo G, et al: A second genetic locus for autosomal dominant polycystic kidney disease. *Lancet* 2:8–11, 1988.
30. Gabow PA, Iklé DW, and Holmes JH: Polycystic kidney disease: Prospective analysis of nonazotemic patients and family members. *Ann Intern Med* 101:238–247, 1984.

31. Delaney VB, et al: Autosomal dominant polycystic kidney disease. Presentation, complications and prognosis. *Am J Kidney Dis* 5:104–111, 1985.
32. Milutinovic J, et al: Clinical manifestations of autosomal dominant polycystic kidney disease in patients older than 50 years. *Am J Kidney Dis* 15:237–243, 1990.
33. Zeier M, et al: Adult dominant polycystic kidney disease. Clinical problems. *Nephron* 49:177–183, 1988.
34. Parfrey PS, et al: The prognosis of autosomal dominant polycystic kidney disease: PKD 1 vs PKD 2. *Kidney Int* 37:251A, 1990.
35. Gabow P, et al: Factors relating to renal functional deterioration in autosomal dominant polycystic kidney disease (APKD). *Kidney Int* 37:248A, 1990.
36. Gabow PA and Schrier RW: Pathophysiology of adult polycystic kidney disease. *Adv Nephrol* 18:19–32, 1989.
37. Wilson PD, et al: A new method for studying human polycystic kidney disease epithelia in culture. *Kidney Int* 30:371–378, 1986.
38. Carone FA: Functional changes in polycystic kidney disease are tubulointerstitial in origin. *Semin Nephrol* 8:89–92, 1988.
39. Huseman R, et al: Macropuncture study of polycystic kidney disease in adult human kidneys. *Kidney Int* 18:375–385, 1980.
40. Schwab SJ and Bander SJ: Cyst infection in autosomal dominant polycystic kidney disease. *Am J Med* 82:714–718, 1987.
41. Sklar AH, et al: Renal infections in autosomal dominant polycystic kidney disease. *Am J Kidney Dis* 10:81–88, 1987.
42. Levine E and Grantham JJ: The role of computed tomography in the evaluation of adult polycystic kidney disease. *Am J Kidney Dis* 1:99–105, 1981.
43. Ng RCK and Suki WN: Renal cell carcinoma occurring in a polycystic kidney of a transplant recipient. *J Urol* 124:710–712, 1980.
44. Bennett WM, et al: Reduction of cyst volume for symptomatic management of autosomal dominant polycystic kidney disease. *J Urol* 137:620–622, 1988.
45. Schulman NB, et al: Prognostic value of serum creatinine and effect of treatment of hypertension on renal function. *Hypertension* 13 (Suppl 1):80–93, 1989.
46. Rostand SG, et al: Renal insufficiency in treated essential hypertension. *N Engl J Med* 320:684–688, 1989.
47. Brahm M, et al: Prognosis in glomerulonephritis. *Acta Med Scand* 217:117–125, 1985.
48. Williams PS, Fass G, and Bone JM: Renal pathology and proteinuria determine progression in untreated mild/moderate chronic renal failure. *Q J Med* 252:343–354, 1988.
49. Stenvinkel P, Alvestrand A, and Bergström J: Factors influencing progression in patients with chronic renal failure. *J Intern Med* 226:183–188, 1989.
50. Giminez LF, Solez K, and Walker GW: Relation between renal calcium content and renal impairment in 246 human renal biopsies. *Kidney Int* 31:93–99, 1987.
51. Ibels L, et al: Calcification in end stage kidneys. *Am J Med* 71:33–37, 1980.
52. Ibels L, et al: Preservation of function in experimental renal disease by dietary restriction of phosphate. *N Engl J Med* 298:122–126, 1978.
53. Alfred AC: Effect of dietary phosphate restriction on renal function and deterioration. *Am J Clin Nutr* 47:153–156, 1988.
54. Grützmacher P, et al: Lipoproteins and apolipoproteins during the progression of chronic renal disease. *Nephron* 50:103–111, 1988.
55. Keane WF, Kasiske BL, and O'Donnell MP: Hyperlipidemia and the progression of renal disease. *Am J Clin Nutr* 47:157–160, 1988.

56. Harris PG, et al: Lovastatin ameliorates the development of glomerulo-sclerosis and uremia in experimental nephrotic syndrome. *Am J Kidney Dis* 15:16–23, 1990.

57. Moorhead JF, et al: Lipid nephrotoxicity in chronic progressive glomerular and tubulo-interstitial disease. *Lancet* 2:1309–1311, 1982.

58. Moorhead JF, et al: Injury to rat mesangial cells in culture by low density lipoproteins. *Kidney Int* 35:433A, 1989.

59. Klahr S, Schreiner G, and Ichikawa I: The progression of renal disease. *N Engl J Med* 318:1657–1666, 1988.

60. Anderson S and Brenner BM: Progressive renal disease: A disorder of adaptation. *Q J Med* 70:185–189, 1989.

61. Miller PL, et al: Glomerular hypertrophy aggravates epithelial cell injury in nephrotic rats. *J Clin Invest* 85:1119–1126, 1990.

62. Mitch WE, et al: A simple method for estimating progression of chronic renal failure. *Lancet* 2:1326–1328, 1976.

63. Kirschbaum BB: Analysis of reciprocal creatinine plots in renal failure. *Am J Med Sci* 291:404–407, 1986.

64. Walser M, Drew HH, and LaFrance ND: Reciprocal creatinine slopes often give erroneous estimates of progression of chronic renal failure. *Kidney Int* 36 (Suppl 27):S81–S89, 1989.

65. MDRD Study Group: Creatinine filtration, secretion and excretion during progressive renal disease. *Kidney Int* 36 (Suppl 27):S73–S80, 1989.

66. Blythe WB: Natural history of hypertension in renal parenchymal disease. *Am J Kidney Dis* 5:A50–A56, 1985.

67. Koomans HA, et al: Sodium balance in renal failure: A comparison of patients with normal subjects under extremes of sodium intake. *Hypertension* 7:714–721, 1985.

68. Ritz E, et al: Pathogenesis of hypertension in glomerular disease. *Am J Nephrol* (Suppl 1):85–90, 1989.

69. Maschio G, Oldrizzi L, and Rugiu C: Role of hypertension on the progression of renal disease in man. *Blood Purific* 6:250–257, 1988.

70. Klahr S: The modification of diet in renal disease study. *N Engl J Med* 320:864–866, 1989.

71. Cruickshank JM: Coronary flow reserve and the J curve: Relation between diastolic blood pressure and myocardial infarction. *Br Med J* 297:1227–1230, 1988.

72. Pettinger WA, et al: Long term improvement in renal function after short term strict blood pressure control in hypertensive nephrosclerosis. *Hypertension* 13:766–772, 1989.

73. Brazy PC, Stead WW, and Fitzwilliam JF: Progression of renal insufficiency: Role of blood pressure. *Kidney Int* 35:670–674, 1989.

74. Bergström J, et al: Stockholm clinical study on progression of chronic renal failure. An interim report. *Kidney Int* 36 (Suppl 27):S110–S114, 1989.

75. Rosman JB, et al: Protein-restricted diets in chronic renal failure: A four year follow-up shows limited indications. *Kidney Int* 36 (Suppl 27):S96–S102, 1989.

76. Mogensen CE: Long term antihypertensive treatment inhibiting progression of diabetic nephropathy. *Br Med J* 285:685–688, 1982.

77. Parving HH, et al: Early aggressive antihypertension treatment reduces rate of decline in kidney function in diabetic nephropathy. *Lancet* 1:1175–1177, 1983.

78. Baldwin DS and Neugarten J: Treatment of hypertension in renal disease. *Am J Kidney Dis* 5:57–70, 1985.

79. Keane WF, et al: Angiotensin converting enzyme inhibitors and progressive renal insufficiency. *Ann Intern Med* 111:503–516, 1989.
80. Abrahan PA, et al: Efficacy and renal effects of enalapril therapy for hypertensive patients with chronic renal insufficiency. *Arch Intern Med* 148:2358–2362, 1988.
81. Ruilope LM, et al: Converting enzyme inhibition in chronic renal failure. *Am J Kidney Dis* 13:120–126, 1989.
82. Brazy PC and Fitzwilliam JF: Progressive renal disease: Role of race and antihypertensive medications. *Kidney Int* 37:1113–1119, 1990.
83. Faubert PF and Porush JG: Managing hypertension in chronic renal disease. *Geriatrics* 42:49–59, 1987.
84. Heyka RJ and Vidt DG: Control of hypertension in patients with chronic renal failure. *Clev Clin J Med* 56:65–76, 1989.
85. Pitts TO, et al: Hyperparathyroidism and 1,25 dihydroxyvitamin D deficiency in mild, moderate and severe renal failure. *J Clin Endocrinol Metab* 67:876–881, 1988.
86. Francis RM, Placock M, and Barkworth SA: Renal impairment and its effects on calcium metabolism in elderly women. *Age Aging* 13:14–20, 1984.
87. Lopez-Hilker S, et al: On the mechanism by which phosphate restriction reverses secondary hyperparathyroidism in advanced renal insufficiency. *Clin Res* 37:582A, 1989.
88. Coburn JW, et al: Study of intestinal absorption of calcium in patients with renal failure. *Kidney Int* 3:264–272, 1973.
89. Llach F, et al: Skeletal resistance of endogenous parathyroid hormone in patients with early renal failure: A possible cause for secondary hyperparathyroidism. *J Clin Endocrinol Metab* 41:339–345, 1975.
90. Lloyd HM, et al: The parathyroid glands in chronic renal failure: A study of their growth and other properties made on the basis of findings in patients with hypercalcemia. *J Lab Clin Med* 114:358–367, 1989.
91. Schiller LR, et al: Effect of the time administration of calcium acetate on phosphorus binding. *N Engl J Med* 320:1110–1113, 1989.
92. Malberti F, et al: Efficacy and safety of long term treatment with calcium carbonate as a phosphate binder. *Am J Kidney Dis* 12:487–491, 1988.
93. Nordal KP and Dahl E: Low dose calcitriol versus placebo in patients with predialysis chronic renal failure. *J Clin Endocrinol Metab* 67:929–936, 1988.
94. Coen G, et al: Bone aluminum content in predialysis chronic renal failure and its relation to secondary hyperparathyroidism and 1,25(OH)$_2$D$_3$ treatment. *Min Electrol Metab* 15:295–302, 1989.
95. Baker LRI, et al: 1,25(OH)$_2$D$_3$ administration in moderate renal failure: A prospective double-blind trial. *Kidney Int* 35:661–669, 1989.
96. Widmer B, et al: Serum electrolyte and acid base composition: The influence of graded degrees of chronic renal failure. *Arch Intern Med* 139:1099–1102, 1979.
97. Warnock DG: Uremic acidosis. *Kidney Int* 34:278–287, 1988.
98. Molitoris BA, et al: Citrate: A major factor in the toxicity of orally administered aluminum compounds. *Kidney Int* 36:949–953, 1989.
99. Howard AD, et al: Analysis of the quantitative relationship between anemia and chronic renal failure. *Am J Med Sci* 297:309–313, 1989.
100. Tinetti ME, Schmidt A, and Baum J: Use of ESR in chronically ill, elderly patients wtih a decline in health status. *Am J Med* 80:844–848, 1986.
101. Schusterman N, et al: Factors influencing erythrocyte sedimentation in patients with chronic renal failure. *Arch Intern Med* 145:1796–1799, 1985.

102. Lacombe C, et al: Peritubular cells are the site of erythropoietin synthesis in the murine hypoxic kidney. *J Clin Invest* 81:620–623, 1988.
103. Eckardt KU, et al: Erythropoietin in polycystic kidneys. *J Clin Invest* 84: 1160–1166, 1989.
104. Sun CH, et al: Serum erythropoietin levels after renal transplantation. *N Engl J Med* 321:151–157, 1989.
105. MacDougall IC, et al: Pharmacokinetics of recombinant human erythropoietin in patients on continuous ambulatory peritoneal dialysis. *Lancet* 1:425–427, 1989.
106. Eschbach JW, et al: Treatment of the anemia of progressive renal failure with recombinant human erythropoietin. *N Engl J Med* 321:158–163, 1989.
107. Bankir L, Bouby N, and Tringh-Trang-Tan MM: Possible involvement of vasopressin and urine concentrating process in the progression of chronic renal failure. *Kidney Int* 36 (Suppl 27):S32–S37, 1989.
108. Nath K, Hostetter MK, and Hostetter TH: Ammonia-complement interaction in the pathogenesis of progressive renal injury. *Kidney Int* 36 (Suppl 27): S52–S54, 1989.
109. Mitch WE: Uremia and the control of protein metabolism. *Nephron* 49: 89–93, 1988.
110. Goodship THJ and Mitch WE: Nutritional approaches to preserving renal function. *Adv Intern Med* 33:337–357, 1988.
111. Cianciaruso B, et al: Dietary compliance to a low protein and phosphate diet in patients with chronic renal failure. *Kidney Int* 36 (Suppl 27):S173–S176, 1989.
112. MDRD Study Group: Nutritional status of patients with different levels of chronic renal insufficiency. *Kidney Int* 36 (Suppl 27):S184–S194, 1989.
113. Williams AJ and Antao JAO: Referral of elderly patients with end-stage renal failure for renal replacement therapy. *Q J Med* 268:749–756, 1989.
114. Wing AJ: Can We Afford to Treat Everybody? The UK View. In Oreopoulos DG (ed), *Geriatric Nephrology.* Boston: Martinus Nijhoff, 1986. Pp. 227–229.
115. Rotellar E, et al: Must patients over 65 be hemodialyzed? *Nephron* 41: 152–156, 1985.
116. Ponticelli C: Renal replacement therapy in the elderly. *Q J Med* 268:667–668, 1989.
117. Vollmer WM, Wahl PW, and Blagg CR: Survival with dialysis and transplantation in patients with end-stage renal disease. *N Engl J Med* 308: 1553–1558, 1983.
118. Krakauer H, et al: The recent U.S. experience in the treatment of end-stage renal disease by dialysis and transplantation. *N Engl J Med* 308:1558–1563, 1983.
119. Mailloux LU, et al: Predictors of survival in patients undergoing dialysis. *Am J Med* 84:855–862, 1988.
120. Kjellstrand C, et al: Hemodialysis in the Elderly. In Oreopoulos DG (ed), *Geriatric Nephrology.* Boston: Martinus Nijhoff, 1986. Pp. 135–145.
121. Burton PR and Walls J: Selection-adjusted comparison of life-expectancy of patients on continuous ambulatory peritoneal dialysis, hemodialysis and renal transplantation. *Lancet* 1:1115–1119, 1987.
122. Mion C, et al: Maintenance dialysis in the elderly. A review of 15 years experience in Languedoc-Roussillon. *Proc EDTA-ERA* 21:490–509, 1984.
123. Panarello G, et al: Dialysis for the elderly: Survival and risk factors. *Adv Peritoneal Dialysis* 5:49–51, 1989.

124. Williams AJ, et al: Continuous ambulatory peritoneal dialysis and haemo-dialysis in the elderly. *Q J Med* 274:215–223, 1990.
125. Husebye DJ, et al: Psychological, social and somatic prognostic indicators in old patients undergoing long-term dialysis. *Arch Intern Med* 147:1921–1924, 1987.
126. Cohen SL, Comty CM, and Shapiro FL: The effect of age on the results of regular haemodialysis treatment. *Proc Eur Dial Transplant Assoc* 7:254–258, 1970.
127. Ghaptous WN, et al: Long-term hemodialysis in the elderly. *Trans Am Soc Artif Intern Organs* 17:125–128, 1971.
128. Hinsdale JG, Lipkowitz GS, and Hoover EL: Vascular access for hemo-dialysis in the elderly: Results and perspectives in a geriatric population. *Dialysis Transpl* 14:560–565, 1985.
129. Jindal KK and Goldstein MB: Urea kinetic modelling in chronic hemodialy-sis: Benefits, problems and practical solutions. *Semin Dial* 1:82–85, 1988.
130. Basila C, Casino F, and Lopez T: Percent reduction in blood urea concentra-tion during dialysis estimates K+/V in a simple and accurate way. *Am J Kidney Dis* 15:40–45, 1990.
131. Jacobs C, et al: Maintenance haemodialysis treatment in patients over 60 years. Demographic profile, clinical aspects and outcome. *Proc EDTA-ERA* 21:477–489, 1984.
132. Faubert PF and Porush JG: Unpublished observations, 1989.
133. Arieff AI: Aluminum and the pathogenesis of dialysis encephalopathy. *Am J Kidney Dis* 6:317–321, 1985.
134. Norris KC, et al: Clinical and laboratory features of aluminum-related bone disease: Differences between sporadic and "epidemic" forms of the syn-drome. *Am J Kidney Dis* 6:342–347, 1985.
135. Malluche HH and Faugere MC: Aluminum: Toxin or innocent bystander in renal osteodystrophy. *Am J Kidney Dis* 6:336–341, 1985.
136. Goodman WG: Bone disease and aluminum: Pathogenic considerations. *Am J Kidney Dis* 6:330–335, 1985.
137. Swartz RD: Deferoxamine and aluminum removal. *Am J Kidney Dis* 6:358–364, 1985.
138. Boelaert JR, et al: The role of deferrioxamine in dialysis associated mucor-mycosis: Report of three cases and review of the literature. *Clin Nephrol* 29:261–266, 1988.
139. Kaye M: Parathyroidectomy in endstage renal disease. *J Lab Clin Med* 114:334–335, 1989.
140. Dunlay R, et al: Direct inhibitory effect of calcitriol on parathyroid function (sigmoid curve) in dialysis. *Kidney Int* 36:1093–1098, 1989.
141. Andress DL, et al: Intravenous calcitriol in the treatment of refractory os-teitis fibrosa of chronic renal failure. *N Engl J Med* 321:274–279, 1989.
142. Blackely JD, et al: Uremic pruritus skin divalent ion content and response to ultraviolet therapy. *Am J Kidney Dis* 5:237–241, 1985.
143. Stähle-Vackdahl M: Uremic pruritus. Clinical and experimental studies. *Acta Derm Venereol* (Suppl 145) 1:38, 1989.
144. Taylor R, et al: A placebo-controlled trial of UV-A phototherapy for the treatment of uraemic pruritus. *Nephron* 33:14–16, 1983.
145. Gilchrist BA, et al: Relief of uremic pruritus with ultraviolet phototherapy. *N Engl J Med* 297:136–138, 1977.
146. Schaefer K, et al: Optimum dialysis treatment for patients over 60 years with primary renal disease. Survival data and clinical results from 242 pa-

tients treated either by hemodialysis or hemofiltration. *Proc EDTA-ERA* 21:510–523, 1984.

147. Westlie J, et al: Mortality, morbidity and life satisfaction in the very old dialysis patient. *Trans Am Soc Artif Intern Organs* 30:21–30, 1984.

148. Carlson DM, et al: Hospitalization in dialysis patients. *Mayo Clin Proc* 59: 769–775, 1984.

149. Zuckerman GR, et al: Upper gastrointestinal bleeding in patients with chronic renal failure. *Ann Intern Med* 102:588–592, 1985.

150. Almond MK: Laser therapy for lesions of the bronchial tree and gastrointestinal tract in the elderly. *Internal Medicine* 8:53–58, 1987.

151. Remuzzi G: Bleeding in renal failure. *Lancet* 1:1205–1208, 1988.

152. Vigano G, et al: Dose-effect and pharmacokinetics of estrogens given to correct bleeding time in uremia. *Kidney Int* 34:853–858, 1988.

153. Bronner MK, et al: Estrogen-progesterone therapy for bleeding gastrointestinal telangiectasias in chronic renal failure. An uncontrolled trial. *Ann Intern Med* 105:371–374, 1986.

154. Camana RJ, et al: Heparin free dialysis: Comparative data and results in high risk patients. *Kidney Int* 31:1351–1355, 1987.

155. McKevitt PM, Jones JF, and Marion RR: The elderly on dialysis: Physical and psychosocial functioning. *Dialysis Transpl* 15:130–137, 1986.

156. O'Keefe, Schultz K, and Powers MJ: Adjustment of older patients to hemodialysis. *Dialysis Transpl* 16:234–241, 1987.

157. Neu S and Kjellstrand CM: Stopping long-term dialysis. An empirical study of withdrawal of life-supporting treatment. *N Engl J Med* 314:14–20, 1986.

158. Nissenson AR, et al: Peritoneal Dialysis in the Elderly. In Oreopoulos DG (ed), *Geriatric Nephrology*. Boston: Martinus Nijhoff, 1986. Pp. 147–156.

159. Nichols AJ, et al: Impact of continuous ambulatory peritoneal dialysis on treatment of renal failure in patients aged over 60 years. *Br Med J* 288: 18–19, 1984.

160. Gokal R, et al: Peritonitis in continuous ambulatory peritoneal dialysis. *Lancet* 2:1388–1391, 1982.

161. Keene WF, et al: CAPD related peritonitis management and antibiotic therapy recommendations. *Peritoneal Dialysis Bull* 7:55–68, 1987.

162. Nolph KD, Lindblad AS, and Novak JW: Continuous ambulatory peritoneal dialysis. *N Engl J Med* 318:1595–1600, 1988.

163. Paterson AD, et al: Removal and replacement of Tenckhoff catheter at a single operation: Successful treatment of resistant peritonitis in continuous ambulatory peritoneal dialysis. *Lancet* 2:1245–1247, 1986.

164. Selgas R, et al: Comparative study of two different routes for insulin administration in CAPD diabetic patients. A multicenter study. *Adv Peritoneal Dialysis* 5:182–190, 1989.

165. Delmonico F, Cosimi BA, and Russell PS: Renal transplantation in the older age groups. *Arch Surg* 110:1107–1109, 1975.

166. Ost L, et al: Cadaveric renal transplantation in patients of 60 years and above. *Transplantation* 30:339–340, 1980.

167. Taube DH, et al: Successful treatment of middle aged and elderly patients with end stage renal disease. *Br Med J* 286:2018–2020, 1983.

168. Schulak JA, et al: Kidney transplantation in patients aged sixty years or older. *Surgery* 108:726–733, 1990.

169. Kjellstrand CM: Age, sex and race inequality in renal transplantation. *Arch Intern Med* 148:1305–1308, 1988.

170. Jordon ML, et al: Renal transplantation in the older recipient. *J Urol* 134: 243–246, 1985.
171. Sommer BG, et al: Renal Transplantation in the Middle Aged and Elderly Uremic Patient: The Recent United States Experience and Results from a Single Institution. In Oreopoulos DG (ed), *Geriatric Nephrology*. Boston: Martinus Nijhoff, 1986. Pp. 157–168.
172. Cardella CJ: Renal Transplantation in the Elderly: The Canadian Experience. In Oreopoulos DG (ed), *Geriatric Nephrology*. Boston: Martinus Nijhoff, 1986. Pp. 169–173.
173. Myers BD, et al: Cyclosporine-associated chronic nephropathy. *N Engl J Med* 311:699–705, 1984.
174. Pirsch JD, et al: Cadaveric renal transplantation with cyclosporine in patients more than 60 years of age. *Transplantation* 47:259–261, 1989.
175. Fauchald P, et al: Renal replacement therapy in elderly patients. *Transplant Intern* 1:131–134, 1988.
176. Foster MC, et al: Use of older patients as cadaveric kidney donors. *Br J Surg* 75:767–769, 1988.

12 HYPERTENSION

AGE AND BLOOD PRESSURE

From 60 to 80 years of age systolic blood pressure increases an average of 4 to 7 mm Hg per decade in the male and 6 to 9 mm Hg in the female. After the age of 80, a drop in systolic pressure, averaging 2 to 3 mm Hg per decade, occurs in both males and females. On the other hand, after the age of 50 the diastolic blood pressure decreases in both males and females, averaging 1 to 3 mm Hg per decade [1–5]. In general, both systolic and diastolic blood pressure in the elderly black male and female are 4 to 6 mm Hg higher than in their white counterparts. The rise in systolic pressure seen with age is a reflection of an increase in total peripheral vascular resistance, since cardiac output, the other variable component of the blood pressure, either decreases slightly [6, 7] or remains unchanged with age [8, 9].

Both structural and functional alterations account for the changes in arterial blood pressure seen with aging. The arterial walls of both the aorta and the peripheral arteries thicken and become stiff owing to degeneration of wall elastin and calcium deposition [10, 11]. As a result, the pulse waves reflected from peripheral vascular sites return earlier during ventricular ejection, causing a prolonged increase in intraventricular systolic pressure, the end point being a boost in the systolic and a decrease in the diastolic pressure. In addition, the stress associated with modern living may be playing a role, since blood pressure does not increase with age in nuns living in a monastery and followed over a 20-year period [12].

In addition to structural changes, an alteration in muscular tone may contribute to the increase in peripheral vascular resistance seen with increasing age. Plasma norepinephrine levels increase with age [13], probably as a result of an increase in sympathetic activity mediated by an age-related change in baroreflex sensitivity [14, 15]. Alpha-adrenergic vasoconstrictor function remains intact with age [16], whereas beta vasodilation is attenuated [17]. This imbalance could lead to a state of relative vasoconstriction. It should be added, however, that in most recent studies, the beta-2-adrenergic response in the elderly has been found to be identical to that seen in younger patients [18]. Aging is also associated with a decrease in erythrocyte Na-K-ATPase activity [19]. If a similar defect is present in vascular smooth muscle cells, sodium transport out of these cells will decrease. Since the cellular concentration of calcium is linked to the sodium gradient across the cell membrane through a calcium-sodium exchanger, a small increase in cytoplasmic sodium may result in enough of an increase in intracellular calcium to produce an increase in smooth muscle tone. Although plasma vasopressin levels increase with age (see Chap. 1), the contribution of this change to the age-dependent rise in blood pressure has not yet been adequately studied.

As discussed in Chap. 1, glomerular filtration rate (GFR) tends to decrease with age, which probably contributes to renal sodium retention and expansion of the extracellular fluid volume leading to an increase in blood pressure. It should be cautioned, however, that this paradigm is only theoretical and is not based on direct studies [20]. However, the importance of salt handling is suggested by the absence of an age-related increase in blood pressure in populations that have a low salt intake [21].

The higher blood pressure found in elderly blacks compared to whites may reflect in part their greater sensitivity to salt [22], a trait most likely genetically transmitted [23].

DEFINITIONS AND MEASUREMENT

Hypertension in the elderly is defined as a systolic blood pressure of greater than 160 mm Hg or a diastolic pressure of greater than 90 mm Hg, determined from the mean readings on three consecutive visits [24]. The systolic pressure should be recorded at the first Korotkoff sound and the diastolic at the fifth phase when the sound disappears, using a cuff width that measures 40 to 50 percent of the upper arm circumference. The cuff should be deflated at a rate of 2 to 3 mm Hg per second [25]. Hypertension is classified as mild when the diastolic pressure is 90 to 104 mm Hg, moderate when it is 105 to 114 mm Hg, and severe when it is greater than 115 mm Hg. A systolic pressure of more than 160 mm Hg and a diastolic of less than 90 mm Hg is labeled as isolated systolic hypertension.

ESSENTIAL HYPERTENSION

PREVALENCE
Figure 12-1 depicts the prevalence of hypertension in various age groups in a civilian, noninstitutionalized U.S. population [26]. In the 1976–1980 National Health and Nutrition Examination Survey (NAHNES) [27], hypertension was found in 44 percent of whites and 60 percent of blacks aged 65 to 74 years. Hypertension was more common in white and black females compared to white and black males by 11 percent and 19 per-

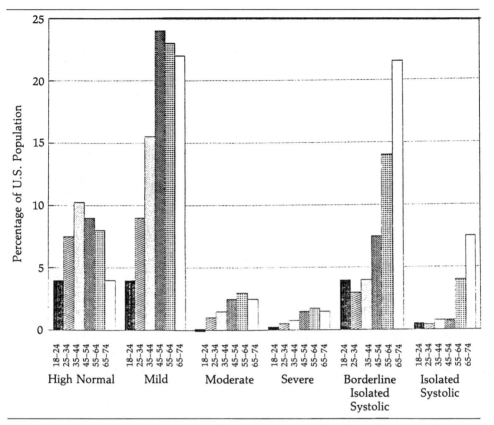

FIGURE 12-1. Percentage of the civilian noninstitutionalized population aged 18 to 74 years with hypertension, categorized by blood pressure (regardless of medication status) and by age, 1976–1980. (From: Final report of the subcommittee on definition and prevalence of hypertension. 1984 Joint National Committee. *Hypertension* 7:457–468, 1985. By permission of the American Heart Association, Inc.)

cent, respectively [28, 29]. As seen in Fig. 12-1, the incidence of mild, moderate, and severe hypertension is similar in the 45- to 54-, 55- to 64-, and 65- to 74-year age groups, whereas isolated systolic hypertension is uncommon before the age of 55 and increases thereafter. Table 12-1 summarizes the prevalence of isolated systolic hypertension as reported from different studies.

HEMODYNAMICS

The hemodynamic parameters of hypertension are quite different in the elderly compared to younger patients. Given an identical mean arterial pressure (MAP), the systolic pressure tends to be higher and the diastolic lower in the elderly. Since the cardiac output in older hypertensives

TABLE 12-1. Prevalence of isolated systolic hypertension in the elderly

Age (yr)	Prevalence (%)	Reference
60–69	6.8 (white males 5.3, black males 6.4, white females 7.4, black females 8.3)	[30]
65–90	14.4 (males) 22.8 (females)	[31]
65–74	7.3	[32]
60–64	3.3	[33]
60–64	12.7	[34]
80+	29.4	[34]
65–75	10–12	[35]

is lower than in younger hypertensives, the elevated blood pressure is maintained by a disproportionately higher total peripheral resistance [36], which is a function of arteriolar tone and, to a lesser degree, blood viscosity.

Pathogenesis of the Enhanced Arteriolar Tone in the Elderly Hypertensive

Potentially reversible as well as irreversible factors are involved in the maintenance of increased arteriolar tone. The irreversible factors include the structural changes that occur with aging such as wall thickening and degeneration of elastin, noted earlier. Not all the structural changes accompanying hypertension are, however, irreversible because significant regression in the thickness of the arterial tunica media may take place following prolonged antihypertensive therapy [37]. This phenomenon results from changes in vascular smooth muscle cells that are identical to the changes in myocardial cells seen in treated hypertensives who manifest reversal of left ventricular hypertrophy [38]. What is not yet evident is whether these arterial changes constitute the primary event leading to the increased vascular resistance or are the result of the hypertension per se. Preliminary evidence showing an increase in the synthesis and release of growth factors by the arterial wall of the hypertensive animal together with the fact that the abnormal vasculature persists despite effective antihypertensive treatment tends to favor the former possibility [39–41]. In addition to structural changes, other potentially reversible factors capable of raising the peripheral resistance in the elderly hypertensive include the sodium and water content of arterial walls, neurohumoral factors, and divalent cations.

SODIUM AND WATER CONTENT OF ARTERIAL WALLS. The role played by an increase in vascular smooth muscle sodium content in the pathogenesis of hypertension is still controversial [42]. To date, there are no data available comparing the sodium content of the arterial wall in elderly normotensive and hypertensive subjects.

NEUROHUMORAL FACTORS. Several circulating vasoactive substances can modify vascular tone. Theoretically, an increase in the activity or sensitivity to a vasoconstrictor not accompanied by a proportional increase in the activity or sensitivity to a vasodilator will increase vascular tone, thereby increasing peripheral vascular resistance. A decrease in the activity or sensitivity to a vasodilator without a similar decrease in the activity or sensitivity to a vasoconstrictor will have the same effect.

As discussed in Chap. 1, plasma renin activity (PRA) decreases with age. Moreover, PRA levels are lower in elderly hypertensives compared with normotensives. On the other hand, plasma aldosterone (PA) is similar in the normotensive and hypertensive elderly, which may be a reflection of an increased sensitivity of the adrenal gland to angiotensin II (AII) in the elderly hypertensive [43]. A similar change in sensitivity of the vasculature to AII may play a pathogenetic role in the hypertension of the elderly as well. The sympathetic nervous system does not appear to be responsible for the increase in peripheral resistance associated with the hypertension of the elderly. Although circulating norepinephrine levels increase with age, they either are no different in normotensive and hypertensive elderly [44], or the levels are higher in normotensives [45, 46]. It should be emphasized, however, that the net effect of the autonomic nervous system on the vasculature is the result of the interaction between the vasoconstrictive effect of the alpha-2 receptor and the vasodilatory effect of the beta-2 receptor. Even though catecholamine levels may be lower in the elderly hypertensive, an increased sensitivity to the constrictive effect of the alpha-2 receptor or a decreased sensitivity to the vasodilatory effect of the beta-2 receptor would result in an increased total peripheral resistance. This issue needs further investigation [47]. Arginine vasopressin, because of its vasoconstrictive property, has been implicated in the pathogenesis of hypertension found in certain experimental models [48] and perhaps also in that associated with chronic renal insufficiency in humans [49]. Information is lacking concerning the contribution of vasopressin to the hypertension seen in the elderly. Plasma vasopressin levels are similar in normotensive and hypertensive white elderly patients but are significantly higher in black hypertensive compared to black normotensive elderly subjects [50].

The concentration of vasodilator peptides such as vasoactive intestinal peptides (VIP) and opioid peptides in the hypertensive animal and plasma substance P in human hypertensives may be reduced [51, 52]. The role played by these substances in the pathogenesis of hypertension remains to be elucidated, however. Although the concentration of kallikreins has been found to be higher in the urine of hypertensive patients compared to normal subjects over the age of 60 [53], the significance of this finding is not clear.

There is data to suggest that some patients with essential hypertension have reduced renal synthesis of prostaglandins (primarily prostaglandin E_2 [PGE_2]) [54]. Similar observations have also been made in elderly hypertensives [55]. Atrial natriuretic peptide (ANP), although closely linked to blood pressure–regulating systems, does not appear to play a role in the pathogenesis of hypertension [56].

DIVALENT IONS.   Both calcium and magnesium have been found to play a role in the pathogenesis of hypertension [57–59]. Significant controversy still exists, however, and the issue is complicated by the fact that serum ionized calcium and magnesium levels vary with PRA in patients with essential hypertension [60, 61]. The higher the PRA, the lower the serum magnesium level and the more magnesium loading lowers the blood pressure [62]. Compared to normotensive subjects, the serum-ionized calcium level is lower in low-renin hypertensives and higher in high-renin patients, suggesting that calcium deficit plays a role in the former group and calcium excess in the latter [63, 64]. Since the prevalence of low-renin hypertension is highest in the elderly [36, 65], it is quite possible that alterations in calcium metabolism due to a basic defect in the plasma membrane contribute to the hypertension seen in this group [66, 67]. The hypotensive effect of oral calcium supplementation in the elderly is rather modest, however [68]. Furthermore, the antihypertensive property of calcium supplementation might be related to its natriuretic property rather than to a direct effect of this cation on total peripheral resistance [69].

OTHER FACTORS.   Endothelium-derived relaxing factor (EDRF) is a substance released by vascular endothelium that mediates relaxation induced by some vasodilators such as acetylcholine, bradykinin, and adenosine 5' diphosphate [70]. It stimulates soluble guanylate cyclase to increase cyclic guanosine monophosphate (GMP) levels in vascular smooth muscle. GMP then mediates relaxation, probably through its actions on intracellular free calcium [71]. In some experimental models of hypertension there is a decrease in EDRF [72]. It is possible that the activity of EDRF may decline with age in humans, as has been reported in the rat [73, 74]. A decrease in EDRF activity would explain some of the structural changes in the vasculature seen in hypertension, since it has an inhibitory effect on smooth muscle growth and proliferation [75]. At the present time, however, there is no direct evidence of a pathogenetic role of this substance in elderly hypertensives.

Endothelin is a potent vasoconstrictor peptide released by endothelial cells in response to various chemical and physical stimuli [76]; it binds specifically to human vascular smooth muscle cells [77]. A possible role for this substance in either the genesis or the maintenance of hypertension is currently under active investigation. It is quite possible, as postulated by Vanhoutte [78], that the increased vascular resistance characteristic of hypertension might result from an imbalance between the vasodilatory effect of EDRF and endothelium-derived constricting factors (endothelin).

As noted earlier, total peripheral resistance is primarily a function of vascular smooth muscle tone and, to a lesser extent, of blood viscosity. The role of blood viscosity has not been specifically studied in the elderly hypertensive, but an increase in blood viscosity proportional to the severity of the hypertension has been found in adult hypertensives (mean age of 45 ± 11 SD) [79]. The higher viscosity was due mainly to an increase in fibrinogen, with hemoconcentration playing a smaller role. The significance of this finding in the elderly hypertensive is not known.

CLINICAL MANIFESTATIONS

As in younger patients, hypertension in the elderly is usually diagnosed during routine physical examination or during evaluation for other unrelated conditions. Occasionally, patients present with headache or vertigo and rarely (fewer than 1 percent in our experience) with accelerated hypertension manifested by encephalopathy or cardiac or renal failure. The presence of a bruit (particularly in diastole) in the abdomen, flank, or costovertebral angle, suggesting the presence of renovascular disease, should always be looked for on physical examination. Components of our baseline laboratory evaluation of the hypertensive elderly are similar to those used in younger patients and include a CBC, BUN, creatinine, electrolytes, glucose, lipid profile, and electrocardiogram [80]. A renal sonogram and a 24-hour urine collection evaluated for protein excretion and creatinine clearance are obtained if renal insufficiency is present. Patients with any suggestion of heart disease undergo an echocardiogram to rule out hypertensive hypertrophic cardiomyopathy so that therapy can be adequately tailored [81, 82].

INDICATIONS FOR THERAPY

It is our opinion that some form of therapeutic intervention (nonpharmacologic or pharmacologic) is indicated in every elderly person with a blood pressure of greater than 160 mm Hg systolic or 90 mm Hg diastolic. This approach is supported by studies demonstrating an increased mortality from stroke and cardiovascular disease in elderly patients aged 60 to 79 with elevated blood pressure, whether systolic or diastolic [83–

TABLE 12-2. Design and outcome of randomized trials of the treatment of diastolic hypertension in the elderly

Study	Type	Age	Blood pressure (mm Hg)	Medication	Outcome
VA (1970)	Randomized double-blind, placebo-controlled study	60–69	90–114 (DBP)	HCTZ and reserpine	Decrease (32%) in cardiovascular morbidity; did not reach significance; magnitude of difference consistent with overall study
HDFP (1979)	Randomized study of special care compared with referred care	60–69	90–115 (DBP)	CTLD and reserpine or alpha-methyldopa	Statistically significant 16.4% reduction in total mortality for special care group
Austr (1980)	Randomized double-blind, placebo-controlled study	60–69	95–109 (DBP)	CTZ and various second-step agents	Reduction (39%) in trial end points for this treatment subgroup; did not reach statistical significance but reduction similar to overall study group
EWPHE (1985)	Randomized double-blind, placebo-controlled study	60–97	90–119 (DBP); 160–239 (SBP)	HCTZ-triamterene and alpha-methyldopa	Significant 38% reduction in cardiac mortality, 32% reduction in cerebrovascular mortality was not quite significant
Coope (1986)	Randomized single-blind, no placebo for controls	60–79	≥ 105 (DBP); ≥ 170 (SBP)	Betablocker and BNFZD	Reduction (30%) in fatal strokes, no effect on myocardial infarction

ABBREVIATIONS: VA = Veterans Administration Cooperative Study; HDFP = Hypertension Detection and Follow-up Program; Austr = Australian Trial on Mild Hypertension; EWPHE = European Working Party on Hypertension in the Elderly; DBP = diastolic blood pressure; SBP = systolic blood pressure; HCTZ = hydrochlorothiazide; CTZ = chlorothiazide; BNFZD = benfluorothiazide; CTLD = chlorthalidone.
SOURCE: Applegate WB: Hypertension in elderly patients. *Ann Intern Med* 110:901–915, 1989.

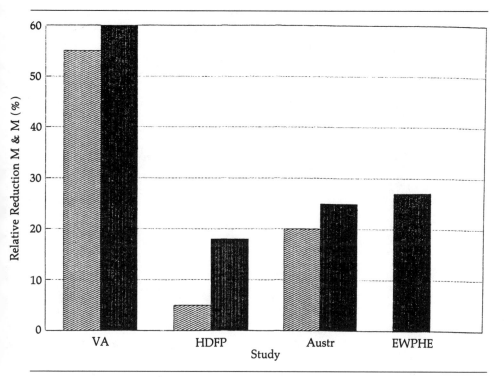

FIGURE 12-2. Impact of antihypertensive therapy on relative reduction (intervention compared with control) of cardiovascular morbidity (VA), mortality (HDFP), and combined cardiovascular morbidity and mortality (M & M) (Austr and EWPHE) for participants younger than age 50 (cross-hatched bars) compared with those older than age 60 (solid bars). VA = Veterans Administration Cooperative Study; HDFP = Hypertension Detection and Follow-up Program; Austr = Australian Trial on Mild Hypertension; EWPHE = European Working Party on Hypertension in the Elderly. Cardiovascular morbidity in each study represents total nonfatal cardiovascular and cerebrovascular events reported. (From: Applegate WB: Hypertension in elderly patients. *Ann Intern Med* 110:901–915, 1989.)

88]. Furthermore, the results of five studies of therapeutic interventions, recently summarized by Applegate (Table 12-2) [89], have shown that therapy reduces the risk of complications in the elderly with systolic and diastolic hypertension. These studies demonstrate that treated elderly patients have the same reduction in cardiovascular mortality as do younger patients (< 50 years of age) (Fig. 12-2). Since the rate of cardiovascular events is generally higher in the elderly, the benefits of treating hypertension are also greater in this group (Fig. 12-3).

It is not yet clear whether lowering the blood pressure in the elderly with isolated systolic hypertension will result in a decrease in cardiovascular complications. An answer may be forthcoming from the ongoing

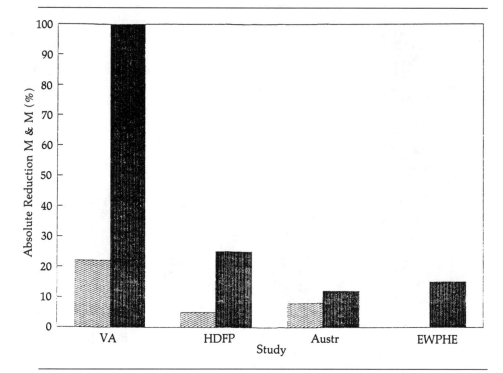

FIGURE 12-3. Impact of antihypertensive therapy on absolute reduction (intervention compared with control) of cardiovascular morbidity (VA), mortality (HDFP), and combined cardiovascular morbidity and mortality (M & M) (Austr and EWPHE) for participants younger than age 50 (cross-hatched bars) compared with those older than age 60 (solid bars). VA = Veterans Administration Cooperative Study; HDFP = Hypertension Detection and Follow-up Program; Austr = Australian Trial on Mild Hypertension; EWPHE = European Working Party on Hypertension in the Elderly. (From: Applegate WB: Hypertension in elderly patients. *Ann Intern Med* 110:901–915, 1989).

Systolic Hypertension in the Elderly Program (SHEP) now in progress [90]. Preliminary data from this study, plus our own experience and that of others, have established that these patients tolerate antihypertensive drugs well [91–98], and therefore our policy is to treat them.

The goal of therapy, as recommended by the working group on hypertension in the elderly [98] and others [99–101], is to reduce the systolic blood pressure to the 140- to 160-mm Hg range and the diastolic to below 90 mm Hg. Some caution should be exercised because a higher incidence of myocardial infarction or mortality has been observed by some authors in elderly patients in whom the diastolic blood pressure was decreased to below 85 mm Hg [87, 102–105]. This phenomenon (the J-shaped curve) may be related to the presence of severe coronary artery disease ($>$ 85 percent stenosis) in many of these patients. Since coronary flow reserves virtually disappear with this degree of stenosis, a fall in diastolic blood pressure below 85 mm Hg would be accompanied by an equivalent fall in coronary flow [106–108]. In the controlled study reported by the European Working Party on High Blood Pressure in the Elderly (EWPHE) [109], an increase in mortality was noted in patients with the lowest blood pressure whether they were taking medicine or placebo. In both groups, patients with the lowest blood pressure were characterized by lower body weight and hemoglobin levels, suggesting that a deterioration of general health was the cause of their higher mortality rather than the drug-induced drop in blood pressure [109]. Controversy also exists about the concept of the J-shaped curve in the treatment of hypertension and coronary artery disease [109a, 109b].

Little information is available on the results of treating either systolic or diastolic hypertension in elderly patients over 80 years of age. In one study involving both male and female Finnish patients over 85, a significantly higher 5-year survival rate was found in hypertensive (59 percent) compared with normotensive (28 percent) subjects [110]. Similar observations have been made by Lauger et al [111] in American men but not in women aged 75 years and over. In the EWPHE study, patients in this older age group did not significantly benefit from therapy, but the number treated was relatively small [112]. At the present time, our approach to therapy in patients over the age of 75 varies according to the functional status of the patient and is similar to that followed by others [113]. In patients who are active and otherwise well, we start with a single drug at a low dose and follow this with a slow titration process to bring the blood pressure to approximately 160/90 mm Hg. The occurrence of any significant side effect is an indication either to stop the medication at the better tolerated dose (even if the blood pressure goal is not achieved) or to discontinue therapy altogether. Frail and severely debilitated elderly patients with multiple other problems are probably better left untreated.

Pseudohypertension

This phenomenon is an artifact in which cuff measurements overestimate the true arterial pressure as assessed by an intra-arterial cannula. This problem can be detected clinically by inflating the blood pressure cuff above the systolic blood pressure and carefully palpatating either the radial or the brachial artery (Osler's maneuver). If either of these vessels remains palpable, the test result is considered positive for pseudohypertension [114]. The automatic infrasonic recorder (IR), which detects subaudible oscillations in the arterial wall under an occluding cuff, may also help in diagnosing pseudohypertension in the elderly [115]. A difference in the diastolic blood pressure of 4 mm Hg or greater between the standard cuff measurements and IR measurements is highly suggestive of pseudohypertension. The incidence of this phenomenon in elderly hypertensives has been variably reported as 0 to 50 percent [116–119]. Osler's maneuver, performed by us in 40 consecutive hypertensive patients over the age of 60, was positive in only one (2.5 percent). Overestimation of the blood pressure by the cuff measurement usually involves the diastolic rather than the systolic pressure [120, 121]. Pseudohypertension should be ruled out in any treated elderly patient who experiences symptoms suggestive of a low pressure such as fainting spells or chronic fatigue when cuff blood pressure readings are still in the hypertensive or even normotensive range.

THERAPY OF HYPERTENSION IN THE ELDERLY
Once the decision to treat hypertension is made, the following factors should be considered.

Postural Hypotension
This condition is present in a significant number of elderly people [122]; therefore, attempts should be made to identify such patients prior to initiating therapy because such knowledge will significantly influence which drugs to use. Also, postprandial drops in blood pressure due to splanchnic vasodilatation and impaired sympathetic reflex reactivity can occur in the elderly [123–125], particularly those 75 years or over. It is not clear at present whether antihypertensive drugs will accentuate this phenomenon.

Drug Interactions
Up to 40 percent of elderly hypertensives have a concomitant medical problem that requires some form of therapy. In one study of 102 elderly hypertensives the average number of medications per patient was 3.6 [126]. The possibility of drug-drug interaction is significant in these patients. Among the most common offenders are the nonsteroidal antiinflammatory drugs (NSAIDs) (with the exception, perhaps, of sulindac), which can interfere with the antihypertensive action of beta blockers, angiotensin-converting enzyme inhibitors, and diuretics [127–131]. Tricyclic antidepressants can interfere with the antihypertensive effect of reserpine and clonidine. Angiotensin-converting enzyme inhibitors may lead to dangerous hyperkalemia in a patient taking supplemental potassium (particularly if the patient is also taking an NSAID).

Price
Most elderly patients live on a rather limited budget and often do not have adequate insurance to cover the cost of drugs. The thiazide diu-

retics are among the cheapest drugs available, followed by central adrenergic inhibitors and vasodilators. The beta blockers are intermediate in price, and the alpha-adrenergic blockers, calcium channel blockers, and converting enzyme inhibitors are the most expensive [89, 132, 133].

Nonpharmacologic Therapy

DIETARY MANAGEMENT. We usually recommend moderate salt restriction (2–3 g Na daily) to our elderly patients with hypertension even though the blood pressure response to this regimen will vary from patient to patient [134–137]. Supplemental potassium (60–65 mEq per day) has been associated with a reduction in blood pressure, but caution should be exercised in elderly patients with superimposed renal insufficiency or those who are taking a converting enzyme inhibitor or NSAID. Since the benefits obtained from potassium supplementation are either moderate or nonexistent, particularly in a patient on a low-sodium diet, we do not routinely advocate potassium supplementation in our elderly hypertensive patients [138–141]. Calcium supplementation (1 g elemental Ca) has been shown to result in a modest decrease in mean arterial pressure in a small number of elderly hypertensives [142]. Because of the preliminary nature of this finding, we do not presently recommend such supplementation, particularly in view of the risk of calcium urolithiasis.

Obese patients are encouraged to lower their weight because a positive correlation has been found between blood pressure and weight in all age groups [5, 143, 144], and weight reduction in the obese leads to a fall in blood pressure [145, 146]. When feasible, the patient should be referred for nutritional counseling because merely instructing the patient to lose weight is not sufficient in most instances [147]. Finally, alcohol consumption should be curtailed in patients who take more than a 1 oz of ethanol per day (two drinks of spirits or their equivalent in wine or beer) [148–150].

EXERCISE. Exercise in the elderly hypertensive is as well tolerated as in the elderly normotensive [151]. Furthermore, low-intensity exercise such as walking 1 hour 3 times weekly has been shown to be associated with a decrease in both systolic and diastolic pressure in the elderly [152].

Pharmacologic Therapy

The drugs that control blood pressure in elderly patients are the same as those used in the treatment of hypertension in all age groups. It should be kept in mind, however, that pharmacokinetics and pharmacodynamics change with age and that other co-morbid states are frequently present in the elderly that require a more considered approach, tailored to the individual's needs and responses, than that used in the usual stepped-care regimens.

DIURETICS. The thiazide diuretics and their equivalents are both safe and effective for treating either isolated systolic or systolic and diastolic hypertension in the elderly [112, 153–155]. It is recommended that therapy be started at the lowest dose with graded increases (Table 12-3). The use of more than 25 mg per day of hydrochlorothiazide or its equivalent is probably not warranted because side effects increase without a significant further drop in blood pressure [156–160]. Initiation of thiazide therapy is associated with a decrease in intravascular volume, which is in part responsible for the antihypertensive effect [161]. The decrease in blood pressure, however, is maintained primarily through a decrease in total peripheral vascular resistance, probably by activating vasodepressor substances such as prostacyclin [162, 163]. Thiazides should not be used in the presence of a serum creatinine of 2.5 mg per dl or greater. One exception, however, is metolazone, which can be added to a loop diuretic (furosemide or bumetanide) to manage elderly hypertensives with chronic renal insufficiency. The most common side effects associated with the thiazides in the elderly are hypokalemia, cardiac arrhythmias, hyponatremia (mainly in females), and hypomagnesemia [164]. Careful attention should be paid to volume status to prevent excessive volume contraction. Indopamide is an indoline diuretic that has been successfully used in treating the elderly. As with the thiazides, normotension is maintained through its effect on total peripheral resistance [165, 166].

ALPHA-2-ADRENORECEPTOR AGONISTS. This group includes methylopa, clonidine, guanadrel sulfate, guanabenz acetate, and guanfacine HCl. They lower blood pressure through either a central or peripheral stimulation of the alpha-2 adrenoreceptor. As a consequence, norepinephrine release is decreased, and sympathetic tone is reduced [167]. Methyldopa can be used in the elderly with mild to moderate hypertension. We usually start with a dose of 125 mg twice a day with slow upright titration, since the drug can decrease cardiac output in the elderly [168] and can induce severe orthostatic hypotension, especially when used in combination with a diuretic [169, 170]. Other common side effects include sleep disturbances and drowsiness [171]. The starting dose for clonidine in 0.05 mg given every 12 hours with slow titration up to 0.6 mg daily [172]. This drug has also been used successfully in combination with a thiazide diuretic. Common side effects are dryness of the mouth and orthostasis. Rebound (overshoot) hypertension and the clonidine withdrawal syndrome (headache, nausea, palpitation, tremor) have been reported within 12 to 48 hours after abrupt discontinuation of the drug. This problem, although uncommon, is important in treating the forgetful elderly patient. Therefore, it would be prudent not to use the drug in these patients [174]. The transdermal patch of the drug is available as TTS-1, TTS-2, and TTS-3 and is programmed to deliver 0.1 mg, 0.2 mg, and 0.3 mg, respectively, of clonidine per day for 7 days. This preparation offers certain advantages for the elderly, including a weekly interval between doses, which facilitates compliance. Blood concentrations are stable, and the incidence of side effects is significantly reduced [175, 176]. The drug is, in our experience, efficient in the elderly with mild hypertension; however, we had to discontinue it in a significant number of our patients because of the development of a bothersome contact dermatitis. The other alpha-2 agonists, guanadrel sulfate, guanabenz acetate, and guanfacine HCl, are long acting and can be used once a day in the elderly with mild to moderate hypertension [177]. Their side effects are identical to those of clonidine.

ALPHA-1-ADRENORECEPTOR ANTAGONISTS.   Prazosin lowers blood pressure by blocking the vasoconstrictive effects of the alpha-1 receptor, thereby decreasing total peripheral resistance. The drug is, in general, well tolerated by the elderly with mild hypertension. Dizziness is the most common side effect [178, 179]. It is recommended that the first dose, usually 1 mg, be given prior to bedtime to minimize the risk of severe postural hypotension that occasionally occurs (so-called first dose response). The drug can be titrated slowly to a maximum of 10 mg twice a day. This drug is advantageous in treatment of the hypertensive elderly male with symptomatic prostatic hypertrophy because it can decrease the frequency of urination in these patients [180]. It may be particularly useful in patients who refuse prostatic surgery or are considered poor surgical risks. The action of terazosin is similar to that of prazosin with the advantage that it can be used once a day. The starting dose is 1 mg, and the maximum is 40 mg per day [181].

BETA-ADRENORECEPTOR ANTAGONISTS.   Several beta antagonists are available in the United States, including nonselective beta-1 and beta-2 antagonists (propranolol, timolol, nadolol); selective beta-1 antagonists (metoprolol, atenolol); nonselective beta-1- and beta-2- and a selective alpha-1-adrenergic antagonist (labetalol). Beta blockers are widely used and well tolerated in elderly hypertensives, in whom the incidence of side effects is similar to that seen in younger patients [182–184]. Mental performance does not appear to be affected [185, 186]. The efficacy of these drugs, however, tends to be reduced in the elderly compared to the younger patient, perhaps because of an age-associated reduction in renin activity and a diminished cardiac performance in elderly hypertensive patients [187].

The antihypertensive action of the beta-adrenergic antagonists depends on their ability to attenuate the effects of catecholamines at the beta adrenoreceptors located in the heart, brain, and presynaptic nerve

TABLE 12-3. Drugs used in the elderly hypertensive patient

Class and drug	Starting dosage	Maintenance dosage	Frequency	Reference
Diuretics				
Hydrochlorothiazide (Hydrodiuril, Esidrix)	25 mg	25–50 mg	Every day	[112, 153–160, 200]
Methylclothiazide (Enduron)	2.5 mg	2.5–5.0 mg	Every day	—
Chlorthalidone (Hygrotin)	12.5 mg	12.5–25 mg	Every day	—
Metolazone (Zaroxolyn, Diulo)	1.25 mg	1.25–10 mg	Every day	[165, 166]
Indapamide (LoZol)	2.5 mg	2.5 mg	Every day	—
Furosemide (Lasix)	40 mg	40–240 mg	Every day	—
Bumetanide (Bumex)	1 mg	1–6 mg	Every day	—
Alpha-2-adrenergic agonists				
Methyldopa (Aldomet)	250 mg	250–1,000 mg	Every day	[168–171]
Clonidine (Catapres)	0.1 mg	0.1–0.3 mg	q8–12h	[172, 173]
Clonidine patch (Clonidine TTS)	TTS-1	TTS-1 to TTS-3	weekly	[175, 176]
Guanadrel sulfate (Hylorel)	5 mg	5–30 mg	Every day	[177]
Guanabenz acetate (Wytensin)	4 mg	4–32 mg	Every day	—
Guanfacine HCl (Tenex)	0.5 mg	0.5–1 mg	Every day	—
Alpha-1-adrenergic antagonists				
Prazosin (Minipress)	2 mg	2–20 mg	q8–12h	[178, 179]
Terazosin (Hytrin)	1 mg	1–40 mg	Every day	[181]

	Starting dose	Dose range	Frequency	References
Beta antagonists				
Propranolol (Inderal)	20 mg	20–40 mg	q12h	—
Propranolol LA (Inderal LA)	40 mg	40–400 mg	Every day	[182]
Timolol (Blocadren)	10 mg	10–60 mg	q12h	[198]
Nadolol (Corgard)	10 mg	10–120 mg	Every day	[199]
Metoprolol (Lopressor)	25 mg	25–300 mg	Every day	[200, 201]
Atenolol (Tenormin)	10 mg	10–60 mg	q12h	[199, 202]
Pindolol (Visken)	10 mg	200–800 mg	Every day	[203, 204]
Acebutolol (Sectral)	200 mg	200–800 mg	Every day	—
Labetalol (Normodyne, Trandate)	200 mg	200–800 mg	Every day	[194, 195, 205, 206]
Vasodilators				
Hydralazine (Apresoline)	25 mg	25–50 mg	q6h	—
Minoxidil (Loniten)	2.5 mg	2.5–10 mg	Every day	[208]
Angiotensin II–converting enzyme inhibitors				
Captopril (Capoten)	12.5 mg	12.5–50 mg	q8–12h	[215–220]
Enalapril (Vasotec)	2.5 mg	2.5–20 mg	q12h	[178, 221, 222]
Lisinopril (Zestril, Prinivil)	20 mg	20–40 mg	Every day	[223, 224]
Calcium channel antagonists				
Nifedipine (Procardia, Adalat)	10 mg	10–20 mg	q8h	[231, 232]
Verapamil (Calan, Calan SR, Isoptin, Isoptin SR)	160 mg	160–240 mg	q12h	[232–234]
Diltiazem (Cardizem, Cardizem SR)	60 mg	60–120 mg	q12h	[235]
Nicardipine (Cardene)	10 mg	10–30 mg	q8h	[236–239]
Nitrendipine	10 mg	10 mg	q12h	[240, 241]
Isradipine	1.25 mg	1.25–10 mg	q12h	[242, 243]

endings of the heart and blood vessels [187]. The net effect is diminished central sympathetic discharge and peripheral norepinephrine release. Acutely, the cardiac output decreases, and the total peripheral vascular resistance increases or remains unchanged. With prolonged therapy, cardiac output returns toward the pretreatment level, and total peripheral resistance decreases [188–190]. The effect of the drug on the vasculature may be secondary to its ability to antagonize AII enhancement of sympathetic nerve stimulation by increasing prostaglandin levels in vascular tissue [191, 192]. The choice of beta blocker should be based on the physician's familiarity with the drug, patient compliance, and co-morbid problems. In general, we try to avoid beta blockers for monotherapy in elderly patients with isolated systolic hypertension because the therapeutic response in our experience and that of others has been rather poor [193]. Good results have been reported with the use of labetalol [194, 195]. Kirkendall [196] has discussed the theoretic advantages of using a beta blocker with intrinsic sympathomimetic activity in the elderly, since less depression of cardiac function should occur. Studies comparing the hemodynamic responses of the elderly to the various beta blockers are lacking, however. Contraindications to the use of these drugs in older hypertensive patients are similar to those operative in younger individuals and include chronic obstructive lung disease, congestive heart failure, heart block, and peripheral vascular disease [197]. The starting and maintenance doses used for the various beta blockers are outlined in Table 12-3.

VASODILATORS. Hydralazine and minoxidil act directly on the vascular smooth muscle through changes in potassium channels to lower total peripheral resistance [207]. Although these drugs are well tolerated in the elderly, they usually cannot be used as monotherapy because they cause tachycardia and salt retention. The starting dose of hydralazine is 25 mg 3 times a day, with upward titration to a maximum of 225 mg per day. Minoxidil is usually reserved for the treatment of severe hypertension and requires the addition of a beta blocker and a diuretic to block the reflex tachycardia and salt retention [208]. Patients in whom a beta blocker is contraindicated should receive clonidine to correct the tachycardia [209]. Minoxidil may also be associated with hypertrichosis, a complication poorly tolerated by females. This problem usually disappears within 2 to 3 weeks after the drug has been discontinued, but occasionally hypertrichosis can persist for months.

ANGIOTENSIN II–CONVERTING ENZYME INHIBITORS (ACEis). These agents exert their antihypertensive effect by lowering total peripheral resistance. They do not have any effect on cardiac output [210]. In addition to reducing angiotensin II activity, the ACEis stimulate prostaglandin synthesis and potentiate the activity of bradykinin resulting from kinase inhibition [211]. The use of a bradykinin inhibitor, aprotinin, or a prostaglandin inhibitor, indomethacin, can blunt the antihypertensive effects of ACEis [212]. These agents are usually well tolerated by the elderly; however, first-dose hypotension has been reported accompanied by reversible renal, cardiac, or cerebral ischemia [213, 214]. Patients at risk for this effect are those taking diuretics as well as those who are hypovolemic, hyponatremic, or who have congestive heart failure. Treatment should be initiated at a low dose and the effect carefully monitored. Acute renal failure can occur in patients with bilateral renal artery stenosis or renal artery stenosis to a solitary kidney (see Chap. 10). Because these drugs can induce hyperkalemia (particularly in patients with renal insufficiency), serum potassium should be measured on a regular basis. Other, less common side effects include skin rash, neutropenia, chronic cough with or without wheezing (more common in females), and angioedema [210]. Captopril and other agents have been successfully used in the elderly with mild to moderate hypertension either as monotherapy or in combination with a diuretic [215–224]. The therapeutic efficacy of the various ACEis in the therapy of isolated systolic hypertension has not been adequately assessed [225]. Our own experience with them has not been good, however. Starting and maintenance doses for the various agents are summarized in Table 12-3.

CALCIUM CHANNEL BLOCKERS. These agents are very efficient in lowering blood pressure in the elderly [226]. A positive correlation has been found between age and the magnitude of the arterial pressure reduction achieved by calcium channel blockers [227]; this might in part be due to the lower PRA that occurs with aging. Indeed, the blood pressure–lowering effect of these drugs is inversely related to pretreatment PRA levels [228]. These drugs lower total peripheral vascular resistance by interfering with calcium influx, which is mediated by the binding of the neurotransmitter norepinephrine to its receptor on the vascular smooth muscle [229]. The drugs currently available in the United States are diltiazem, nifedipine, verapamil, nicardipine, and nimodipine. Others, such as nitrendipine and isradipine, will become available shortly. Despite their similar effect on peripheral vascular resistance, these drugs have different effects on cardiac function. They all affect inotropy and chronotropy, with verapamil, followed by diltiazem, having the most negative effects [226]. Nifedipine and nicardipine have the least effect. These differences should be kept in mind when considering calcium channel blockers in patients with heart failure or atrioventricular conduction defects. The recommended doses in the elderly are described in Table 12-3. The most common side effect in the elderly is constipation, which at times can be quite troublesome. Headaches and pedal edema are not as common [230]. Calcium channel blockers, in our experience, are effective in treating isolated systolic hypertension as well as systolic-diastolic hypertension in the elderly.

Antihypertensive Drugs and Lipids

Recently there has been a great deal of interest in the effects of various antihypertensive drugs on lipid metabolism. The subject has been reviewed extensively [244–248]. To summarize, thiazide diuretics can increase triglycerides, total cholesterol, very low density lipoproteins (VLDL), and low-density lipoproteins (LDL), at least during the short term and possibly during the long term as well (2 years or longer); high-density lipoproteins (HDL), however, are not changed. In the elderly these alterations appear to be dose dependent, since significant hyperlipidemia did not develop at the dose used (25–50 mg per day of chlorthalidone) in the EWPHE study [112]. Similar observations have also been made by others [249]. The effects of beta blockers on plasma lipids depend on the agent used. Nonselective and selective beta-1 antagonists increase triglycerides and total and LDL cholesterol while decreasing HDL (5–19 percent). Pindolol decreases LDL while increasing HDL, whereas labetalol does not affect lipid levels at all. The alpha-1-adrenoreceptor antagonists decrease triglycerides and total cholesterol and increase HDL. The ACEis and calcium channel blockers do not alter plasma lipids. The clinical significance of these observations is not clear. We use a prudent approach in following lipid levels in every patient treated with any of the agents known to affect lipid levels adversely and avoiding them altogehter in patients with significant elevations of total and LDL cholesterol initially.

Effects of Antihypertensive Drugs on Left Ventricular Hypertrophy

Left ventricular hypertrophy (LVH) is commonly found in the elderly at the time of initial diagnosis of hypertension [250]. During the past few years LVH has been shown to be not entirely pressure dependent and has been identified as a major risk factor for sudden death, myocardial infarction, and congestive heart failure [251–253]. Physical examination and the electrocardiogram (ECG), the two most commonly and readily available means of detecting LVH, are relatively insensitive. The echocardiogram is more sensitive but is relatively expensive [254]. In general, its routine use is not warranted in elderly hypertensive patients for evaluating the presence of LVH when the ECG is normal, but it should be done when this information is necessary for appropriate therapy, particularly if the diagnosis of hypertensive hypertrophic cardiomyopathy is being considered [81, 82]. Furthermore, there have been no prospective studies carried out to determine whether reducing or reversing LVH in the elderly will improve its inherent ominous prognosis. Finally, reduction of LVH is carried out in the same way as the reduction of arterial blood pressure using all classes of drugs discussed in Table 12-3 with the possible exception of diuretics and vasodilators (controversial) [255]. The number of patients with unrecognized LVH treated solely with a diuretic or a vasodilator in recent years is probably quite small, so this issue is not a real problem.

HYPERTENSIVE EMERGENCIES AND URGENCIES IN THE ELDERLY

A hypertensive emergency (malignant hypertension) refers to patients with a markedly elevated blood pressure (diastolic pressure usually > 130 mm Hg) associated with concomitant acute end-organ involvement such as grade IV Keith-Wagoner-Barker retinopathy, encephalopathy, left ventricular failure, acute renal failure, or dissecting aortic aneurysm. Blood pressure in such patients must be lowered immediately. Other situations in which blood pressure must be treated aggressively and the patient closely observed are referred to as hypertensive urgencies. The diastolic blood pressure in such patients is generally at least 120 mm Hg. Included in this group are hypertensive patients with acute symptomatic coronary artery disease, those in the immediate pre- or postoperative period or with an intracranial bleed [256]. The incidence of hypertensive emergencies in the elderly is not known, but our own recent experience suggests that it is infrequent. For example, in the period from January 1977 to December 1981 we treated 18 such patients compared to only 5 from January 1982 to December 1986, during a time when the number of elderly hypertensives treated by us increased significantly. Part of the reason for the decline in numbers may be patient education and a more aggressive therapeutic approach to elderly hypertension taken by primary physicians [97].

In patients with hypertensive emergencies the clinical manifestations are usually those of the target organ involved. Patients with CNS involvement may be confused and agitated. The presence of coma or focal neurologic signs suggests an intracerebral bleed. Pulmonary congestion or edema is present in patients with cardiac involvement (LVH is found in virtually every patient). Patients with acute renal failure may be asymptomatic, and the diagnosis is made only after blood chemistries become available. The urine may have red cells and proteinuria, but these are not invariably present. The pathologic lesion characteristic of malignant hypertension is that of fibrinoid necrosis of the arteriolar wall with subsequent endothelial damage. In the kidneys, the glomeruli are relatively spared, apart from some tuft collapse or wrinkling of the glomerular basement membrane [257].

For patients with malignant hypertension we usually initiate therapy with sodium nitroprusside infused at the rate of 0.5 mg per kg per minute and then titrate the dose up to 10 mg per kg per minute, as necessary. The mean dose required to control blood pressure (see earlier discussion) is approximately 1 mg per kg per minute. Labetalol, administered either as a bolus of 20, 40, or 80 mg or as a continuous infusion of 1 to 3 mg per minute, has been used successfully in the elderly [258]. The blood pressure–lowering effect of this agent is not accompanied by reflex tachycardia, making it the drug of choice in the management of the elderly with a dissecting aneurysm. Other parenteral drugs are available and include diazoxide, enalaprilat, tremethaphan camsylate, and phentolamine. Diazoxide is given as a bolus of 50 to 100 mg, repeated every 10 to 15 minutes until a maximum of 300 mg has been administered. Enalaprilat is administered as a bolus of 1.25 mg, which can be repeated every 6 hours. Trimethaphan camsylate is used as a continuous infusion of 1 mg per minute, and phentolamine is given at 0.1 to 0.5 mg per minute. This last drug is reserved for patients with pheochromocytoma. We generally try to avoid diazoxide in patients with heart failure and dissecting aneurysm, since tachycardia and salt retention are common side effects [259]. Whenever possible, oral therapy should be started concomitant with parenteral therapy, preferably with short-acting agents to facilitate rapid changes.

It is not presently clear what constitutes a safe target blood pressure in the elderly with malignant hypertension. We aim for a mean arterial pressure of 120 mm Hg (approximately 160/100 mm Hg), based on evidence recently reviewed by Ledingham [260]. Once the blood pressure has been brought under control, the prognosis for reversal of target organ dysfunction is usually good. We routinely evaluate elderly patients with malignant hypertension for the presence of renovascular disease. The yield in our experience has been more than 70 percent. Three of the seven patients reported by Given et al [261], and one of the three reported by Cressman et al [258] had renovascular disease, a significantly higher percentage than that found in the general hypertensive population.

The goal in lowering the blood pressure in hypertensive urgencies is the same as that outlined above. Hypertensive urgencies are encountered more frequently in a geriatric practice than malignant hypertension. The majority of our patients have had severe hypertension in the pre- or postoperative period. The other clinical situations referred to earlier have been encountered less frequently. In these patients, unless absolutely contraindicated (in which case parenteral therapy should be used), the oral route is the preferred method of controlling the blood pressure. Clonidine and nifedipine are the most commonly used drugs [262]. The starting dose of clonidine is 0.1 or 0.2 mg, followed by 0.1 mg every hour, with a maximum dose of 0.7 mg [263, 264]. Nifedipine can be either chewed and swallowed, or the capsule can be punctured and placed under the tongue. The onset of action is probably faster with the former method [265–267]. Ten milligrams is the usual dose, which can be repeated every 20 to 40 minutes, if necessary, up to a maximum of 40 mg every 4 to 6 hours [268–270]. Both drugs are usually well tolerated and have minimum side effects in the elderly. Other regimens have been recommended, but clinical experience with them in the elderly is limited. These include captopril, 25 to 50 mg every 4 to 6 hours [271]; labetalol, 200 to 400 mg every 6 to 12 hours [272]; and a combination of minoxidil, 2.5 to 10 mg every 4 to 6 hours, with a beta blocker and a diuretic [273]. In contrast to patients with malignant hypertension, the overwhelming majority of elderly people with hypertensive urgencies have essential hypertension, and therefore a routine search for renovascular disease is not warranted.

SECONDARY HYPERTENSION

Renovascular hypertension and hypertension of renal insufficiency are the two most common forms of secondary hypertension in the elderly and are dealt with in Chapters 11 and 13. The other forms of secondary hypertension seen in the elderly include pheochromocytoma, primary hyperaldosteronism, and other adrenocortical diseases.

PHEOCHROMOCYTOMA

This entity is seen in 0.2 to 0.7 percent of patients with hypertension [274]. Approximately 22 percent of reported cases were in patients 60 years or older [275–282]. These tumors are located intra-adrenally in 75 percent of cases and extra-adrenally in the remainder. Common extra-adrenal sites (medullary zone) include the abdomen, peripheral nerves, and intrathoracic and intravesical sites. In addition to hypertension, which is present in 92 percent of elderly patients with pheochromocytoma (sustained in 50 percent and paroxysmal in 42 percent), patients may complain of headaches, diaphoresis, palpitations, and various gastrointestinal symptoms [279, 281, 283]. Orthostatic hypotension is seen occasionally, and hyperglycemia is observed quite frequently. Because of the nonspecific nature of these findings, the diagnosis is often made only at autopsy (31 percent of the time) [278]. It is not clear whether this finding is applicable to the elderly. Hypercalcemia or evidence of pituitary dysfunction, suggestive of multiple endocrine neoplasia, is rare in the elderly. The presence of neurofibromatosis and hypertension should raise the suspicion of this disease.

The hypertension seen in patients with pheochromocytoma, as in those with essential hypertension, is associated with an increase in total peripheral resistance. Since no strong correlation exists between blood pressure and the level of catecholamines in patients with pheochromocytoma, other modulating factors are probably at play [284, 285]. The state of the patient's circulating blood volume, which may be reduced because of the catecholamine-induced venoconstriction, is probably important [286]. A generalized increase in sympathetic nervous system activity is also present because clonidine, an inhibitor of central sympathetic outflow as well as presynaptic receptors, decreases blood pressure in patients with pheochromocytoma without changing plasma catecholamines [287]. Vasodilators (dopamine, prostaglandins) secreted by the tumor may also modulate the blood pressure, since a negative correlation has been found between the ratio of dopamine-norepinephrine and blood pressure, suggesting that the blood pressure is determined by a balance of vasoconstrictor and vasodilator substances [288]. Finally, the high level of circulating catecholamines is likely to be associated with down-regulation of the vascular smooth muscle cell receptors, thereby decreasing their sensitivity to these agents [289]. Furthermore, aging itself has been shown to induce a state of relative insensitivity to catecholamines [290].

The laboratory investigation of pheochromocytoma usually starts with a 24-hour urinary collection for metanephrine levels. The upper limit of normal in our elderly patients is similar to that reported in the essential hypertensive population at large, 1.8 mg per 24 hours. This test is quite reliable [291]. The major drawback is that urine has to be collected over a 24-hour period, which may lead to major errors in some elderly patients. In such patients, plasma catecholamines should be determined. The patient should be in a fasting state, and a large-bore needle is then inserted into a vein at least 30 minutes prior to the test, while the patient is kept supine in a quiet room. The plasma norepinephrine (NE) level in both normotensive and essential hypertensive elderly is less than 700 pg per ml, and plasma epinephrine (E) is less than 150 pg per ml [14, 44, 292]. Values for plasma NE or E in our elderly patients with proved pheochromocytomas have been greater than 2,000 pg per ml. Patients with values of less than 2,000 pg per ml but higher than normal in whom there is a high clinical suspicion for pheochromocytoma should be considered for the clonidine suppression test. This consists of measuring NE and E prior to and 2 to 3 hours after oral administration of 0.3 mg of clonidine. A fall of NE and E to a level below 500 pg per ml is evidence against the presence of a pheochromocytoma [291].

Once the diagnosis of a pheochromocytoma has been confirmed biochemically, an abdominal CT scan should be obtained. In patients with tumors larger than 1.0 cm this test has a localizing precision of 96 percent [293, 294]. Nuclear magnetic resonance imaging (NMRI) is no more accurate or sensitive and is much more expensive [295]. Since the CT scan may miss small adrenal and extra-adrenal tumors, patients with clinical and biochemical evidence of a pheochromocytoma and a negative CT scan should be referred for radioisotopic imaging, using ^{131}I meta-iodobenzylguanidine (mIBG), which is a guanethidine analogue possessing an affinity for chromaffin tissue. It is actively concentrated in pheochromocytoma cells, providing a functional means of tumor localization. Images are recorded 24, 48, and 72 hours after intravenous injection of 0.5 to 1.0 mCi. This test has a diagnostic sensitivity of about 85 percent and a specificity of about 98 percent [296, 297]. Other diagnostic tests such as measurement of platelet catecholamines, arteriography, and catecholamine venous sampling can be tried. Their usefulness, however, is limited.

The management of pheochromocytoma in the elderly is surgical. One or two weeks prior to surgery, alpha-adrenergic blockade should be initiated to reduce operative morbidity and mortality [298]. Phenoxybenzamine blocks both postsynaptic alpha-1 and presynaptic alpha-2 receptors. The starting dose is 10 mg every 12 hours, which can be slowly increased every 48 to 72 hours until the blood pressure is controlled. The average daily dose required in the elderly varies from 40 to 100 mg. Orthostatic hypotension is the most common side effect. Because the drug increases the rate as well as the contractile force of the heart, angina may be precipitated in patients with marginal coronary perfusion, a common finding in the elderly [281]. In such patients careful addition of a beta blocker to control heart rate should be considered but only after the pressor effect of the phenoxybenzamine has been established. Prazosin, a specific postsynaptic alpha-1 blocker, is an alternative to phenoxybenzamine. One major advantage is the lower incidence of tachycardia that occurs with this agent. The starting dose is 1 mg every 8 hours. The average daily dose varies between 8 and 12 mg. Labetalol, which is both an alpha and a beta blocker, the calcium channel blockers [299, 300], and adenosine (100–500 μg per kg), an antagonist of the cardiovascular effects of catecholamines [301], have been advocated as alternatives to phenoxybenzamine and prazosin. Experience with these drugs in the elderly is rather limited at the present time.

Despite a higher incidence of symptomatic heart disease in older compared with younger patients, the perioperative mortality is similarly low, approximately 1 percent [281, 283]. Surgical excision is curative in 65 to 70 percent of patients. In the remaining patients, hypertension persists despite a return of plasma catecholamines to normal. The frequency of neurologic or cardiac disability in such patients has been high [281, 302]. Persistent elevation of catecholamines despite excisional surgery suggests either multiple primary lesions or metastases from a malignant pheochromocytoma. Clues to malignancy include large tumors, extensive areas of necrosis, and a predominance of small cells [303]. The correct approach to these patients is performance of a whole body mIBG scan. Patients with metastatic disease should be referred to an oncologist for appropriate management [299]. Elderly patients who are judged unfit for surgery can be managed with long-term blocking agents, as outlined earlier.

PRIMARY ALDOSTERONISM

This form of secondary hypertension is seen in 0.3 to 0.4 percent of the general hypertensive population [274]. Six percent of these patients are 60 years or older [304, 305]. Although the disease is rare, it should be considered in an elderly hypertensive patient presenting with significant hypokalemia (serum K < 3.1 mEq per liter) that either is unprovoked or that follows conventional diuretic therapy, an elevated serum bicarbonate level, and a high urinary potassium (> 30 mEq per liter). The hallmark of the diagnosis is an elevated plasma aldosterone level associated with hyporeninemia. The autonomous secretion of aldosterone is, in the majority of cases, secondary to a unilateral adrenocortical adenoma; occasionally bilateral adrenal hyperplasia or an adrenocarcinoma is found [306, 307].

The hypertension of primary aldosteronism is associated with a hyperkinetic cirulatory state—a higher cardiac output, higher heart rate, and an expanded intravascular volume compared with patients of the same sex and age with essential hypertension [305, 308]. The hypokalemia resulting from urinary K losses and the increase in urinary hydrogen losses resulting in the alkalosis are due to the effects of aldosterone on the distal part of the nephron (see Chap. 3). Whereas increased aldosterone production in patients with a unilateral lesion is due to a primary increase in biosynthesis of aldosterone by the adenoma cells, in those with bilateral adrenal hyperplasia the increased secretion of a glycoprotein of probable pituitary origin may be the stimulus for the cells of the adrenal zona glomerulosa to overproduce aldosterone [309].

Since the therapy for an adenoma is surgery and that of bilateral hyperplasia is pharmacologic intervention, it is important to differentiate these two entities, a task made easy by the use of a CT scan of the adrenal gland that takes very thin (5 mm) tomographic views [306, 310]. False-negative results occur in about 10 percent of the patients. Therefore, in those patients in whom biochemical findings suggest the presence of an adenoma but in whom the CT scan results are not definitive, adrenal venous sampling from both veins during continuous ACTH infusion should be attempted. Specimens are assayed for mineralocorticoids and glucocorticoids. Once collection has been completed, venography is performed to confirm the location of the catheter tip [311]. This procedure, if successfully completed, is very accurate. A major problem is the difficulty in cannulating the right adrenal vein. Adrenal scans using ^{131}I-iodocholesterol can be used. This test provides both anatomic and functional information, but the sensitivity is less than that of a CT scan (72 percent). Furthermore, the isotope is expensive and is not readily available [312]. A diagnostic role for NMRI in patients with primary hyperaldosteronism remains to be determined.

Hypertension associated with hypokalemia, an increase in urinary K, or metabolic alkalosis can occur in patients ingesting compounds with mineralocorticoid-like activity such as licorice, carbenoxolone, or certain nasal sprays [313]. In these patients the plasma aldosterone, in contrast to that in patients with primary aldosteronism, is either within normal limits or low.

The treatment of an aldosterone-producing adenoma is surgical. Patients are usually prepared with spironolactone (100–800 mg per day) or amiloride (20–40 mg per day) to correct hypokalemia. Spironolactone may also control the hypertension. The prognosis following adrenalectomy is usually good, with 70 to 80 percent of the patients achieving normotension [306, 314]. In the elderly the prognosis is probably not as good, but no definitive information is available. Patients unable to tolerate surgery or those with idiopathic hyperaldosteronism can be managed with spironolactone, 100 to 400 mg per day given in three to four divided doses. Amiloride, 10 to 40 mg per day in a single dose, may also be used [315]. Although this drug does control hypokalemia, additional agents are usually required to control the blood pressure. Triamterene, 100 mg twice a day, has also been used successfully when given with a thiazide diuretic [316, 317]. Nifedipine and enalapril have been tried in a small number of patients [318, 319].

CUSHING'S SYNDROME

Cushing's syndrome is present in 0.1 to 0.3 percent of the hypertensive population [274]. This entity as a cause of hypertension in the elderly is very rare [320, 321]. As in younger patients, the presence of a cushingoid appearance (moon face, truncal obesity, proximal muscle weakness, increase in facial hair) in a hypertensive elderly patient should raise the possibility of this syndrome, particularly if the patient is also diabetic. The diagnosis can be confirmed by serum measurements of ACTH, daily urine free cortisol excretion, and a low-dose (2 mg) dexamethasone suppression test together with radiologic evaluation (magnetic resonance imaging in patients in whom a pituitary lesion is suspected, or computed tomography if an adrenal tumor is suspected) [322]. The pathogenesis of hypertension in this syndrome is most likely multifactorial and includes an imbalance between the activity of various vasoconstrictive and vasodilatory agents as well as abnormalities in the renin-angiotensin axis

[323]. The treatment is usually surgical. Metyrapone, 750 mg every 4 hours, may be tried in patients who are considered poor surgical risks [321].

REFERENCES

1. Boe J, Hummerfelt S, and Wedervang F: The blood pressure in a population. Blood pressure readings and height and weight determinations in the adult population of the city of Bergen. *Acta Med Scand* (Suppl) 321:1–336, 1957.
2. Dyer AR, et al: Hypertension in the elderly. *Med Clin North Am* 61:513–529, 1977.
3. Avolio AP, et al: Effects of aging on changing arterial compliance and left ventricular load in a Northern Chinese urban community. *Circulation* 68:50–58, 1983.
4. Kotchen JM, McKean HE, and Kotchen TA: Blood pressure trends with aging. *Hypertension* 4 (Suppl III):128–134, 1984.
5. Phillips SJ, O'Fallon WM, and Whisnant JP: A population-based model for predicting blood pressure. *Mayo Clin Proc* 63:700–706, 1988.
6. Amery A, L, et al: Hypertension in the elderly. *Acta Med Scand* 210:221–229, 1981.
7. Gordon JM, et al: Echocardiographic measurements in normal subjects: Evaluation of an adult population without clinically apparent heart disease. *Journal of Clinical Ultrasound* 7:439–447, 1979.
8. Rodeleffer RJ, et al: Exercise cardiac output is maintained with advancing age in healthy human subjects: Cardiac dilatation and increased stroke volume compensate for a diminished heart rate. *Circulation* 69:203–215, 1984.
9. Walsh RA: Cardiovascular effects of the aging process. *Am J Med* 82 (Suppl 1B):34–40, 1987.
10. Gozna ER, et al: Age related changes in the mechanics of the aorta and pulmonary artery of man. *J Appl Physiol* 36:407–411, 1974.
11. O'Rourke M: Arterial stiffness, systolic blood pressure and logical treatment of arterial hypertension. *Hypertension* 15:339–347, 1990.
12. Timio M, et al: Age and blood pressure changes. *Hypertension* 12:457–461, 1988.
13. Sowers JR, Rubenstein LZ, and Stern N: Plasma norepinephrine responses to posture and isometric exercise increase with age in the absence of obesity. *J Gerontol* 38:315–317, 1983.
14. Pfeifer MA, et al: Differential changes of autonomic nervous system function with age in man. *Am J Med* 75:249–258, 1983.
15. Shinada K, et al: Age-related changes of baroreflex function, plasma norepinephrine and blood pressure. *Hypertension* 7:113–117, 1985.
16. Buehler FR, et al: Plasma catecholamines and cardiac, renal and peripheral vascular adrenoreceptor mediated responses in different age groups of normal and hypertensive subjects. *Clin Exp Hypertens* 2:409–426, 1980.
17. Van Brummelen P, Buhler FR, and Kiowski W: Age related decrease in cardiac and peripheral vascular responsiveness to isoprenaline: Studies in normal subjects. *Clin Sci* 60:571–577, 1981.
18. Klein C, et al: Age does not alter human vascular and nonvascular β_2-adrenergic responses to isoproterenol. *Clin Pharmacol Ther* 44:573–578, 1988.
19. Gambert SR and Duthie EH: Effect of age on red-cell membrane sodium po-

tassium dependent adenosine triphosphatase (Na$^+$–K$^+$-ATPase) activity in healthy man. *Gerontology* 38:23–28, 1983.

20. Brenner BM, Garcia DL, and Anderson S: Glomeruli and blood pressure. Less of one, more the other? *Am J Hypertens* 1:335–347, 1988.
21. Corvalho JJM, et al: Blood pressure in four remote populations. *Hypertension* 14:238–246, 1989.
22. Bowers JR, et al: Salt sensitivity in blacks. Salt intake and natriuretic substances. *Hypertension* 12:485–490, 1988.
23. Luft FC, et al: Differences in response to sodium administration in normotensive white and black subjects. *J Lab Clin Med* 90:555–562, 1977.
24. National Health and Nutrition Examination Survey: Working group on hypertension in the elderly: Statement on hypertension in the elderly. *JAMA* 256:70–74, 1986.
25. Kirkendall WM, et al: Recommendations for human blood pressure determinations by sphygmomanometers. Subcommittee of the AHA postgraduate education committee. *Circulation* 62:1146A–1155A, 1980.
26. Joint National Committee: Hypertension prevalance and the status of awareness, treatment and control in the United States. *Hypertension* 7:457–468, 1985.
27. National Health and Nutrition Examination Survey: Working group on hypertension in the elderly: Statement on hypertension in the elderly. *JAMA* 256:70–74, 1986.
28. Cohen CE: Prevalence of hypertension among the elderly in an urban community. *J Amer Geriatr Soc* 23:165–168, 1975.
29. Curb DJ, et al: Determinants of isolated systolic hypertension. *Am J Epidemiol* 121:371–376, 1985.
30. Hypertension detection and follow-up program (HDFP): Isolated systolic hypertension in 14 communities. *Am J Epidemiol* 121:362–370, 1985.
31. Wilking SVB, et al: Determinants of isolated systolic hypertension. *JAMA* 260:3451–3455, 1988.
32. Shekelle RB, Ostfeld AM, and Klawans HL Jr: Hypertension and risk of stroke in an elderly population. *Stroke* 5:71–75, 1974.
33. Garland C and Barrett-Connor E: Isolated systolic hypertension and mortality after age 60 years: A prospective population-based study. *Am J Epidemiol* 118:365–376, 1983.
34. Smith WM, et al: Blood pressure characteristics of a population aged 60 to 90 years: SHEP *J Hypertens* 4 (Suppl 5):64A, 1986.
35. Harlan WR, et al: High blood pressure in older Americans. The first national health and nutrition examination survey. *Hypertension* 6:802–809, 1984.
36. Messerli FH, et al: Essential hypertension in the elderly: Hemodynamics, intravascular volume, plasma renin activity and circulating catecholamine levels. *Lancet* 2:983–986, 1983.
37. Heagerty AM, Bund SJ, and Aalkjaer C: Effects of drug treatment on human resistance arteriole morphology in essential hypertension: Direct evidence of structural remodeling of resistance vessels. *Lancet* 2:1209–1211, 1988.
38. Fouad-Tarazi FM and Liebson PR: Echocardiographic studies of regression of left ventricular hypertrophy in hypertension. *Hypertension* 9 (Suppl II):65–68, 1987.
39. Sarzani R, Brecher P, and Chobanian AV: Growth factor expression in aorta of normotensive and hypertensive rats. *J Clin Invest* 83:1404–1408, 1989.
40. Naftilan AJ, Pratrt RE, and Dzau J: Induction of platelet-derived growth factor: A-chain and C-myc gene expressions by angiotensin II in cultured rat vascular smooth muscle cells. *J Clin Invest* 83:1419–1424, 1989.
41. Aalkjaer C, et al: Abnormal structure and function of isolated subcutaneous

resistance vessels from essential hypertensive patients despite antihypertensive treatment. *J Hypertens* 7:305–310, 1989.

42. Simon G: Is intracellular sodium increased in hypertension? *Clin Sci* 76: 455–461, 1989.

43. Stern N, et al: Circadian rhythm of plasma renin activity in older normal and essential hypertensive man: Relation with inactive renin, aldosterone, cortisol and REM sleep. *J Hypertens* 4:643–550, 1986.

44. Kawamoto A, et al: Cardiovascular regulatory functions in elderly patients with hypertension. *Hypertension* 13:401–407, 1989.

45. Goldstein DS, et al: Age-dependence of the hypertensive-normotensive differences in plasma norepinephrine. *Hypertension* 5:100–107, 1983.

46. Stern N, et al: Dissociation of 24-hour catecholamine levels from blood pressure in older men. *Hypertension* 7:1023–1029, 1985.

47. Yamada Y, et al: Age-related changes in muscle sympathetic nerve activity in essential hypertension. *Hypertension* 13:870–877, 1989.

48. Crofton JT, et al: Importance of vasopressin in the development and maintenance of DOC-salt hypertension in the rat. *Hypertension* 1:31–38, 1979.

49. Gavras J, et al: Effects of a specific inhibitor of the vascular action of vasopressin in humans. *Hypertension* 6 (Suppl I):156–160, 1984.

50. Burztyn M, et al: Pressor hormones in elderly hypertensive persons. Racial differences. *Hypertension* 15 (Suppl I):88–92, 1990.

51. Said Sami I: Vasoactive peptides. State-of-the-art review. *Hypertension* 5 (Suppl I):17–26, 1983.

52. Faulhaber HE, et al: Evidence of decreased plasma P levels in human essential hypertension and influence of prazosin treatment. *Biomed Biochem Acta* 42:1019–1025, 1983.

53. Naka O, et al: The effect of aging on urinary kallikrein excretion in normotensive subjects and in patients with essential hypertension. *J Clin Endocrinol Metab* 52:1023–1026, 1981.

54. Tan SY, Bravo E, and Mulrow PJ: Impaired renal prostaglandin E_2 biosynthesis in human hypertensive states. *Postgrad Med* 1:76–75, 1978.

55. Mackenzie T, et al: The importance of age on prostaglandin E_2 secretion in normal and hypertensive men. *Nephron* 38:178–182, 1984.

56. Lang RE, Unger T, and Genten D: Atrial natriuretic peptide: A new factor in blood pressure control. *J Hypertens* 5:255–271, 1987.

57. Kesteloot H and Geboers J: Calcium and blood pressure. *Lancet* 1:813–815, 1982.

58. McCarron DA: Low serum concentrations of ionized calcium in patients with hypertension. *N Engl J Med* 307:226–228, 1982.

59. Altura BM, et al: Magnesium deficiency and hypertension: Correlation between magnesium-deficiency diets and microcirculatory changes in situ. *Science* 223:1315–1317, 1984.

60. Resnick LM, et al: Divalent cations in essential hypertension. Relations between serum ionized calcium, magnesium and plasma renin activity. *N Engl J Med* 309:888–891, 1983.

61. Kesteloot H and Joossens JV: Relationship of dietary sodium, potassium, calcium and magnesium with blood pressure. *Hypertension* 12:594–599, 1988.

62. Resnick LM, Gupta RK, and Laragh JH: Intracellular free magnesium in erythrocytes of essential hypertension: Relation to blood pressure and serum divalent cations. *Proc Natl Acad Sci USA* 81:6511–6515, 1984.

63. Resnick LM, Muller FB, and Laragh JH: Calcium-regulating hormones in es-

sential hypertension: Relation to plasma renin activity and sodium metabolism. *Ann Intern Med* 105:649–654, 1986.

64. Resnick LM, et al: Dietary calcium modifies the pressor effects of dietary salt intake in essential hypertension. *J Hypertens* 4 (Suppl 6):679–681, 1986.

65. Niarchos AP and Laragh JH: Renin dependency in isolated systolic hypertension. *Am J Nephrol* 77:407–414, 1984.

66. Postnov YV and Orlov SN: C11 membrane alterations as a source of primary hypertension. *J Hypertens* 2:1–6, 1984.

67. Bohr DF and Webb RC: Vascular smooth muscle membrane in hypertension. *Ann Rev Pharmacol Toxicol* 28:389–409, 1988.

68. Tabuchi Y, et al: Hypotensive effect of a long-term oral calcium supplementation in elderly patients with essential hypertension. *J Clin Hypertens* 2:254–256, 1986.

69. Lasaridis AN, et al: Increased natriuretic ability and hypotensive effect during short term high calcium intake in essential hypertension. *Nephron* 51:517–523, 1989.

70. Gryglewski RJ, Botting RM, and Vane Jr: Mediators produced by the endothelial cell. *Hypertension* 12:530–548, 1988.

71. Griffith TM, et al: Endothelium-derived relaxing factor. *J Am Coll Cardiol* 12:797–806, 1988.

72. Van de Voorde J and Leusen I: Endothelium-dependent and independent relaxation of aortic rings from hypertensive rats. *Am J Physiol* 250:H711–H717, 1986.

73. Shiraski Y, et al: Endothelial modulation of vascular relaxation to nitrovasodilators in aging and hypertension. *J Clin Pharm* 239:861–866, 1986.

74. Koga T, et al: Age and hypertension promote endothelium-dependent contractions to acetylcholine in the aorta of the rat. *Hypertension* 14:542–548, 1989.

75. Garg UC and Hassid A: Nitric oxide-generating vasodilators and 8-bromocyclic guanosine monophosphate inhibit mitogenesis and proliferation of cultured rat vascular smooth muscle cells. *J Clin Invest* 83:1774–1777, 1989.

76. Yanagisawa M, et al: A novel potent vasoconstrictor peptide produced by vascular endothelial cells. *Nature* 332:411–415, 1988.

77. Clozel M, Fischli W, and Guilly C: Specific binding of endothelin on human vascular smooth muscle cells in culture. *J Clin Invest* 83:1758–1761, 1989.

78. Vanhoutte PM: Endothelium and control of vascular function. State of the art lecture. *Hypertension* 13:658–667, 1989.

79. Letcher RL, et al: Direct relationship between blood pressure and blood viscosity in normal and hypertensive subjects. Role of fibrinogen and concentration. *Am J Med* 70:1195–1202, 1981.

80. Gifford RS Jr, et al: Office evaluation of hypertension. A statement for health professionals by a writing group of the council for high blood pressure research, American Heart Association. *Hypertension* 13:283–293, 1989.

81. Topol EJ, Traill TA, and Fortrein NJ: Hypertensive hypertrophic cardiomyopathy of the elderly. *N Engl J Med* 312:277–283, 1985.

82. Pearson AC, Gudipati CV, and Labovitz AJ: Systolic and diastolic flow abnormalities in elderly patients with hypertensive hypertrophic cardiomyopathy. *J Am Coll Cardiol* 12:989–995, 1988.

83. Shekelle RB, Ostfeld AM, and Klawans HL Jr. Hypertension and risk of stroke in an elderly population. *Stroke* 5:71–74, 1974.

84. Kannel WB, Dawber TR, and McGee DL: Perspective on systolic hypertension. The Framingham Study. *Circulation* 61:1179–1182, 1980.

85. Borhani NO: Prevalence and prognostic significance of hypertension in the elderly. *J Am Geriatr Soc* 34:112–114, 1986.
86. Landahl S, Lernfelt B, and Sundh V: Blood pressure and mortality in old age. Eleven years' followup of a 70 year old population. *J Hypertens* 5:745–748, 1987.
87. Coope J, Warrender TS, and McPherson K: The prognostic significance of blood pressure in the elderly. *J Hum Hypertens* 2:79–88, 1988.
88. Ueda K, et al: Prognosis and outcome of elderly hypertensives in a Japanese community: Results from a long term prospective study. *J Hypertens* 6:991–997, 1988.
89. Applegate WB: Hypertension in elderly patients. *Ann Intern Med* 110:901–915, 1989.
90. Hulley SB, et al: Systolic hypertension in the elderly program (SHEP): Antihypertensive efficacy of chlorthalidone. *Am J Cardiol* 56:913–920, 1985.
91. Gifford RW Jr: Isolated systolic hypertension in the elderly. Some controversial issues. *JAMA* 247:781–785, 1982.
92. Seligman AW, Alderman MH, and Davis TK: Systolic hypertension: Occurrence and treatment in a defined community. *J Am Geriatr Soc* 27:135–138, 1979.
93. Vardan S, et al: Systolic hypertension in the elderly. Hemodynamic response to long term thiazide diuretic therapy and its side effects. *JAMA* 250:2807–2813, 1983.
94. Garland BJ, et al: Effects of treatment for isolated systolic hypertension on cognitive status and depression in the elderly. *J Am Geriatr Soc* 36:1015–1022, 1988.
95. Goldstein G, et al: Treatment of hypertension in the elderly: II. Cognitive and behavioral function. Results of a Department of Veterans Affairs cooperative study. *Hypertension* 15:361–369, 1990.
96. Dustan HP: Isolated systolic hypertension: A long-neglected cause of cardiovascular complications. *Am J Med* 86:368–369, 1989.
97. Breckenridge MB and Kostis JB: Isolated systolic hypertension in the elderly: Results of a statewide survey of clinical practice in New Jersey. *Am J Med* 86:370–375, 1989.
98. National Health and Nutrition Examination Survey: Working group on hypertension in the elderly: Statement on hypertension in the elderly. *JAMA* 256:70–74, 1986.
99. Larochella P, et al: Recommendation from the Consensus Conference on Hypertension in the Elderly. *Can Med Assoc J* 135:741–745, 1986.
100. Davidson RA and Caranasos GJ: Should the elderly hypertensive be treated? *Arch Intern Med* 147:1933–1937, 1987.
101. McFate Smith W: The case for treating hypertension in the elderly. *Am J Hypertens* 1:173S–178S, 1988.
102. Applegate WB, et al: Control of systolic blood pressure in elderly black patients. *J Am Geriatr Soc* 30:391–392, 1983.
103. Applegate WB, Dismuke SE, and Runyan JW: Treatment of hypertension in the elderly: A time for caution? *J Am Geriatr Soc* 32L21–23, 1984.
104. Cruickshank JM, Thorp JM, and Zacharies FJ: Benefits and potential harm of lowering high blood pressure. *Lancet* 1:581–584, 1987.
105. Alderman MH, et al: Treatment-induced blood pressure reduction and the risk of myocardial infarction. *JAMA* 262:920–924, 1989.
106. Cruickshank JM: Coronary flow reserve and the J curve relation between diastolic blood pressure and myocardial infarction. *Br Med J* 297:1227–1230, 1988.

107. Strandgaard S and Hannso S: Why does antihypertensive treatment prevent stroke but not myocardial infarction? *Lancet* 2:658–660, 1987.
108. Editorial: How far to lower blood pressure? *Lancet* 2:251–252, 1987.
109. Staessen J, et al: Relation between mortality and treated blood pressure in elderly patients with hypertension: Report of the European Working Party on High Blood Pressure in the Elderly. *Br Med J* 298:1552–1556, 1989.
109a. MacMahon, S, et al: Blood pressure, stroke and coronary heart disease. Part 1, prolonged difference in blood pressure: Prospective observational studies corrected for the regression dilution bias. *Lancet* 335:765–774, 1990.
109b. Collins R, et al: Blood pressure, stroke and coronary heart disease. Part 2, short-term reductions in blood pressure: Overview of randomised drug trials in their epidemiological context. *Lancet* 335:827–838, 1990.
110. Mattilea K, et al: Blood pressure and five-year survival in the very old. *Br Med J* 296:887–889, 1988.
111. Lauger RD, Ganiats TG, and Barrett-Connor E: Paradoxical survival of elderly man with high blood pressure. *Br Med J* 298:1356–1358, 1989.
112. Amery A, et al: Mortality and morbidity results from the European Working Party on High Blood Pressure in the Elderly trial. *Lancet* 2:1349–1354, 1985.
113. Weber MA, Neutel JM, and Cheung DG: Hypertension in the aged: A pathophysiologic basis for treatment. *Am J Cardiol* 63:25H–32H, 1989.
114. Messerli FH, Ventura HO, and Amodes C: Osler's maneuver and pseudohypertension. *N Engl J Med* 312:1548–1551, 1985.
115. Hla KM and Feussner JR: Screening for pseudohypertension. A qualitative non-invasive approach. *Arch Intern Med* 148:673–676, 1988.
116. O'Callaghan WG, et al: Accuracy of indirect blood pressure measurement in the elderly. *Br Med J* 286:1545–1546, 1983.
117. Hla KM, Vokaty KA, and Feussner JR: Overestimation of diastolic blood pressure in the elderly: Magnitude of the problem and a potential solution. *J Am Geriatr Soc* 33:659–663, 1985.
118. Pitlik SD, et al: Overestimation of blood pressure in the elderly. *Isr J Med* 22:435–437, 1986.
119. Prochazka AV and Martel R: Osler's maneuver in outpatient veterans. *J Clin Hypertens* 3:554–558, 1987.
120. Spence JD, Sibbald WJ, and Cape RD: Pseudohypertension in the elderly. *Clin Sci Mol Med* 55:399S–402S, 1978.
121. Varder S, et al: Systolic hypertension: Direct and indirect blood pressure measurements. *Arch Intern Med* 143:935–938, 1983.
122. Mader SL: Aging and postural hypotension: An update. *J Am Geriatr Soc* 37:129–137, 1989.
123. Lipsitz LA, et al: Postprandial reduction in blood pressure in the elderly. *N Engl J Med* 309:81–83, 1983.
124. Lipsitz LA and Fullerton KJ: Postprandial blood pressure reduction in healthy elderly. *J Am Geriatr Soc* 34:267–279, 1986.
125. Peitzman SJ and Berger SR: Postprandial blood pressure decrease in well elderly persons. *Arch Intern Med* 149:286–288, 1989.
126. Anderson RJ, Reed G, and Kirk LM: Therapeutic considerations for elderly hypertensives. *Clin Ther* 5:25–38, 1982.
127. Swartz SL, et al: Captopril-induced changes in prostaglandin production: Relationship to vascular responses in normal man. *J Clin Invest* 65:1257–1264, 1980.

128. Webster J: Interactions of NSAIDs with diuretics and beta-blockers. Mechanisms and clinical implications. *Drugs* 30:32–41, 1985.
129. Ebel DL, Rhymer AR, and Stahl E: Effect of sulindac, piroxicam and placebo on the hypotensive effect of propranolol in patients with mild to moderate essential hypertension. *Adv Ther* 2:131–142, 1985.
130. Wong DG, et al: Effect of non-steroidal anti-inflammatory drugs on control of hypertension by beta-blockers and diuretics. *Lancet* 1:997–1001, 1986.
131. Oates JA: Antagonism of antihypertensive drug therapy by non-steroidal anti-inflammatory drugs. *Hypertension* 11 (Suppl II): 4–6, 1988.
132. Dustan HP: Calcium channel blockers. Potential medical benefits and side-effects. *Hypertension* 13 (Suppl I):137–140, 1989.
133. Stason WB: Cost and quality trade-offs in the treatment of hypertension. *Hypertension* 13 (Suppl I): 145–148, 1989.
134. Richards AM: Blood-pressure response to moderate sodium restriction and to potassium supplementation in mild essential hypertension. *Lancet* 1:757–761, 1984.
135. Weinberger MH, et al: Dietary sodium restriction as adjunctive treatment of hypertension. *JAMA* 259:2561–2565, 1988.
136. Luft FC and Weinberger MH: Review of salt restriction and the response to antihypertensive drugs. *Hypertension* 11 (Suppl I):299–232, 1988.
137. Australian National Health and Medical Research Council Dietary Salt Study Management Committee: Fall in blood pressure with modest reduction in dietary salt intake in mild hypertension. *Lancet* 1:399–402, 1989.
138. MacGregor GA, et al: Moderate potassium supplementation in essential hypertension. *Lancet* 2:567–570, 1982.
139. Kaplan, NM, et al: Potassium supplementation in hypertensive patients with diuretic-induced hypokalemia. *N Engl J Med* 312:746–749, 1985.
140. Krishna GG, Miller E, and Kapoor S: Increased blood pressure having potassium depletion in normotensive men. *N Engl J Med* 320:1177–1182, 1989.
141. Grimm RH Jr, et al: The influence of oral potassium chloride on blood pressure in hypertensive men on a low-sodium diet. *N Engl J Med* 322:569–574, 1990.
142. Morris CD and McCarron DA: Calcium supplementation reduces blood pressure in older systolic hypertensives. *J Hypertens* 4 (Suppl 5):S562A, 1986.
143. Berchtold P, et al: Obesity and hypertension: Cardiovascular response to weight reduction. *Hypertension* 4 (Suppl III):50–55, 1982.
144. Smith WCS, et al: Urinary electrolyte excretion, alcohol consumption and blood pressure in the Scottish Heart Health Study. *Br Med J* 297:329–330, 1988.
145. Rouse IL, et al: Blood-pressure lowering effect of a vegetarian diet: Controlled trial in normotensive subjects. *Lancet* 1:5–9, 1983.
146. Weight reduction in hypertension (editorial). *Lancet* 1:1251–1252, 1985.
147. Ramsay LE, et al: Weight reduction in a blood pressure clinic. *Br Med J* 2:244–245, 1978.
148. Saunders JB, Beevers DE, and Paton A: Alcohol-induced hypertension. *Lancet* 2:653–656, 1981.
149. Subcommittee on Nonpharmacological Therapy of the 1984 Joint Committee on Detection, Evaluation and Treatment of High Blood Pressure. Nonpharmacological approaches to the control of high blood pressure. *Hypertension* 8:444–467, 1986.

150. Trevisan M, et al: Alcohol consumption, drinking pattern and blood pressure: Analysis of data from the Italian National Research Council Study. *Int J Epidemiol* 16:520–527, 1987.
151. Mountain SJ, et al: Altered hemodynamics during exercise in older essential hypertensive subjects. *Hypertension* 12:479–484, 1988.
152. Hagberg JM, et al: Effect of exercise training in 60- to 69-year-old persons with essential hypertension. *Am J Cardiol* 64:348–353, 1989.
153. Myers MG: Hydrochlorothiazide with or without amiloride for hypertension in the elderly. *Arch Intern Med* 147:1026–1030, 1987.
154. Freis ED: Age and antihypertensive drugs (hydrochlorothiazide, bendromethiazide, nadolol and captopril). *Am J Cardiol* 61:117–121, 1988.
155. Leehay DJ and Hartman E: Comparison of diltiazem and hydrochlorothiazide for treatment of patients 60 years of age or older with systemic hypertension. *Am J Cardiol* 62:1218–1223, 1988.
156. Vardan S, et al: Systolic hypertension in the elderly: Hemodynamic response to long term diuretic therapy and its side effects. *JAMA* 250:2807–2813, 1983.
157. Gifford RW Jr: Management of isolated systolic hypertension in the elderly *J Am Geriatr Soc* 34:106–111, 1986.
158. Morledge JH, et al: Isolated systolic hypertension in the elderly. A placebo-controlled, dose response evaluation of chlorthalidone. *J Am Geriatr Soc* 34:199–206, 1986.
159. Medical Research Council's trials of treatment of mild hypertension: comparison of the antihypertensive efficacy and adverse reactions to two doses of bendrofluazide and hydrochlorothiazide and the effect of potassium supplementation on the hypotensive action of bendrofluazide. *J Clin Pharmacol* 27:271–277, 1987.
160. Materson BJ, et al: Treatment of hypertension in the elderly. I: Blood pressure and clinical changes. Results of a Department of Veterans Affairs Cooperative Study. *Hypertension* 15:348–360, 1990.
161. Freis ED, Reda DJ, and Materson BJ: Volume (weight) loss and blood pressure response following thiazide diuretics. *Hypertension* 12:244–250, 1988.
162. Webster J, et al: Antihypertensive action of bendroflumethiazide: Increased prostacyclin production? *Clin Pharmacol Ther* 28:751–754, 1980.
163. O'Connor DT: Response of the renal kallikrein-kinin system, intravascular volume and renal hemodynamics to sodium restriction and diuretic treatment in essential hypertension. *Hypertension* 4 (Suppl III):72–78, 1982.
164. MacLennan WJ: Diuretics in the elderly: How safe? *Br Med J* 296:1550, 1988.
165. Plante GE and Dessurault DL: Hypertension in elderly patients. A comparative study between indapamide and hydrochlorothiazide. *Am J Med* 84 (Suppl IB): 98–103, 1988.
166. Werning C, Weitz T, and Ludwig B: Assessment of indapamide in elderly hypertensive patients with special emphasis on well-being. *Am J Med* 84 (Suppl IB):104–108, 1988.
167. Langer SZ, Cavero I, and Massingham R: Recent developments in noradrenergic neurotransmission and its relevance to the mechanism of action of certain antihypertensive agents. *Hypertension* 2:372–382, 1980.
168. Messerli FH, et al: Antiadrenergic therapy: Special aspects in hypertension in the elderly. *Hypertension* 3 (Suppl II):226–229, 1981.
169. Jackson G, et al: Inappropriate antihypertensive therapy in the elderly. *Lancet* 2:1317–1318, 1976.
170. Jansen PAF, et al: Contribution of inappropriate treatment for hypertension to pathogenesis of stroke in the elderly. *Br Med J* 293:914–917, 1986.

171. Applegate WB, et al: Comparison of the use of reserpine versus alpha-methyldopa for the second step treatment of hypertension in the elderly. *J Am Geriatr Soc* 33:109–115, 1985.

172. Thananopavarn C, Golub MS, and Sambhi MP: Clonidine in the elderly hypertensive. Monotherapy and therapy with a diuretic. *Chest* 83:410–411, 1983.

173. Weber MA, Drayer JIM, and Gray DR: Combined diuretic and sympatholytic therapy in elderly patients with predominant systolic hypertension. *Chest* 83:416–418, 1983.

174. Whitsett TL, et al: Abrupt cessation of clonidine administration: A prospective study. *Am J Cardiol* 41:1285–1290, 1978.

175. Klein C, et al: Transdermal clonidine therapy in elderly mild hypertensives: Effects on blood pressure, plasma norepinephrine and plasma glucose. *J Hypertens* 3 (Suppl 4): 81–84, 1985.

176. Schmidt GR, Schuna AA, and Goodfriend TL: Transdermal clonidine compared with hydrochlorothiazide as monotherapy in elderly hypertensive males. *J Clin Pharmacol* 29:133–139, 1989.

177. Owens SD and Dunn MI: Efficacy and safety of guanadrel in elderly hypertensive patients. *Arch Intern Med* 148:1515–1518, 1988.

178. Cheung DG, et al: Mild hypertension in the elderly. A comparison of prazosin and enalapril. *Am J Med* 86 (Suppl 1B):87–99, 1989.

179. Ram CVS, et al: Antihypertensive therapy in the elderly. Effects on blood pressure and cerebral blood flow. *Am J Med* 82 (Suppl 1A):53–57, 1987.

180. Kirby RS, et al: Prazosin in the treatment of prostatic obstruction. A placebo-controlled study. *Br J Urol* 60:136–142, 1987.

181. Dauer AD: Terazosin: An effective once-daily monotherapy for the treatment of hypertension. *Am J Med* 80 (Suppl 5B):29–34, 1986.

182. Hamdy C, et al: Use of long-acting propranolol (Inderal LA) in the management of elderly hypertensive patients. *Eur J Clin Pharmacol* 22:379–381, 1982.

183. Wikstrand J and Berglund G: Antihypertensive treatment with beta blockers in patients aged over 65. *Br Med J* 285:850, 1982.

184. Forrest WA: The treatment of hypertension in older patients: A comparative study between a diuretic, a beta receptor antagonist and their fixed combination. *Practitioner* 226:777–778, 1982.

185. Frohlich ED: Beta-blockers and mental performance. *Arch Intern Med* 148:777–778, 1988.

186. Gango FM, et al: The effect of beta-blockers on mental performance on older hypertensive patients. *Arch Intern Med* 148:779–784, 1988.

187. Buhler FR, Hulthen VL, and Kiowskiw: Beta blockers and calcium antagonists: Cornerstone of antihypertensive therapy. *Drugs* 25 (Suppl 2): 50–57, 1983.

188. Frohlich ED, et al: The paradox of beta-adrenergic blockade in hypertension. *Circulation* 37:417–421, 1968.

189. Wikstrand J, et al: Increased cardiac output and lowered peripheral resistance during metoprolol treatment. *Acta Med Scand* (Suppl) 672:105–110, 1983.

190. Hartford M, et al: Cardiovascular and renal effects of long-term antihypertensive therapy. *JAMA* 259:2553–2557, 1988.

191. Jackson EK and Campbell WB: A possible antihypertensive mechanism of propranolol: Antagonism of angiotensin II enhancement of sympathetic nerve transmission through prostaglandins. *Hypertension* 3:23–33, 1981.

192. Beckmann, ML, et al: Propranolol increases prostacyclin synthesis in patients with essential hypertension. *Hypertension* 12:582–588, 1988.
193. Cressman MD, Gifford RW Jr, and Vidt DG: Geriatric hypertension controversies: Uses of newer agents. *Geriatrics* 40:53–68, 1985.
194. Giles TD, et al: Treatment of isolated systolic hypertension with labetalol in the elderly. *Arch Intern Med* 150:974–976, 1990.
195. DeQuattro V, et al: Labetalol blunts morning pressor surge in systolic hypertension. *Hypertension* 11 (Suppl 1):198–201, 1988.
196. Kirkendall WM: Treatment of hypertension in the elderly. *Am J Cardiol* 57:63C–68C, 1986.
197. Roberts DH, et al: Placebo-controlled comparison of captopril, atenolol, labetalol and pindolol in hypertension complicated by intermittent claudication. *Lancet* 2:650–653, 1987.
198. Hosie J, Vallé-Jones JC, and Clifford PD: Long term usage of Prestim (Timolol/bendrofluazide) in the management of mild to moderate hypertension in general practice. *Br J Clin Pract* 11/12:393–396, 1983.
199. O'Callaghan WG, et al: Antihypertensive and renal hemodynamic effects of atenolol and nadolol in elderly hypertensive patients. *Br J Clin Pharmacol* 16:417–421, 1983.
200. Wikstrand J, et al: Antihypertensive treatment with metoprolol or hydrochlorothiazide in patients aged 60 to 75 years. *JAMA* 255:1304–1310, 1986.
201. Wikstrand J: New concepts in the treatment of elderly hypertensive patients. *Am Heart J* 116:296–304, 1988.
202. Andersen GS: Atenolol versus bendroflumethiazide in middle-aged and elderly hypertensives. *Acta Med Scand* 218:165–172, 1985.
203. Perrson I: Treatment of hypertension in the elderly with pindolol and clopamide. *J Am Geriatr Soc* 26:337–340, 1978.
204. Marks AD, et al: An office-based primary care trial of pindolol (Visken) in essential hypertension. *Curr Med Res Opin* 10(S):297–307, 1986.
205. Eisalo A and Virta P: Treatment of hypertension in the elderly with labetalol. *Acta Med Scand* (Suppl) 665:129–133, 1982.
206. Abernathy DR, et al: Pharmacodynamics and disposition of labetalol in elderly hypertensive patients. *J Clin Pharmacol* 25:468A, 1985.
207. Meisheri KD, Cipkus KLA, and Taylor CA: Mechanism of action of minoxidil-sulfate induced vasodilation: A role for increased K permeability. *J Pharmacol Exp Ther* 245:751–760, 1988.
208. Spitalewitz S, Porush JG, and Reiser IW: Minoxidil, nadolol and a diuretic. Once-a-day therapy for resistant hypertension. *Arch Intern Med* 146:882–886, 1986.
209. Velasco M, et al: Cardiovascular hemodynamic interactions between clonidine and minoxidil in hypertensive patients. *Chest* 83 (Suppl 3): 360–364, 1983.
210. Williams GH: Converting-enzyme inhibitors in the treatment of hypertension. *N Engl J Med* 319:1517–1525, 1988.
211. Zusman RM: Renin and non-renin mediated antihypertensive actions of converting enzyme inhibitors. *Kidney Int* 25:969–983, 1984.
212. Mimran A, Targhetta R, and Laroche B: The antihypertensive effect of captopril: Evidence for an influence of kinins. *Hypertension* 2:732–737, 1980.
213. Reid JL, et al: Angiotensin-converting enzyme inhibitors in the elderly. *Am Heart J* 117:751–754, 1989.
214. Chobanian AV: The use of angiotensin-converting enzyme inhibitors in elderly patients with hypertension. *J Am Geriatr Soc* 35:269–270, 1987.

215. Jenkins AC, Knill JR, and Dreslinski GR: Captopril in the treatment of the elderly hypertensive patient. *Arch Intern Med* 145:2029–2031, 1985.

216. Tuck ML, et al: Low-dose captopril in mild to moderate geriatric hypertension. *J Am Geriatr Soc* 34:693–696, 1986.

217. Creisson C, Baulac L, and Lenfant B: Captopril/hydrochlorothiazide combination in elderly patients with mild-moderate hypertension. A double-blind, randomized, placebo-controlled study. *Postgrad Med J* 62 (Suppl 1): 139–141, 1986.

218. Ambrosio GB, Zamboni S, and Botta G: Captopril in elderly hypertensive patients. Results from a multicenter Italian trial. The Study Group on Captopril in the Elderly. *Am J Med* (Suppl 3A):152–154, 1988.

219. Cox JP, et al: A double blind evaluation of captopril in elderly hypertensives. *J Hypertens* 7:299–303, 1989.

220. Woo J, et al: Single-blind randomized, cross-over study of angiotensin converting enzyme inhibitor and triamterene and hydrochlorothiazide in the treatment of mild to moderate hypertension in the elderly. *Arch Intern Med* 1471:1386–1389, 1987.

221. Woo J, Woo KS, and Valalance-Owen J: The use of the angiotensin-converting enzyme (ACE) inhibitor enalapril in the treatment of mild to moderate hypertension in the elderly. *Br Clin Pract* 41:845–847, 1987.

222. Cooper WD, Glover DR, and Kimber GR: The influence of age on the blood pressure response to enalapril. *Gerontology* 33 (Suppl 1): 48–54, 1987.

223. Laher MS, et al: Antihypertensive and renal effects of lisinopril in older patients with hypertension. *Am J Med* 85 (Suppl 3B):38–43, 1988.

224. Gomez HJ, Smith SG, and Moncloa F: Efficacy and safety of lisinopril in older patients with essential hypertension. *Am J Med* 85 (Suppl 3B):35–37, 1988.

225. Giles TD: Treatment of isolated systolic hypertension in the older patient. *Pract Cardiol* 15:1–8, 1989.

226. Piepho RW and Sowers JR: Antihypertensive therapy in the geriatric patient. I: A review of the role of calcium channel blockers. *J Clin Pharmacol* 29:193–200, 1989.

227. Bolli P, et al: Using Age and Plasma Renin to Design Antihypertensive Therapy. In Epstein SE (ed): *Current Status of Calcium Channel Blockers in Hypertension*. New York: USA Biomedical Information Corp, 1986.

228. Resnick LM, Nicholson JP, and Laragh JH: Calcium metabolism and the renin-aldosterone system in essential hypertension. *J Cardiovasc Pharmacol* 7 (Suppl 6):187–193, 1985.

229. Van Zweiten PA, Van Meel JC, and Timmermans P: Pharmacology of calcium entry blockers: Interaction with vascular alpha-adrenoceptors. *Hypertension* 5 (Suppl II): 8–17, 1983.

230. Krebs R: Adverse reactions with calcium antagonists. *Hypertension* 5 (Suppl II): 125–129, 1983.

231. Ben-Ishay D, Liebel B, and Stessman J: Calcium channel blockers in the management of hypertension in the elderly. *Am J Med* 81 (Suppl 6A):30–34, 1986.

232. Erne P, et al: Factors influencing the hypotensive effects of calcium antagonists. *Hypertension* 5 (Suppl II):97–102, 1983.

233. Rotolo V, Lombardo F, and Ciccittini L: Long term effect of oral antihypertensive treatment with verapamil in elderly patients. *Clin Ther* 15:1–4, 1985.

234. Abernathy DR, et al: Verapamil pharmacodynamics and disposition in younger and elderly hypertensive patients. *Ann Intern Med* 105:328–336, 1986.

235. Schwartz JB and Abernathy DR: Responses to intravenous and oral diltiazem in elderly and younger patients with systemic hypertension. *Am J Cardiol* 59:1111–1117, 1987.

236. Leonetti G and Zamchetti A: Antihypertensive efficacy of nicardipine-based treatment in patients of different age and in patients with isolated systolic hypertension. *J Hypertens* 6 (Suppl 4):655–657, 1988.

237. Krakoff LR: Nicardipine monotherapy in ambulatory elderly patients with hypertension. *Am Heart J* 117:250–254, 1989.

238. Forette F, et al: Nicardipine in elderly patients with hypertension: A review of experience in France. *Am Heart J* 117:255–261, 1989.

239. Littler E: Nicardipine in the elderly hypertensive: A review of experience in the United Kingdom. *Am Heart J* 117:262–265, 1989.

240. Byyny RL, LoVerde M, and Mitchell W: Treatment of hypertension in the elderly with a new calcium channel blocking drug, nitrendipine. *Am J Med* 86:49–55, 1989.

241. Jansen RWMM, VanLier HJJ, and Hoefnagels WHL: Nitrendipine versus hydrochlorothiazide in hypertensive patients over 70 years of age. *Clin Pharmacol Ther* 45:291–298, 1989.

242. Rowe JW: Approach to the treatment of hypertension in older patients. Preliminary results with isradipine. *Am J Med* 84 (Suppl 3B):46–50, 1988.

243. The British Isradipine Hypertension Group. Evaluation of the safety and efficacy of isradipine in elderly patients with essential hypertension. *Am J Med* 86 (Suppl 4A):110–114, 1989.

244. Weinberger MH: Antihypertensive therapy and lipids: Evidence, mechanisms and implications. *Arch Intern Med* 145:1102–1105, 1985.

245. Weinberger MH: Antihypertensive therapy and lipids. Paradoxical influences on cardiovascular disease risk. *Am J Med* 80 (Suppl 2 A):64–70, 1986.

246. Weidman P, Gerber A, and Mordasini R: Effects of antihypertensive therapy on serum lysoproteins. *Hypertension* 5 (Suppl III):120–131, 1986.

247. Amery A and Lijnen P: Alterations in lipid metabolism induced by antihypertensive therapy. *Drugs* 36 (Suppl 2):1–5, 1988.

248. Pollare T, Lithell H, and Berne C: A comparison of the effects of hydrochlorothiazide and captopril on glucose and lipid metabolism in patients with hypertension. *N Engl J Med* 321:868–873, 1989.

249. Thakur N, Kochar MS, and Thakur RK: Comparison of hypertension control in elderly black and white males. *J Clin Pharmacol* 28:910A, 1988.

250. Devereux RB, et al: Left ventricular hypertrophy in hypertension. Prevalence and relationship to pathophysiologic variables. *Hypertension* 9 (Suppl II):53–60, 1987.

251. Kannel WB: Prevalence and natural history of electrocardiographic left ventricular hypertrophy. *Am J Med* 75 (Suppl 3A):4–11, 1983.

252. Messerli FH, et al: Hypertension and sudden death increased ventricular ectopy activity in left ventricular hypertrophy. *Am J Med* 77:18–22, 1984.

253. Kannel WB, Levy D, and Cupples LA: Left ventricular hypertrophy and risk of cardiac failure. The Framingham Study. *Circulation* 74 (Suppl 2):76A, 1986.

254. Devereux RB, et al: Cost-effectiveness of echocardiography and electrocardiography for detection of left ventricular hypertrophy in patients with systemic hypertension. *Hypertension* 9 (Suppl II):69–76, 1987.

255. Messerli F, Losem CJ, and Kaesser VR: Left ventricular hypertrophy. Effect of antihypertensive therapy. *Drug Ther* 7:34–43, 1989.

256. Anderson RJ and Read WG: Current concepts in treatment of hypertensive urgencies. *Am Heart J* 111:211–219, 1986.

257. Isles CG, McLay A, and Boulton Jones JM: Recovery in malignant hypertension presenting as acute renal failure. *Q J Med* 53:439–452, 1984.
258. Cressman MD, et al: Intravenous labetalol in the management of severe hypertension and hypertensive emergencies. *Am Heart J* 107:980–985, 1984.
259. DeQuattro V: Treating hypertensive crisis: Which drug for which patient. *J Crit Illness* 2:24–35, 1987.
260. Ledingham JGG: Management of hypertensive crisis. *Hypertension* 5 (Suppl 3):114–1198, 1983.
261. Given BD, et al: Nifedipine in severely hypertensive patients with congestive heart failure and preserved ventricular systolic function. *Arch Intern Med* 145:281–285, 1985.
262. Jaker M, et al: Oral nifedipine versus oral clonidine in the treatment of urgent hypertension. *Arch Intern Med* 149:260–265, 1989.
263. Anderson RJ, et al: Oral clonidine loading in hypertensive urgencies. *JAMA* 246:848–850, 1981.
264. Spitalewitz S, Porush JG, and Oguagha C: Use of oral clonidine for rapid titration of blood pressure in severe hypertension. *Chest* 83 (Suppl):404–407, 1983.
265. Haft J and Litterer WE: Chewing nifedipine to rapidly treat hypertension. *Arch Intern Med* 144:2356–2359, 1984.
266. McAllister RG: Kinetics and dynamics of nifedipine after oral and sublingual doses. *Am J Med* 81 (Suppl 6A): 2–5, 1986.
267. Harten JV, et al: Negligible sublingual absorption of nifedipine. *Lancet* 2:1363–1365, 1987.
268. Conen D and Bertel O: Oral calcium antagonist for treatment of hypertensive emergencies. *J Cardiovasc Pharmacol* 4:S378–382, 1982.
269. Lacche A and Bagagglia P: Hypertensive emergencies: Effects of therapy by nifedipine administered sublingually. *Curr Ther Res* 34:879, 1973.
270. Houston MC: Treatment of hypertensive urgencies and emergencies with nifedipine. *Am Heart J* 111:963–969, 1986.
271. Case DB, et al: Acute and chronic treatment of severe and malignant hypertension with the oral converting enzyme inhibitor captopril. *Circulation* 64:765–771, 1981.
272. Davies AB, et al: Rapid reduction of blood pressure with acute oral labetalol. *Br J Clin Pharmacol* 3:705–710, 1982.
273. Campese WM, Stein D, and DeQuattro V: Treatment of severe hypertension with minoxidil: Advantages and limitations. *J Clin Pharmacol* 19:231–241, 1979.
274. Danielson M and Dammström BG: The prevalence of secondary and curable hypertension. *Acta Med Scand* 209:451–455, 1981.
275. Melicow MM: One-hundred cases of pheochromocytoma (107) tumors at the Columbia Presbyterian Medical Center 1926–1976. *Cancer* 40:1987–2004, 1977.
276. Modlin IM, et al: Pheochromocytomas in 72 patients: Clinical and diagnostic features, treatment and long term results. *Br J Surg* 66:456–465, 1979.
277. Ganguly A, et al: Diagnosis and localization of pheochromocytoma. *Am J Med* 67:21–26, 1979.
278. St. John Sutton MG, Sheps SG, and Lie JT: Prevalence of clinically unsuspected pheochromocytoma. *Mayo Clin Proc* 56:354–360, 1981.
279. Stenström G and Svärdsudd K: Pheochromocytoma in Sweden 1958–1981. *Acta Med Scand* 220:225–232, 1986.

280. Shub C, et al: Echocardiographic findings in pheochromocytoma. *Am J Cardiol* 57:971–975, 1986.
281. Stenström G, Ernest I, and Tisell LE: Long-term results in 64 patients operated upon for pheochromocytoma. *Acta Med Scand* 223:345–352, 1988.
282. Havlik RJ, Cahow EC, and Kinder BK: Advances in the diagnosis and treatment of pheochromocytoma. *Arch Surg* 123:626–630, 1988.
283. Cooper ME, et al: Pheochromocytoma in the elderly: A poorly recognised entity? *Br Med J* 293:1474–1475, 1986.
284. Bravo EL, et al: Circulating and urinary catecholamines in pheochromocytoma. *N Engl J Med* 301:682–686, 1979.
285. Bravo E, et al: A reevaluation of the hemodynamics of pheochromocytoma. *Hypertension* 15 (Suppl I):128–131, 1990.
286. Brunjes S, Johns VJ Jr, and Crane MG: Pheochromocytoma. Postoperative shock and blood volume. *N Engl J Med* 262:393–396, 1960.
287. Bravo EL, et al: Blood pressure regulation in pheochromocytoma. *Hypertension* 4 (Suppl II):193–199, 1982.
288. Pruyo A, et al: Total plasma dopamine and norepinephrine ratio in catcholamine-secreting tumors. *Hypertension* 11 (Suppl I):202–206, 1988.
289. Tsujimoto G, Manger WM, and Hoffman BB: Desensitization of beta adrenergic receptors by pheochromocytoma. *Endocrinology* 114:1272–1278, 1984.
290. Lakatta ED: Age-related alterations in the cardiovascular response to adrenergic mediated stress. *Fed Proc* 39:3172–3177, 1980.
291. Bravo EL and Gifford RW Jr: Pheochromocytoma diagnosis, localization and management. *N Engl J Med* 311:1298–1302, 1984.
292. Young JB, et al: Enhanced plasma norepinephrine response to upright posture and oral glucose administration in elderly human subjects. *Metabolism* 29:532–539, 1980.
293. Ganguly A, et al: Diagnosis and localization of pheochromocytoma. Detection by measurement of urinary norepinephrine excretion during sleep, plasma norepinephrine concentration and computerized axial tomography (CAT scan). *Am J Med* 67:21–26, 1979.
294. Levine SN and McDonald JC: The evaluation and management of pheochromocytomas. *Adv Surg* 17:281–331, 1984.
295. Schultz CL, et al: Magnetic resonance imaging of the adrenal glands: A comparison with computed tomography. *AJR* 143:1235–1240, 1980.
296. McEwan AJ, et al: Radioiodobenzylguanidine for the scintigraphic location and therapy of adrenergic tumors. *Semin Nucl Med* 15:132–153, 1985.
297. Iodobenzylguanidine for location and treatment of pheochromocytoma (editorial). *Lancet* 2:905–907, 1984.
298. Hull CJ: Pheochromocytoma. Diagnosis, preoperative preparation and anaesthetic management. *Br J Anaesth* 58:1453–1468, 1986.
299. Shapiro B and Fig LM: Management of pheochromocytoma. *Endocrinol Metab Clin North Am* 18:443–447, 1989.
300. Proye C, et al: Exclusive use of calcium channel blockers in preoperative and intraoperative control of pheochromocytomas: Hemodynamics and free catecholamine assay in ten consecutive patients. *Surgery* 106:1149–1154, 1989.
301. Gröndel S, et al: Adenosine: A new antihypertensive agent during pheochromocytoma. *World J Surg* 12:581–585, 1988.
302. Faubert PF and Porush JG: Unpublished observations, 1988.
303. Nadeiros JL, et al: Adrenal pheochromocytoma: A clinico-pathologic review of 60 cases. *Hum Pathol* 16:580–589, 1985.

304. Streeten DHP, Tomycz N, and Anderson GH Jr: Reliability screening methods for the diagnosis of primary aldosteronism. *Am J Med* 67:403–413, 1979.

305. Bravo EL, et al: Clinical implications of primary aldosteronism with resistant hypertension. *Hypertension* 11 (Suppl 1):207–211, 1988.

306. Lim RC Jr, et al: Primary aldosteronism: Changing concepts in diagnosis and management. *Am J Surg* 152:116–121, 1986.

307. Artaega E, et al: Aldosterone-producing adrenocortical carcinoma. Preoperative recognition and course in three cases. *Ann Intern Med* 101:316–321, 1984.

308. Tarazi RC, et al: Hemodynamic characteristics of primary hyperaldosteronism. *N Engl J Med* 289:1330–1335, 1973.

309. Carey RM, et al: Idiopathic hyperaldosteronism. A possible role for aldosterone-stimulating factor. *N Engl J Med* 311:94–100, 1984.

310. White EA, et al: Use of computed tomography in diagnosing the cause of primary aldosteronism. *N Engl J Med* 303:1503–1507, 1980.

311. Dunnick NR, et al: Localization of functional adrenal tumors by computed tomography and venous sampling. *Radiology* 142:429–433, 1982.

312. Young WR Jr and Klee GG: Primary aldosteronism, diagnostic evaluation. *Endocrinol Metab Clin North Am* 17:367–377, 1988.

313. Mantero F, et al: Mineralocorticoid-hypertension due to a nasal spray containing 9 alpha-fluoroprednisolone. *Am J Med* 71:352–357, 1981.

314. Lins PE and Adamson V: Primary aldosteronism. A follow-up study of 28 cases of surgically treated aldosterone-producing adenomas. *Acta Clin Scand* 221:275–282, 1987.

315. Hofnagels WHL, et al: Spironolactone and amiloride in hypertensive patients with or without aldosterone excess. *Clin Pharmacol Ther* 27:317–323, 1980.

316. Ganguly A and Weinberger MH: Triamterene-thiazide combination: Alternative therapy for primary aldosteronism. *Clin Pharmacol Ther* 30:246–250, 1981.

317. Griffing GT, et al: Amiloride in primary aldosteronism. *Clin Pharmacol Ther* 31:56–61, 1982.

318. Nadler JL, Hsueh W, and Horton R: Therapeutic effect of calcium channel blockade in primary aldosteronism. *J Clin Endocrinol Metab* 60:896–899, 1985.

319. Griffing GT and Melby JC: The therapeutic effect of a new angiotensin converting enzyme inhibitor, enalapril maleate, in idiopathic hyperaldosteronism. *J Clin Hypertens* 1:265–268, 1985.

320. Bertagna C and Orth DN: Clinical and laboratory findings and results of therapy in 58 patients with adrenocortical tumors admitted to a single medical center (1951–1978). *Am J Med* 71:855–875, 1981.

321. Donckier J, et al: Successful control of Cushing's disease in the elderly with long-term metyrapone. *Postgrad Med J* 62:727–730, 1986.

322. Kaye TB and Crapo L: The Cushing syndrome: An update on diagnostic tests. *Ann Intern Med* 112:434–444, 1990.

323. Saruta T, et al: Multiple factors contribute to the pathogenesis of hypertension in Cushing's syndrome. *J Clin Endocrinol Metab* 62:275–279, 1986.

13 VASCULAR DISEASE OF THE KIDNEY

Vascular disease of the kidney is the most common cause of renal insufficiency in the elderly. Both the arterial and venous systems can be involved, as summarized in Table 13-1.

ARTERIAL DISEASE

INFLAMMATORY DISEASE (VASCULITIS)
Vasculitis is discussed in Chap. 7.

ARTERIOSCLEROTIC RENAL ARTERY DISEASE
Renal artery stenosis secondary to atheromatous disease is rather common in subjects over the age of 50 years [1, 2]. In one study of 200 consecutive patients (mean age 57 years) undergoing coronary and abdominal angiography, renal artery stenosis (> 50 percent luminal narrowing) was found in 21 (11 percent) [3]. The incidence is even higher (52 percent) in patients with known aortoiliac occlusive diseases or other forms of peripheral vascular disease [4, 5]. Fifteen to thirty percent of patients with renal artery disease are 60 years or over [1, 2]. The patient with renovascular disease may present with hypertension only, hypertension together with renal insufficiency, or renal insufficiency only.

Renovascular Hypertension
Aside from chronic renal disease, renovascular hypertension is the most common cause of secondary hypertension in the elderly. The diagnosis of renovascular hypertension should be considered in the elderly hypertensive with (1) recent onset of hypertension; (2) worsening of hypertension that was previously controlled (after the age of 50 to 55); (3) malignant hypertension (particularly in whites); (4) recurrent pulmonary edema [6]; (5) evidence of peripheral vascular disease elsewhere (particularly if the patient is a smoker) [7, 8]; and (6) a rapid decrease in renal function as the BP is being controlled [9]. In addition to these criteria, azotemia and hypertension that is refractory to drug therapy in elderly patients are highly suspicious, since approximately 50 percent of these patients will have renovascular disease [10].

On physical examination, a high-pitched bruit may be heard in the periumbilical area anteriorly or paravertebrally posteriorly with radiation

TABLE 13-1. Classification of
vascular disease of the kidney in the elderly

Arterial disease
  Inflammatory: vasculitis
  Atherosclerotic
  Embolic disease
  Nephrosclerosis
Venous disease
  Renal vein thrombosis

---

laterally. Bruits over carotid or femoral vessels or an aortic aneurysm are commonly present. In addition, evidence of end-organ damage (retinopathy or left ventricular enlargement) is frequently found.

Urinalysis is generally unremarkable. Renal insufficiency is present in more than 50 percent of patients. On kidney-uretero-bladder (KUB) films or tomograms, a discrepancy (of > 1.5 cm) in kidney size may be found.

Our understanding of the pathogenesis of renovascular hypertension is based mainly on experimental data [11]. During the initiation phase of the hypertension, stimulation of angiotensin II (AII) will result in an increase in peripheral resistance. Stimulation of aldosterone by AII results in an increase in renal sodium (Na) reabsorption followed by volume expansion, which contributes to the sustained blood pressure elevation. During the maintenance phase, other factors such as an increase in central pressor mechanisms, most likely linked to AII and central sympathetic activation [12], and structural changes in systemic blood vessels probably become operative.

Several screening methods such as a rapid sequence intravenous pyelogram (IVP), isotope renography, plasma renin activity, and digital-subtraction angiography have been used with limited diagnostic accuracy [13]. The plasma renin activity (PRA) response to the oral administration of 25 to 50 mg of captopril is unsatisfactory as a screening tool because of its limitation in the presence of renal insufficiency, commonly found in the elderly [14, 15]. Baseline and captopril-stimulated ^{131}I-orthoiodohippurate and ^{99m}Tc-diethylene-triaminepentacetic acid (DTPA) renography, with or without split glomerular filtration rate (GFR) determinations, offers promise in the diagnosis of unilateral renal artery disease as well as in predicting response to interventional therapy (surgery or percutaneous transluminal angioplasty). More information is needed, however, before this technique can be universally recommended [16].

Since the definitive diagnosis of renal artery disease requires arteriography, in selected patients when the clinical evaluation is strongly suggestive one should proceed directly to the arteriogram [17]. Given the increased risk of nephrotoxicity due to contrast agents in the elderly with vascular disease and associated renal insufficiency, it is necessary to take precautions to avoid renal failure by preventing dehydration, correcting heart failure if present, and administering either furosemide or mannitol immediately after the dye injection (see Chap. 10).

The presence of a stenotic lesion on the arteriogram does not necessarily indicate that the lesion is causing hypertension [18]. In an autopsy study of 114 elderly patients with renal artery stenosis reported by Holley et al [19], 66 patients had moderate disease (more than one-third and less than two-thirds involvement of the intimal surface by atheromatous plaques). Five (8 percent) of the patients with moderate disease were hypertensive, and four of these (80 percent) had bilateral disease. Fifteen (31 percent) of the patients with severe disease were hypertensive, 13 of whom (87 percent) had bilateral disease. Physicians have relied on renal vein renin determinations to predict cure or improvement in blood pressure following surgical or angioplastic intervention [20]; a ratio of 1.5:1 or greater has been accepted as highly predictive of success. This technique, however, has a significant false-negative rate and therefore cannot be adopted as the sole criterion in making the decision to intervene [21].

In patients with unilateral renal artery stenosis and hypertension three choices of therapy are available: drug therapy, surgery, and percutaneous transluminal angioplasty (PCTA). The choice of treatment should be tailored to the individual patient. Since 88 percent of elderly patients with renal artery disease have generalized atherosclerosis and there is also a high incidence of renal insufficiency or renovascular hypertension superimposed on essential hypertension, a prudent approach is to reserve invasive interventions (surgery, PCTA) for patients whose blood pressure cannot be controlled with an appropriate drug regimen [22]. The percentage of patients requiring intervention for blood pressure control alone has decreased from 42 percent during 1975–1980 to 26 percent during 1981–1984 [23]. Patients who fail to respond to medical therapy and those who have complete occlusion of the renal artery with postocclusion retrograde filling may benefit from either surgery or PCTA. Surgery may consist of either endarterectomy or revascularization (aortorenal, splenorenal, or hepatorenal bypass). In some patients simultaneous aortic surgery (aneurysm repair) may be necessary. Those with a small atrophied kidney (< 8 cm in length) that has little or no function as assessed by differential nuclear scanning should probably have a nephrectomy [24, 25]. Surgery in the elderly does not appear to be associated with a higher risk compared to younger patients if patients are carefully selected. Therefore, criteria such as co-morbid conditions and surgical expertise rather than age per se should be taken into consideration when making a decision about operating [1, 2, 8, 24, 25].

PCTA consists of a controlled disruption of the arterial wall, performed with a fluoroscopically placed balloon. The latter is inflated to a diameter approximately 1 or 2 mm greater than the internal diameter of the healthy portion of the renal artery. Dilation occurs by splitting the atheroma and making radial and longitudinal tears between the intima and media of the artery, with the adventitia (the portion of the vessel wall most resistant to dilatation) stretched and ballooned outward [26, 27]. This technique has been used successfully in the elderly with renovascular hypertension by several groups [28–31]. The overall technical success rate is 40 to 65 percent, and improvement in blood pressure is noted in approximately 55 percent, but cure is achieved in only 8 to 14 percent [31–33]. The lowest success rate was found in patients with ostial lesions. We share Vidt's recommendation that PCTA should be restricted to patients with focal, nonostial lesions [34]. Complications include acute renal failure (which is not always reversible), hematomas (either retroperitoneal or at the puncture site), and microembolization of the kidneys, bowel, and lower extremities by atheromatous fragments. Renal artery occlusion and rupture have been reported; thus the surgical team should be prepared to intervene on an emergency basis whenever PCTA is attempted [35, 36]. Recurrent stenosis does occur, the incidence varying from 0 to 23 percent in various series [37].

Renovascular Disease and Renal Insufficiency

Renovascular disease in the elderly is bilateral in 50 to 80 percent of patients [1, 2, 24, 38, 39], or it may be present in a solitary kidney [40]. An incidence of renal insufficiency of over 80 percent was reported in one series [38], which is similar to our own experience. Although no large prospective study has compared the long-term outcome with the three therapeutic options discussed previously, a variety of retrospective series suggest that despite good blood pressure control, patients managed medically have poorer long-term renal function and survival than their counterparts treated with either surgery or angioplasty [41–43]. The poor prognosis in these patients is probably explained by the progressive nature of the atherosclerotic disease but may be augmented by cholesterol embolization [40, 44]. In a group of 85 medically treated patients with renal artery stenosis followed by Schreiber and associates [45], serial arteriograms indicated progression of the stenosis in 44 percent. In patients with less than 50 percent stenosis, progression was noted in 31 percent (5 percent developed complete occlusion). In lesions with greater than 75 percent stenosis, approximately 40 percent progressed to complete occlusion. Progression tends to occur relatively early, usually within 2 years following the initial arteriography, and is usually manifested clinically by a reduction in kidney size and a decrease in renal function in those with bilateral disease [46].

At the present time, the best approach to management of patients with bilateral renal artery disease or stenosis in a solitary kidney with renal insufficiency remains to be determined. In patients with collateral circulation (which may be visualized by angiography) that is adequate to maintain organ survival but insufficient to maintain adequate excretory function, renal function may be improved by PCTA or surgery even when the renal disease has reached end-stage [47–52]. The mortality rate following the first two postoperative months in such patients is 15 to 20 percent [50, 51]. Data on the long-term natural history of elderly patients who successfully undergo renovascularization are not available.

The choice between surgery or PCTA is influenced by such considerations as the presence of a significant contraindication to surgery (advanced coronary disease, poor general condition), the local expertise and technical success rate for each approach, and the location of the lesion or lesions; as noted, ostial lesions for the most part should not be treated by PCTA.

In general, the better the kidney function prior to intervention, the greater the likelihood of improvement in blood pressure control and increase in kidney function [38, 53]. No data comparing the long-term results between these two approaches are available. In our experience and that of others [2], surgery appears to be superior to PCTA. Following either procedure, patients should be followed on a regular basis with periodic determination of serum creatinine or creatinine clearance, nephrotomographic studies to follow kidney size, or renal scan/flow studies. Deterioration in kidney function or a reduction in kidney mass is an indication for repeat angiography to determine the need for further intervention.

EMBOLIC DISEASE
Renal Artery Embolism of Cardiac Origin
Renal artery embolism has been found in 1.4 percent of 4,411 autopsies reported by Hoxie and Coggin [54]. The true incidence in the elderly is not known, but this age group makes up approximately 36 percent of reported cases [55, 56]. Seventy percent of the patients have atrial fibrillation at the time of diagnosis. In the remaining 30 percent renal artery embolization was associated with recent acute myocardial infarction, cardiomyopathy with associated congestive heart failure, or bacterial endocarditis. The disease usually presents with a sudden onset of flank pain associated with nausea and vomiting. On physical examination, low-grade fever, costovertebral angle tenderness, moderate guarding, and hypoactive bowel sounds are universally present. Hypertension is also quite frequent. Patients with bilateral embolization or embolization to a solitary kidney (50 percent of patients) may be oliguric or anuric. Mild to moderate leukocytosis and an elevated serum lactic de-

hydrogenase (LDH) are present in most patients. Renal insufficiency is found in 90 percent. On urinalysis, proteinura (1–4+) and hematuria are usually found. On renal scan there is absence of blood flow to an entire kidney or segment of a kidney.

The differential diagnosis of renal artery embolization includes acute pyelonephritis, which most often presents with pyuria and bacteriuria, and acute nephrolithiasis, which can usually be ruled out by a KUB and sonographic studies. The definitive diagnosis is made angiographically [57–60]. Once the diagnosis has been made, therapy should be initiated with intra-arterial streptokinase at a dose of 9,000 U per hour for the first hour followed by a maintenance dose of 5,000 U per hour until the clot lyses or 36 hours (whichever comes first) [61]. Higher doses have been used by others—200,000 U intravenously given over 20 to 30 minutes followed by 100,000 U per hour given by a constant infusion pump for 8 hours [62]. Once the desired therapeutic effect has been achieved, intra-venous heparin at the usual dose followed by oral warfarin is indicated [63]. The kidney salvage rate with this approach is approximately 75 per-cent, which compares well to the 83 percent salvage rate reported with embolectomy. Therefore, transluminal angioplasty or surgery should be reserved for patients who fail to improve with "medical" therapy [64]. Long-term anticoagulation should be continued in every patient.

Cholesterol Embolization
Cholesterol embolism is part of the entity referred to as atheromatous renal disease by Meyrier and colleagues [40], in which the renal disease is due either to atheromatous stenosis of the renal artery solely (69 per-cent of cases) or cholesterol emboli solely (6 percent of cases), or to a combination of both (25 percent of cases). In another study of 24 patients with biopsy-proven renal cholesterol emboli, renal artery stenosis (either unilateral or bilateral) was found in 19 (79 percent) [44]. The true inci-dence of cholesterol embolism–induced renal failure in the elderly is not known, but this age group comprises 63 percent of the reported cases, with males outnumbering females by a ratio of 8.6 : 1.4 [44, 65–70]. Renal cholesterol embolization usually develops in patients with extensive atherosclerosis of the aorta as well as clinical and laboratory evidence of vascular disease elsewhere. It may occur following spontaneous detach-ment of atheromatous plaques from the aorta [71] or following aortic surgery [72, 73], aortography [74–76], or percutaneous transluminal angioplasty of coronary [77] or renal vessels [78]. Renal cholesterol em-boli were found at autopsy in 30 percent of patients who died within 6 months following aortography [79]. Embolization occurs in 25 percent of patients undergoing repair for an aortic aneurysm [78] and in 1.4 to 3.0 percent of patients following angioplasty [78]. Spontaneous cho-

lesterol embolization occurs in 0.8 to 4.2 percent of the general population [79, 80].

The diagnosis of cholesterol embolism should be suspected whenever renal failure develops in an elderly patient subjected to any of the procedures described above, particularly if other systemic manifestations are present such as skin discoloration (purple toes, livido reticularis), retinal embolism, and multiple visceral involvement including the small and large bowel and the pancreas. The central nervous system and the spinal cord may also be involved as part of the so-called multiple cholesterol embolization syndrome [81].

Renal dysfunction may become manifest anytime from hours to 2 to 6 weeks following the initial event. The kidney disease tends to be progressive, and most patients require dialysis, however in some patients the disease follows a more indolent course, and there is subsequent improvement in function, occasionally even after maintenance dialysis has been initiated [65, 68]. In the majority of elderly hypertensive patients with cholesterol emboli, acute worsening of hypertension occurs that is often difficult to control, probably related to activation of the renin-angiotensin system [82]. The erythrocyte sedimentation rate and white blood cell count are usually elevated. Eosinophilia has been reported [83] as well as hypocomplementia [67]. It is postulated that atheromatous emboli activate complement either directly by surface contact or indirectly through enzymes of the coagulation system. The eosinophilia may be related to activation of the complement system, since C5a is chemotactic for eosinophils [84]. Proteinuria, when present, is minimal (1+), and the urinary sediment is nonspecific. Definitive diagnosis of renal cholesterol embolization depends on the demonstration of the biconcave, needle-shaped clefts (which remain after dissolution of the cholesterol crystals during routine histologic preparation) in the arcuate or interlobular arteries or glomerular tufts associated with corresponding ischemic changes in the renal parenchyma [85]. In patients with livido reticularis and renal failure, a punch biopsy of the affected skin may reveal similar intravascular clefts [68], obviating the need for a kidney biopsy.

In patients who present with hypertension, multiple organ involvement, and eosinophilia, cholesterol embolization may mimic polyarteritis nodosa or other vasculitides involving the kidneys. An active urinary sediment (hematuria, RBC casts) favors the diagnosis of vasculitis; otherwise, angiographic or histologic confirmation is necessary. Contrast media–induced acute renal failure must be ruled out in patients who have undergone angiography. Dye-induced renal failure, in contrast to cholesterol embolism, is not accompanied by systemic manifestations and follows a shorter and more benign course, with recovery generally taking place within 7 to 14 days (see Chap. 10). Left atrial myoma and bacterial endocarditis may occasionally present a clinical picture similar to that of cholesterol embolization. These conditions usually can be evaluated by physical examination, echocardiography, and blood culture.

The management of renal failure in patients with cholesterol embolization is similar to that of other forms of renal disease. Anticoagulation is of no benefit and may even be harmful, since inhibition of thrombus formation on ulcerated or traumatized atheromatous plaques may render them more brittle and prone to release even more cholesterol crystals [65]. Patients who develop symptoms and signs of vascular occlusion at the time of the procedure do very poorly, and the majority of them die with multiple organ infarction. Those who manifest a more subacute or chronic course do better and, as noted earlier, may recover enough kidney function to discontinue maintenance dialysis if it has been started [65, 69].

NEPHROSCLEROSIS

Nephrosclerosis, or arteriolarnephrosclerosis, is a histologic diagnosis made when occlusive changes, consisting of hyaline thickening of the walls of the afferent arterioles, are found in the kidney of a hypertensive patient [86]. Clinically, this diagnosis is entertained in a patient with long-standing hypertension who presents with renal insufficiency and proteinuria of less than 1 g per 24 hours after other causes of renal disease such as bilateral renovascular disease, obstructive uropathy, congenital disease (polycystic kidney disease), and various tubulointerstitial nephritides have been ruled out. Primary glomerulopathies are usually recognized by the presence of relatively large amounts of protein in the urine (> 2 g per 24 hours). Occasionally, patients with biopsy-proven nephrosclerosis may have similar amounts of proteinuria [87].

Lindeman et al [88] have shown a significant correlation between the mean arterial blood pressure and the rate of decline in creatinine clearance with time in subjects aged 22 to 97 years who have been followed serially. Also, the prevalence of serum creatinine concentrations equal to or greater than 1.5 mg per dl increases with age in the hypertensive population [89].

Even though nephrosclerosis appears to constitute the leading cause of chronic renal insufficiency in the elderly (see Chap. 11), there is controversy about whether clinically significant renal insufficiency occurs in patients with essential hypertension in the absence of malignant or accelerated hypertension [90]. The problem exists because most patients with the diagnosis of nephrosclerosis do not undergo a kidney biopsy, and often renovascular disease is not adequately eliminated [40, 91]. Furthermore, even when a biopsy has been performed, arteriolarnephrosclerosis may be seen in conjunction with other forms of advanced renal disease, which are no longer diagnosable because of severe glomerulosclerosis, tubular atrophy, and intersitial fibrosis (end-stage kidney). Thus, there is little doubt that nephrosclerosis is overdiagnosed in the elderly, but this entity still remains the most common cause of progressive renal disease in the elderly (particularly among blacks).

The management of the elderly with renal insufficiency secondary to nephrosclerosis includes aggressive blood pressure control and other approaches geared toward slowing the progression of the renal failure, as discussed in Chap. 11. In our experience the disease tends either to stabilize or to follow a very slow course once BP has been controlled, even when advanced renal insufficiency is present. In some patients, primarily elderly black males, rapid deterioration in renal function occurs despite good blood pressure control [92]. The mechanism responsible for this phenomenon is not clear but appears to be related to the general problem of increased renal failure in blacks with hypertension compared to other ethnic groups [93].

VENOUS DISEASE

RENAL VEIN THROMBOSIS

Renal vein thrombosis may be associated with severe volume contraction, extension of thromboembolic diseases from the vena cava, involvement of the vascular pedicle by cancer or other retroperitoneal disease, and various glomerular diseases associated with nephrotic syndrome [94]. The association of renal vein thrombosis with the nephrotic syndrome is important because it may alter acutely the natural history of the various glomerulopathies and may add significantly to morbidity, as discussed in Chap. 6.

REFERENCES

1. Delin K, et al: Surgical treatment of renovascular hypertension in the elderly patient. *Acta Med Scand* 211:169–174, 1982.
2. Olin JW, et al: Renovascular disease in the elderly: An analysis of 50 patients. *J Am Coll Cardiol* 5:1232–1238, 1985.
3. Vetrovec GW, et al: Frequency of renal artery stenosis in hypertensive patients undergoing coronary angiography. *Clin Res* 34:205A, 1986.
4. Crawford ES, et al: Aortoiliac occlusive disease: Factors influencing survival and function following reconstructive operation over a 25-year period. *Surgery* 90:1055–1066, 1981.

5. Holley KE, et al: Renal artery stenosis. A clinical-pathologic study in normotensive and hypertensive patients. *Am J Med* 37:14–22, 1964.
6. Pickering TG, et al: Recurrent pulmonary oedema in hypertension due to bilateral renal artery stenosis. Treatment by angioplasty or surgical revascularization. *Lancet* 2:551–552, 1988.
7. Nicholson JP, et al: Cigarette smoking and renovascular hypertension. *Lancet* 2:765–766, 1983.
8. Van Bockel JH, et al: Surgical treatment of renovascular hypertension caused by arteriosclerosis. II. Influence of preoperative risk factors and postoperative blood pressure response on late patient survival. *Surgery* 101:468–477, 1987.
9. Textor SC, et al: Critical perfusion pressure for renal function in patients with bilateral atherosclerotic renal vascular disease. *Ann Intern Med* 102:308–314, 1985.
10. Ying CY, et al: Renal revascularization in the azotemic hypertensive patient resistant to therapy. *N Engl J Med* 311:1070–1075, 1984.
11. Dietz R: Renovascular hypertension. *Contr Nephrol* 43:129–143, 1984.
12. Oparil S: The sympathetic nervous system in clinical and experimental hypertension. *Kidney Int* 30:437–452, 1986.
13. Havey RJ, et al: Screening for renovascular hypertension. *JAMA* 254:388–393, 1985.
14. Muller FB, et al: The captopril test for identifying renovascular disease in hypertensive patients. *Am J Med* 80:633–644, 1986.
15. Idrissi A, Fournier A, and Renaud N: The captopril challenge test as a screening test for renovascular hypertension. *Kidney Int* 34 (Suppl 25): S138–S141, 1988.
16. Nally JV: The captopril test: A new concept in detecting renovascular hypertension? *Clev Clin J Med* 56:395–401, 1989.
17. Carmichael DJS, et al: Detection and investigation of renal artery stenosis. *Lancet* 1:667–670, 1986.
18. Eyler WR, et al: Angiography of the renal areas including a comparative study of renal artery stenosis in patients with and without hypertension. *Radiology* 78:879–891, 1962.
19. Holley KE, et al: Renal artery stenosis: A clinical-pathologic study in normotensive and hypertensive patients. *Am J Med* 37:14–22, 1964.
20. Vaughan JED: Renovascular hypertension. *Kidney Int* 27:811–827, 1985.
21. Pickering TG, et al: Differing patterns of renal veins renin secretion in patients with renovascular hypertension and their role in predicting the response to angioplasty. *Nephron* 44 (Suppl 1):8–11, 1986.
22. Lawrie GM, et al: Renovascular reconstruction. Factors affecting long term prognosis in 919 patients follow-up to 31 years. *Am J Cardiol* 63:1085–1092, 1989.
23. Novick AC: Trends in surgical revascularization for renal artery disease. Ten years experience. *JAMA* 257:498–501, 1987.
24. Geyske GG, et al: Renovascular hypertension: The small kidney updated. *Q J Med* 251:203–217, 1988.
25. Anderson GS, et al: Treatment of renovascular hypertension by unilateral nephrectomy: A follow-up study in patients above 60 years of age. *Scand J Urol Nephrol* 20:51–56, 1986.
26. Sos TA, et al: Technical aspects of percutaneous transluminal angioplasty in renovascular disease. *Nephron* 44 (Suppl):45–50, 1986.
27. Kinney TB, et al: Transluminal angioplasty: A mechanical-pathophysiological correlation of its physical mechanisms. *Radiology* 153:85–89, 1984.

28. Canzanello VJ, et al: Percutaneous transluminal renal angioplasty in management of atherosclerotic renovascular hypertension: Results in 100 patients. *Hypertension* 13:163–172, 1982.
29. Grim CE, et al: Percutaneous transluminal dilatation in the treatment of renal vascular hypertension. *Ann Intern Med* 95:439–442, 1981.
30. Kuhlman U, et al: Renovascular hypertension: Treatment by percutaneous transluminal dilatation. *Ann Intern Med* 92:1–6, 1980.
31. Sos TA, et al: Percutaneous transluminal renal angioplasty in renovascular hypertension due to atheroma or fibromuscular dysplasia. *N Engl J Med* 309:274–279, 1983.
32. Brown LA and Ramsay LE: Is improvement real with percutaneous transluminal angioplasty in the management of renovascular hypertension? *Lancet* 2:1313–1316, 1987.
33. Ramsey LE and Waller OPC: Blood pressure response to percutaneous transluminal angioplasty for renovascular hypertension: An overview of published series. *Br Med J* 300:569–572, 1990.
34. Vidt DG: Geriatric hypertension of renovascular origin: diagnosis and management. *Geriatrics* 42:59–70, 1987.
35. Tegtmeyer CJ, Kellum CD, and Ayers C: Percutaneous transluminal angioplasty of the renal artery. Results and long term follow-up. *Radiology* 153:77–84, 1984.
36. Mahler F, et al: Complication in percutaneous transluminal dilatation of renal arteries. *Nephron* 44 (Suppl):60–63, 1986.
37. Wise KL, et al: Renovascular hypertension. *J Urol* 140:911–924, 1988.
38. Bedoya L, et al: Baseline renal function and surgical revascularization in atherosclerotic renal arterial disease in the elderly. *Clev Clin J Med* 56:415–421, 1989.
39. Faubert PF and Porush JG: Unpublished observations, 1987.
40. Meyrier A, et al: Atheromatous renal disease. *Am J Med* 85:139–146, 1988.
41. Hunt JC, et al: Renal and renovascular hypertension: A reasoned approach to diagnosis and management. *Arch Intern Med* 133:988–999, 1974.
42. Dean RH, et al: Renovascular hypertension: Anatomic and renal function changes during drug therapy. *Arch Surg* 116:1408–1415, 1981.
43. Chiarni C, et al: The time problem in renovascular hypertension (RVH): Renal ischemia. *Kidney Int* 28:247A, 1985.
44. Vidt DG, et al: Atheroembolic renal disease: Association with renal artery stenosis. *Clev Clin J Med* 56:407–413, 1989.
45. Schreiber MJ, Pohl MA, and Novick AC: The natural history of atherosclerotic and fibrous renal artery disease. *Urol Clin North Am* 11:383–392, 1984.
46. Scarpelli PT, et al: Chronic total renal artery occlusion: A diagnostic challenge. *Eur Urol* 10:178–182, 1984.
47. Zinman L and Libertino JA: Revascularization of the chronic totally occluded renal artery with restoration of renal function. *J Urol* 118:517–521, 1977.
48. Schefft P, et al: Renal revascularization in patients with total occlusion of the renal artery. *J Urol* 124:184–186, 1980.
49. Elmore JR, et al: Renal failure and advanced atherosclerotic lesions. Salvage by vascular reconstruction. *Arch Surg* 123:610–613, 1988.
50. Jamieson GG, et al: Reconstructive renal vascular surgery for chronic renal failure. *Br J Surg* 71:338–340, 1984.
51. Bilfinger TW, Gore DC, and Wolma FJ: Renal revascularization in anuric patients. Determinants of outcome. *South Med J* 82:558–562, 1989.

52. Kaylor WM, et al: Reversal of end stage renal failure with surgical revascularization in patients with atherosclerotic renal artery occlusion. *J Urol* 141:486–488, 1989.
53. Sicard G, et al: Improved renal function after renal artery revascularization. *J Cardiovasc Surg* 26:157–161, 1985.
54. Hoxie HJ and Coggin CB: Renal infarction. Statistical study of two hundred and five cases and a detailed report of an unusual case. *Arch Intern Med* 65:587–594, 1940.
55. Moyer JD, et al: Conservative management of renal artery embolus. *J Urol* 109:138–143, 1973.
56. Lessman RK, et al: Renal artery embolism. Clinical features and long-term follow-up of 17 cases. *Ann Intern Med* 89:477–482, 1978.
57. Selli C, Turini D, and Berni G: Embolism in a single functioning kidney: Report of two cases. *Br J Urol* 48:419–425, 1976.
58. Buckspur MB and Goldberg MR: Renal artery embolism: Diagnosis and treatment. *Can J Surg* 21:362–366, 1978.
59. Barry JM and Hodges CV: Revascularization of totally occluded renal arteries. *J Urol* 119:412–415, 1978.
60. Fletcher S, et al: Acute embolic bilateral renal artery occlusions in an elderly patient. Case report: Importance of early diagnosis. *Gerontology* 30:178–181, 1984.
61. Rudy DC, et al: Segmental renal artery emboli treated with low dose intraarterial streptokinase. *Urology* 19:410–413, 1982.
62. Zucchelli P, et al: Acute Renal Failure due to Renal Artery Occlusion. In Eliahou E (ed), *Clinical Acute Renal Failure.* London: John Libbey, 1982. Pp. 152–255.
63. Wu KK: New pharmacologic approaches to thromboembolic disorders. *Hosp Pract* 20:101–120, 1985.
64. Nicholas GG and DeMuth WE: Treatment of renal artery embolism. *Arch Surg* 119:278–281, 1984.
65. Smith MC, Ghose MK, and Henry AR: The clinical spectrum of renal cholesterol embolization. *Am J Med* 71:174–180, 1981.
66. Drost H, et al: Cholesterol embolism as a complication of left heart catheterization. *Br Heart J* 52:339–342, 1984.
67. Cosio FG, Zager RA, and Sharma HM: Atheroembolic renal disease causes hypocomplementemia. *Lancet* 2:118–121, 1985.
68. McGowan JA and Greenberg A: Cholesterol atheroembolic renal disease. *Am J Nephrol* 6:135–139, 1986.
69. Siemons L, et al: Peritoneal dialysis in acute renal failure due to cholesterol embolization: Two cases of recovery of renal function and extended survival. *Clin Nephrol* 28:205–208, 1987.
70. Hendell RC, et al: Multiple cholesterol emboli syndrome. *Arch Intern Med* 149:2371–2374, 1989.
71. Gore J and Collins DP: Spontaneous atheromatous embolization. Review of the literature and a report of 16 additional cases. *Am J Clin Pathol* 33:416–426, 1960.
72. Thurbeck WM and Castleman B: Atheromatous emboli to kidneys after aortic surgery. *N Engl J Med* 257:442–447, 1957.
73. McCombs PR: Acute renal failure following resection of abdominal aortic aneurysm. *Surg Gynecol Obstet* 148:175–179, 1977.
74. Harrington JT, Sommers SG, and Kassirer JP: Atheromatous emboli with progressive renal failure. *Ann Intern Med* 68:152–159, 1968.
75. Gaines PA, et al: Cholesterol embolisation: A lethal complication of vascular catheterisation. *Lancet* 1:168–170, 1988.

76. Colt HG, et al: Cholesterol emboli after cardiac catheterization. *Medicine* 67:389–400, 1988.
77. Tilley WS, et al: Renal failure due to cholesterol emboli following PCTA. *Am Heart J* 110:1301–1302, 1985.
78. Weitz Z, et al: Cholesterol emboli in atherosclerotic patients: Report of five cases occurring spontaneously or complicating angioplasty and renal bypass. *J Am Geriatr Soc* 35:357–359, 1987.
79. Ramirez G, et al: Cholesterol embolization, a complication of angiography. *Arch Intern Med* 138:1430–1432, 1978.
80. Kealy WF: Atheroembolism. *J Clin Pathol* 31:984–989, 1978.
81. Rosansky SJ and Deschamps EG: Multiple cholesterol emboli syndrome after angiography. *Am J Med Sci* 288:45–48, 1984.
82. Delakos TG, et al: Malignant hypertension resulting from atheromatous embolization predominantly of one kidney. *Am J Med* 57:135–138, 1974.
83. Kasinath BS, et al: Eosinophilia in the diagnosis of atheroembolic renal disease. *Am J Nephrol* 7:173–177, 1987.
84. Kay AB, Shin HS, and Austen KF: Selective attraction of eosinophils and synergism between eosinophil chemotactic factor of anaphylaxis (ECF-A) and a fragment cleaved from the fifth component of complement (C_{5a}). *Immunology* 24:969–976, 1973.
85. Jones DB and Iannaccone PM: Atheromatous emboli in renal biopsies. *Am J Pathol* 78:261–276, 1975.
86. Tracy RE, et al: The evolution of benign arterionephrosclerosis from ages 6 to 70 years. *Am J Pathol* 136:429–439, 1990.
87. Mujais SK, et al: Marked proteinuria in hypertensive nephrosclerosis. *Am J Nephrol* 5:190–195, 1985.
88. Lindeman RD, Tobin JD, and Shock NW: Association between blood pressure and the rate of decline in renal function with age. *Kidney Int* 26:861–868, 1984.
89. Shulman NB, et al: Prognostic value of serum creatinine and effect of treatment of hypertension on renal function. *Hypertension* 13 (Suppl I) 8:I80–I93, 1989.
90. Baldwin DS and Neugarten J: Treatment of hypertension in renal disease. *Am J Kidney Dis* 5:A57–A70, 1985.
91. Kasiske BL: Relationship between vascular disease and age-associated changes in the human kidney. *Kidney Int* 31:1153–1159, 1987.
92. Rostand SG, et al: Renal insufficiency in treated essential hypertension. *N Engl J Med* 320:684–688, 1989.
93. Kirk KA, Rutsky EA, and Pate BA: Racial differences in the incidence of treatment for end-stage renal disease. *N Engl J Med* 306:1276–1279, 1982.
94. Keating MA and Althansen AF: The clinical spectrum of renal vein thrombosis. *J Urol* 133:938–945, 1985.

INDEX